The Wilderness First Responder:

a text for the recognition, treatment and prevention of wilderness emergencies

by *Buck Tilton, M.S.*
with Frank Hubbell, D.O.

The Globe Pequot Press

Old Saybrook, Connecticut

The Wilderness First Responder
©1998 Buck Tilton

Illustrations by Bethany "P" Crittendon, except as otherwise noted.
Illustrations in Chapter 36 by Marc Bohne
Photography by Melissa Bugg Gray
Cover photos by Melissa Bugg Gray
Book design by Matthew Midnight Gaylen w/Buck Tilton

LIBRARY OF CONGRESS CATALOGING-IN-PUBLICATION DATA
Tilton, Buck,
The Wilderness First Responder / by Buck Tilton
p. cm.
Includes Index, comprehensive table of contents

ISBN 0-7627-0392-X

Printed and bound in the United States of America
1st Printing / 1st Edition

♻ Printed on recycled paper

ACKNOWLEDGMENTS

This book would not have been possible without the tremendous efforts of Shana Tarter who read and re-read, Bethany Crittendon who drew and re-drew, and Tom Burke, MD, who added a final and critical touch of medical science and art. Deepest thanks to you three.

Several others contributed wisely and generously, and to them go great thanks:

Melissa "Bugg" Gray, WEMT

Joe Costello, MS, CSCS, CMT

Mark Crawford, WEMT-P

Dan De Kay RN, WEMT

Kate Dernocoeur, EMT-P

William Forgey, MD

Charles Gregg, ESQ

Colin Grissom, MD

Murray Hamlet, DVM

Linda Lindsey, RN

Tod Schimelpfenig EMT-I

Richard Sugden, MD

Ken Thompson, WEMT

To these people, and to all those who have helped make wilderness medicine so much more than a couple of words, this book is gratefully dedicated.

Contents

Chapter 12: Fractures

Chapter 13: Dislocations

Chapter 14: Athletic Injuries

Chapter 15: Soft Tissue Injuries 125

Chapter 16: Cold-induced Emergencies 138

Chapter 17: Heat-induced Emergencies 148

Chapter 18: Altitude Illnesses 154

Chapter 29: Abdominal Emergencies

Chapter 30: Communicable Diseases

Chapter 31: Common Simple Wilderness Medical Problems

Chapter 32: Gender-specific Emergencies 249

Chapter 33: Obstetrical Emergencies 256

Chapter 34: Psychological And Behavioral Emergencies 264

Chapter 35: Emergency Procedures For Outdoor Groups 271

List of Figures

The Wilderness First Responder:

a text for the recognition, treatment and prevention of wilderness emergencies

Chapter 1: *Wilderness Emergency Medical Care*

You should be able to:

1. Describe the need for well trained providers of wilderness medicine.

2. Outline a brief history of wilderness medicine.

3. Describe the practical context of wilderness medicine.

It could happen to you

After two days of late summer hiking under heavy backpacks into the Bighorn Crags of Idaho, you and three friends near the point on the map where an unnamed lake supposedly abounds with fine fishing and pleasant campsites tucked into the shadows of a dense forest. Clouds that collected over the afternoon start to spill a thin shower, and you stop to put on rain gear. With only a short series of switchbacks separating you from your destination, your group arrives at the scene of an accident. A lone hiker sits against a tree, pack by his side, face wearing a grimace of pain. He complains of lower right leg pain, and the inability to bear weight on the injury. Your patient states he slipped on a wet rock while descending the trail. He wears a cotton T-shirt and shorts, and you note his lower right leg appears bloody and bruised. Occasional shivers disrupt his ability to speak.

Introduction

Welcome to the world of wilderness medicine! It's an extraordinary world, a world filled with mountains and deserts, lakes and rivers, broad expanses of tundra and serpentine canyons, fields of ice and fields of flowers, deep oceans with distant shorelines, and undeveloped lands where English is a foreign language. It's a world of cold and heat, wet and dry, high and low, dark and light, rushing noise and immense quiet, and, sometimes, utter aloneness. It takes an hour to hike to this place, or a day of paddling, or a week of climbing, or a month of sailing. What common thread weaves through the world of wilderness medicine? *The Wilderness Medical Society Practice Guidelines for Wilderness Emergency Care* states you are "more than one hour from definitive medical care." Hospitals and, usually, physicians are far enough away that the closest thing to anything definitively medical is You.

Even though the accidents and sudden illnesses seen in remote places are often much the same as those seen in urban and hospital settings, there are distinct differences in the management requirements for patients in isolated areas where rapid access to a hospital or medical center is delayed or impossible. Distinct challenges inherent in wilderness medicine can be divided into three general areas:

1) Contact time with the patient which may extend over hours, overnight, or for days, and which may require the use of long-term management principles, e.g., wound cleaning and closure, reduction of dislocations, and the long-term management of the patient's basic needs such as food and water.

2) A remote and possibly hostile environment which may create a challenge to patient and rescuers alike, e.g., cold, hot, wet, and which may create unusual emergencies, e.g., altitude illness.

3) Limited and non-specialized equipment which often requires creative improvisation by the rescuer.

One of the greatest challenges of wilderness medicine, however, is the variety of situations the rescuer may find, unique circumstances which often defy a "cookbook" approach to medicine. In order to choose the treatment "recipe," the Wilderness First Responder (WFR) needs training and common sense as a foundation for making decisions.

Another unique aspect of wilderness medicine is this: The decisions made and treatment provided by a WFR often enable the patient to remain in the field enjoying a wilderness experience.

First Response And Responsibility

Wilderness medicine is often difficult and demanding. The wilderness can turn little emergencies into big emergencies. There is a smaller margin for error than in an urban environment. The Wilderness First Responder must be able to recognize, treat, and, whenever possible, prevent problems created by and within a wilderness environment. Anticipating and preventing problems and managing the risks that are inherent in wilderness travel are at least as important as recognizing and treating problems. Indeed, taking action to prevent emergencies, especially emergencies related to the wilderness environment such as heat, cold, altitude, hygiene, and blisters, is a particular responsibility of the WFR. The best guideline for the WFR might well be stated as this: Plan Ahead and Prepare.

To travel beyond the trailhead or put-in is to accept responsibility for your health and well-being and the health and well-being of those you lead. The WFR must know how to travel in wilderness, how to dress and eat and drink, how to choose and care for gear—in short, how to live properly and safely in wilderness.

Whatever the terms you choose to define wilderness, broad or narrow, physical or spiritual, all tracts of the world's wildlands share two common truths: They are decreasing in size and increasing in value. To journey into wilderness is to accept the responsibility to leave what you find as untouched by your passing as possible, to Leave No Trace (SEE APPENDIX A).

A Brief History Of Wilderness Medicine

Before there was any medicine there was "wilderness medicine," if we use that term to describe care given people far from a hospital. Evidence indicates that even in prehistoric skeletal remains broken bones were set and adequate healing occurred. Almost every culture which has left record of its existence has left signs that some form of medicine was practiced, often well outside of a medicine man's or woman's "office."

In the frigid winter of 1811-12, Napoleon's Surgeon General Baron Larrey trained soldiers to care for their wounded comrades at the battle front. Here was the first known orchestrated effort to keep participants in action by providing immediate attention in the field. Hypothermia and frostbite drove Larrey and the remainder of Napoleon's troops out of Russia without the defenders having to fire too many shots, but the precedent had been set, and pre-hospital emergency medicine took its initial organized leap forward.

During the early years of the United States, almost all medicine was wilderness medicine, care provided in remote environments. Doctors were few, self-reliance was necessary for survival, and people learned to provide treatment for themselves and others when it was required. To early American pioneers, wilderness was a constant presence and medicine was a regular activity. When this nation went to war, management of injuries in the field continued to be an immediate necessity, our battlegrounds were another type of wilderness, and much of the modern growth in emergency medicine originated with the U. S. military.

As populations congregated in cities, medical needs were met more and more by physicians and hospitals, but accidents and sudden illnesses remained a major health problem. The American Red Cross, founded in 1905, began teaching first aid classes that continue today, classes that have affected hundreds of thousands of people. First aid, then and now, has been designed to provide care over a relatively short time span, until a physician can be reached.

The next official leaps in urban pre-hospital care waited until 1966, a year that was important for two significant developments: 1) The United States Government passed the National Highways Safety Act, giving the Department of Transportation (DOT) the responsibility of developing an Emergency Medical Services (EMS) system. From this act came the first Emergency Medical Technician (EMT) course. The EMT program became extremely popular but was designed, and remains today, oriented to the "Golden Hour" and the goal of getting the patient to the hospital within 60 minutes. 2) The American Heart Association (AHA) began to teach cardiopulmonary resuscitation (CPR) courses to the public.

After World War II, with the appearance of more and more leisure time, people began to return to remote areas for recreation. Their medical problems followed them. Prior to 1966 a significant unofficial realization had taken place: an awareness of the inadequacy of Red Cross First Aid courses to prepare outdoor enthusiasts for extended wilderness ventures. In the 1950s training programs were initiated that adapted the growing knowledge of medicine to wilderness settings. These early "mountaineering first aid" programs were written by physicians and managed by outdoor organizations such as The Mountaineers in Seattle. A grand addition to the almost nonexistent literature of wilderness medicine appeared in 1967, the first edition of *Medicine for Mountaineering*, edited by James Wilkerson, MD.

In 1976 Stan Bush, a wilderness search-and-rescue director in Colorado, proposed the first Wilderness EMT course. In 1977 the Appalachian Search and Rescue Conference (ASRC) began offering wilderness-oriented EMT classes at the University of Virginia, and the National Outdoor Leadership School (NOLS) began to offer advanced first aid courses designed especially to meet the needs of their instructors. In February 1977, Stonehearth Open Learning Opportunities (SOLO), a training center in Conway, NH, began offering "wilderness first aid" courses, specializing in the needs of outdoor leaders. The first edition of *Wilderness Medicine* by William Forgey, MD, the "Father of Wilderness Medicine," was published in 1979. Founded in 1983, the Wilderness Medical Society (WMS), a physician-oriented group, began to offer wilderness medical training through conventions and scientific meetings. The first edition of *Management of Wilderness and Environmental Emergencies*, edited by Auerbach and Geehr, both MDs, the definitive piece of wilderness medicine literature to date, also appeared in 1983. In 1984 SOLO developed the first Wilderness First Responder curriculum, and, in January 1985, taught the first WFR course to Outward Bound instructors in Florida. In 1990 the first edition of *Medicine for the Backcountry* was published, a book written by Buck Tilton and Frank Hubbell, cofounder of SOLO, to provide the first practical guide for WFR students.

The last decade has seen the birth of many wilderness prehospital emergency medicine training organizations such as Wilderness Medical Associates and the Wilderness Medicine Institute, which originated as the western representative of SOLO. And the list keeps growing.

Research and development in wilderness medicine continues to be a dynamic area of the medical world. Providers of wilderness medical treatment and prevention are reaching out further and further into the field to save lives and limit suffering. To be the best possible Wilderness First Responder will require you to learn well now, and to keep up with the steady advancement of wilderness medicine.

Practical Context Of Wilderness Medicine

Wilderness medicine involves standard medical principles provided in a context, as stated earlier, that requires attention to extended contact time with the patient, environmental extremes, and treatment with limited and non-specialized equipment which may necessitate improvisation.

1) Extended Contact Time

Patient needs change over time. Problems may become worse and the patient's life or limb may be threatened by the changes. Open fractures, for instance, require little additional attention from the urban First Responder since they are handled by the hospital, typically within an hour. In the wilderness, an open fracture may lead to life-threatening infection or complications resulting in loss of limb before an evacuation can be accomplished. Applying long-term management principles to a patient becomes your responsibility.

Over hours, through nights, and sometimes for days, attention to the patient's general wellbeing must be considered: urination, defecation, hydration, thermoregulation, as well as physical and psychological comfort. This phase of a patient's care, which usually takes place in a hospital, becomes your responsibility.

2) Environmental Extremes

Cold, heat, wind, rain, snow, ice, rough terrain, high altitude, and other environmental extremes may become hazards to the patient and to the rescuers. In addition to the physical risk, harsh conditions may complicate even the most simple care. Dealing with the environment and its effect on the patient and the rescuers becomes your responsibility.

3) Limited Equipment

In the wilderness there is often little or no medical equipment available. The principles of treatment do not change, but care may have to be provided with improvised gear. Deciding what can be used and how it can be used becomes your responsibility.

WFR Training

What a Wilderness First Responder needs to know is well-established. Training should include the underlying general anatomy and physiology, and the foundational skill of a thorough patient assessment. The recognition, treatment and, where applicable, the prevention of all the most likely traumatic, medical, and environmental problems needs to be addressed. Students need to be trained in the management of these emergencies over a long period of time, and such training should include cleaning and closing of wounds; reduction of dislocations and angulated fractures; long-term care of cold, heat, and other environment-related problems; and, when appropriate, "clearing" the spine, to name a few priority consider-

ations. Instruction should include the handling of minor as well as major complications. In addition, students need to learn general patient care over hours to days which includes keeping a patient warm, clean and comfortable; attention to nutrition and hydration needs; and maintenance of body functions. The course should include basic rescue considerations from a wilderness environment, i.e., when and how do you get a patient "out of the woods."

The first aid "kit" that saves lives, prevents disability, and eases suffering is carried, for the most part, in the human brain. The safest plan for anyone who works or plays far from definitive medical intervention is to be well trained in wilderness medicine.

Conclusion

After a quick initial survey, you determine that your patient in the Bighorn Crags has no immediate threats to life. Within a few minutes, you've helped ease him off the wet ground onto his sleeping pad. You've dug dry clothing and rain gear from his pack, and, protected from the environment, his shivering begins to subside.

A focused survey reveals no concerns other than the lower right leg and the potential for moderate to severe hypothermia. Your assessment of the leg reveals the possibility of a fracture. With the wound thoroughly

cleaned and bandaged, you and one of your friends immobilize the leg using extra clothing for padding and a Crazy Creek® chair for rigid support.

While you're treating the patient, your two other companions have set camp as close as comfortably possible. It's no problem for the four of you to carry the patient into the tent. You help him into his sleeping bag, and begin dinner preparations.

Over dinner you and your group decide the best plan of action includes going out for help. You write, complete with

details concerning the status of the patient, a request for aid. Two of your friends will start out with the message tomorrow morning.

Note: All this, and much more, is the stuff of wilderness medicine. The instruction offered by this book will help you learn to provide care in urban and wilderness settings, but the emphasis in every case remains on response to the sick or injured when definitive treatment is far away, and, whenever possible, on steps to take in order to prevent emergencies.

Chapter 2:   *Legal Issues In Wilderness Medicine*

You should be able to:

1. *Describe the legal principles involved in wilderness pre-hospital care.*

2. *Describe specific legal issues important to the wilderness care provider.*

3. *Describe legal protection for the Wilderness First Responder.*

It could happen to you

On a trek in Nepal, one of your clients, Mr. Brown, slips on a treacherous stretch of trail, tumbles a couple of dozen feet, and ends up looking as if he was trampled by a herd of yaks. Most of the damage is superficial-- except the dislocation of his left shoulder. According to the protocols written by your medical advisor, supported by your training and current certification, you reduce the dislocation and evacu-ate Mr. Brown under his own power. During the walk out, the patient complains of numbness in the affected arm. Back in the States, Mr. Brown's physician diagnoses lingering nerve damage, mild but bothersome, a result of your reduction.

Mr. Brown had signed a pre-trip assumption of risk and release from liability and indemnity agreement which stated 1) he understood injury was one of the dangers of the trek, and he assumed that risk, and 2) he released you from all liability, claims and causes of action connected with his participation in the trek. Despite the release, Mr. Brown sues you, claiming negligence in your failure to properly care for his dislocated shoulder. You move to have the claim dismissed, arguing Mr. Brown understood the risk and signed a valid release.

Introduction

"Reasonable and prudent actions" should describe the medical care you provide in wilderness settings. The conscientious and responsible Wilderness First Responder will concentrate on the opportunities to be of service and not let a concern for liability affect his or her performance. The law requires only what rational patients should require and protects those care providers who do their jobs well.

You could find yourself, however, defending a lawsuit which claims that you should have done more, or less, for a patient. Failure to defend such a claim successfully can hurt you professionally and financially. You should, therefore, understand the legal issues involved in this new and important field of medicine of which you have chosen to be a part.

This chapter will deal with general legal concepts, not the laws of particular states. You should seek legal advice regarding the applicable laws of your state and consult with your medi-cal advisor, if you have one, regarding the medical aspects of the discussion which follows. A medical advisor is a licensed physician who advises an unlicensed medical practitioner.

The areas of the law which are most important to the care provider, whether in the city or the wilderness, are contract and tort law. These are branches of civil law, as opposed to criminal law.

Contract Law

Contracts are promises which are expressed or implied, written or oral. A person can be sued to enforce these promises or to pay money if they are broken. All parts of a contract should be clearly expressed and understood: Who is to do what for whom, when, and for what consideration or payment, and the remedy if a person does not perform as promised. At some time in your career, you will have a contract with someone, perhaps your employer or a person in your care. Some states might consider that you have entered into an implied oral contract as soon as you or someone on your behalf causes another to believe you will give medical help if needed. Other contracts with which you may be involved are "releases," whereby a person forgives you in advance for a wrong you might later commit, and contracts of insurance which allow you to acquire protection from claims of persons who may be injured by you.

Tort Law

The other area of the law, the one in which you will probably be involved if you are ever named in a suit, is tort law, which deals with wrongs to people and property not usually involving contracts. The word *tort* comes from a French word meaning "wrong" or "harm." While the most familiar of these torts are intentional bodily injuries and fraud, the focus of our discussion will be the tort of "negligence," that is, the careless, unintentional act which harms another person to whom you owe a duty of care.

Negligence

The good news is that, generally, you will be protected from legal liability for negligence if you do your job well and in accordance with the standards of your profession. Typically, and in your favor, persons who participate in outdoor ventures are more likely than others to accept responsibility for a risky activity and, therefore, are less likely to sue. Nevertheless this area of the law is of considerable interest to the wilderness care provider, whose scope of responsibility and authority may vary from state to state and whose role in a particular situation may not always be well defined by law.

The elements of a claim of negligence are 1) a duty of care, 2) a failure to perform that duty, and 3) a loss or injury that was 4) contributed to by the failure.

Duty Of Care

In most states you have a duty to act if you have a prior relationship with the injured or ill person. If the person is in your direct care, or is a participant in an activity (a summer camp or outdoor program activity, for example) for which you have been hired to provide medical care services as all or part of your job, you clearly have a duty to that person. If you know a person is relying on you for assistance, you, once again, have a duty to that person. You have a special relationship with that person, who is no longer a "stranger."

The Good Samaritan

To encourage trained people to offer care, most states have laws called "Good Samaritan" laws which provide that a person who voluntarily gives emergency assistance will not be liable for "simple" carelessness, i.e., negligence. There is no such protection for "gross" negligence, which is carelessness that is so extreme that it appears you had complete disregard for the person injured. Note that Good Samaritan care must be *voluntary* and performed in an *emergency*. In a wilderness setting, such a statute might control your voluntary care of a stranger found injured on the trail, but if you have a duty to act the Good Sam laws do not protect you.

Consent

Before care is given, the *informed* consent of an adult, or the parent or guardian of a minor, is required by law and should be in writing or at least witnessed by a third party whenever possible. Informed consent means the patient is advised of the problem, the proposed treatment, and what to expect if no treatment is given; and the patient gives consent, actual or implied. Failure to acquire informed consent could possibly result in a suit against you for assault and/or battery. Fortunately, the law recognizes *implied* consent in emergency situations when it can be reasonably assumed that the patient, if conscious and reliable (or a parent, if the patient is a minor), would have agreed to the assistance offered. If you work with minors, which means, in most cases, any- one under 18 years of age, you are well advised to carry a document signed by the parent or guardian allowing you to provide medical care in an emergency. If you find yourself in an emergency involving a minor and without pre-arranged consent, go ahead and treat to the best of your ability.

Standard Of Care

The standard of care in pre-hospital medicine is largely determined by the specific training you have been given, the training that has provided you with the skills and knowledge of how to do what, and when. If your patient assessment, for instance, reveals the possibility of a fractured leg, the standard of care, generally, is to appropriately splint the leg in question and monitor the patient.

Because wilderness medicine is a newer profession, the standards may be less clear than for those operating in ambulances, emergency rooms, and other city situations. *What* you are allowed to do will depend on the laws of the state where you work and/or the medical protocols written for you by your medical advisor, if you have one. Be sure you are operating within those laws and protocols as you consider reducing a dislocation, for example. *How well* you perform will be measured by standards which are much broader. Never do more, or less, than you are trained to do.

Be sure to stay well informed and well trained up to the standards of your level of certification in order to act in the best interest of your patient--with or without the possibility of a lawsuit.

Failure To Perform The Duty

The second element of negligence is a violation, or breach, of the duty of care. A breach can be an act (commission) or the failure to act (omission). In most cases that have gone to court, wilderness medicine providers have been sued for failure to act.

Generally speaking, the law will consider you at fault and liable for payment of damages to the injured person, if you have not performed as would a reasonable person with your background and training, acting in the same or similar circumstances.

Examples might be the misreading of obvious vital signs or the failure to splint a fracture. *Gross* negligence might be attempting to provide care when you are under the influence of drugs or alcohol.

Loss Or Injury Caused By The Failure

The third and fourth elements of a negligence claim are a loss or injury of which the breach of duty or wrongful act is a contributing cause. The "loss" can include fright and other emotional trauma and certainly includes loss of property, personal injury, and death. You will not be liable if another person or event is shown to have caused the injury--for example, a qualified person to whom you transfer the patient acts negligently. Also, the loss must have been a reasonably foreseeable result of the breach of duty. You should not be liable if a person, because of some pre-existing condition of which you could not have been aware, reacts badly to a regular procedure applied by you. In this event, a person with your training could not have foreseen the result and should not be liable.

The Wilderness First Responder   7

Abandonment

You may be liable to a patient, or to a patient's family, for abandonment when you terminate care prematurely and the patient suffers harm later, or you transfer care to a less qualified or unqualified person and the patient suffers harm later.

Example One: You, the Wilderness First Responder, stop on a steep trail to aid an out-of-shape hiker "dead on his feet" from extreme fatigue and nausea, a hiker who begins to depend on your assistance. You know this to be a busy trail, and you leave the hiker unattended because you want to make it over the next pass before dark. Arguably, you have abandoned a patient who may suffer harm.

Example Two: You, the Wilderness First Responder, stop to aid the hiker in Example One and leave him in the care of the next passerby who happens to have no medical training. Arguably, you have abandoned a patient who may suffer harm.

Example Three: You, the Wilderness First Responder, stop to aid the hiker in Example One, and you decide the hiker will not be able to continue on his own. Your decision is to leave him unattended in order to hike out for more help. You leave him well supplied with food, water, and extra clothing. Arguably, you have *not* abandoned a patient because you have acted in a reasonable and prudent manner.

Defenses

If you are sued for negligence, you have defenses. These defenses include the absence of one or more of the four necessary elements: Duty, failure to perform the duty, loss or injury, and causation. The negligence of others, including the person injured, also can reduce or eliminate your liability. In many states, the judge or jury is allowed to compare, on a percentage basis, the fault of all who may have contributed to the injury. This is usually referred to as "comparative negligence" or "comparative fault" and assures that you are obligated only for that part of the loss that you caused.

Documentation

You have heard the saying, "If it isn't written down, it didn't happen." This means that, in a lawsuit, if an important event is not recorded by the care provider, the judge and jury probably will assume that it did not occur. It is important, therefore, in order to avoid guessing about what happened in the field, that you make a written record at the time of the event or shortly thereafter. The record should include at least dates and times, patient history, a description of the scene, your physical assessment and treatment, and changes in the patient while in your care. It is also important to document, with a witness if possible, a refusal of treatment by an informed patient.

The Care Provider as an Employee

The fact that you are an employee is no protection from liability, except to the extent the employer's insurance may take care of your legal liability and expenses. Insurance is a matter you should carefully consider, whether you are acting independently or for an employer. It is your responsibility to know whether or not you are insured and how well the insurance protects you.

Damages

You will have to pay damages to the injured person if you are found to be negligent. These damages are the best estimate by the judge or jury of what you should pay to make up for the loss you caused including pain and suffering, medical and other expenses, lost earnings, and even penalty or "exemplary" damages if your negligence was gross.

The Law And The Wilderness Care Provider

What is the practical legal effect of all this? The care provider, as we know, assesses the emergency; removes the patient from harm; stabilizes the patient; provides other limited, essential care; and prepares proper reports and records. As a wilderness care provider you probably will have more responsibilities (for expedition medicines, for example) and provide more treatments that might not be indicated if hospital care were more available.

Most of the issues facing the care provider on wilderness expeditions will relate to athletic injuries, environmental emergencies, and hygiene-related problems, but there is always the possibility of severe trauma or illness, a difficult-to-diagnose stomach cramp, a diabetic reac-tion, or a severe laceration. Such occurrences, an hour or longer from the attention of a licensed physician, are much more serious than if encountered in Your Home Town, USA. If you accept the responsibility of care in the wilderness, you must be prepared with appropriate training, equipment, and medical protocols.

You are well advised, then, if you work for an outdoor program or search-and-rescue team to seek out and work under the authority of a medical advisor. The medical advisor or base-station physician will share responsibility with you for the adequacy (or inadequacy) of your performance if he or she authorizes you to administer drugs or reduce dislocations, close wounds, or otherwise engage in procedures that might exceed the customary role of the city First Responder. If it is done well, there will be no complaint. If done improperly, questions of training, technique, authority, consent and alternative remedies will be carefully examined by investigators, lawyers, experts, and a judge and jury.

In a wilderness or outdoor program setting, additional issues important to you as a staff-person will include 1) the screening and supervision of participants, 2) the adequacy of equipment and supplies, and 3) the presence of a carefully designed plan for medication administration, evacuation, and other emergencies.

Conclusion

The court determines it is reasonable to assume that you, as a leader of a trek to Nepal, would have knowledge of reducing dislocations in the field. An expert witness explains to the court that the protocols written by your medical advisor were precise, and that your documentation indicates you followed them precisely. Another expert witness explains that the future of Mr. Brown's shoulder looks far better than it would if it had remained dislocated. The pre-trip form Mr. Brown signed, says the court, indicates he understood an injury of this nature could occur and that he assumed that risk. You go back to work in the wilderness.

Charles R. Gregg, Esq., contributed his expertise to this chapter.

Chapter 3: Patient Assessment

You should be able to:

1. *Describe how to immediately establish control of the scene.*

2. *Describe how to establish a safe scene including the use of body substance isolation.*

3. *Define mechanism of injury (MOI) and describe why it is important as a factor in patient assessment.*

4. *Describe the importance of and methods of establishing an effective relationship with the patient.*

5. *Demonstrate how to do an initial assessment and a focused assessment, which will include performing a physical examination, measuring vital signs, obtaining a patient history, and documenting the event.*

It could happen to you

Only the rocks know what happened, maybe a couple of trees, but they aren't talking. Spring warms the air, the cotton-woods have sprouted new leaves, and this quiet section of the lower Green River you and a friend are canoeing, the river that now passes beneath a high sandstone cliff, has carried you within sight of a young man sprawled on the ground near the water's edge. In the stern of the canoe, you back paddle while your friend in the bow draws. The canoe eases to shore.

The young man lies face up, unmoving, a smear of blood from mouth to ear. No other people are evident. Stillness reigns. What happened? What do you do? There are clues everywhere, but where is Sherlock Holmes when you need him?

Introduction

The ability to adequately manage an emergency is founded on your ability to properly assess the scene and the patient. The patient assessment, the actual medical skill, is made through the gathering of information, or "clues," in a series of surveys. The surveys include a scene size-up, an initial assessment of the patient, and a focused history and exam of the patient. Imagine the ineffable Mr. Holmes, pipe clamped between his teeth, eyes missing nothing, mind shifting into high gear. But this is not Baker Street, Dr. Watson. This is the wild outdoors.

Assessment provides the foundation of all medicine, but assessment is far more than a medical skill. When you watch someone who does an excellent job of assessing, you watch someone who does an excellent job of relating to people. Your assessment will come easiest and best for all concerned if you establish control of the people at the scene, establish an effective relationship with the patient, and maintain a healthy working relationship with co-workers and others for whom you have responsibility.

On the scene, a rush of adrenaline may threaten to alter your abilities. To help you, consider stopping momentarily in your assessment to take a deep calming breath. Stop! Breathe. Go.

Stop! Size-up The Scene

Establish Control

Emergencies are often charged with emotion and confusion. Even minor chaos increases the risk of injury to rescuers and bystanders, and the risk of inadequate care for the patient. Someone needs to establish control of the scene. Someone needs to take charge. This is best accomplished if you have discussed leadership in case of an emergency with coworkers, and others for whom you have responsibility, prior to a critical situation.

Two qualities describe the best Wilderness First Responder in an emergency: 1) Competence. You know your stuff. You are capable and ready to act. 2) Confidence. You appear able to deal with the situation. You don't have to feel confident, but you should appear confident and sound confident. Avoid shouting. Speak with quiet authority.

Your goals should be to 1) provide the greatest good for the greatest number in the shortest time, and 2) do no harm.

Survey The Scene For Hazards

Every assessment should start before you ever reach the patient's side: An assessment of the scene for hazards. Is there immediate danger from the environment, e.g., rockfall, thin ice over water, carbon monoxide filling the tent? Have you taken precautions to prevent being a giver or taker of communicable diseases (SEE BELOW BODY SUBSTANCE ISOLATION)?

Your desire to rush in and help as soon as possible must be tempered with your need to maintain 1) your own personal safety, 2) the safety of other members of your party, and 3) the safety of the patient, in order to prevent further injury. A second patient is always a tragedy, not to mention a dramatic increase in the difficulty of the situation. In the wilderness a second patient is not only tragic but also represents a loss of resources. Every person in a wilderness situation is an irreplaceable resource, someone who can help carry and care for the patient. Protect your resources.

Never create a second patient! Hazards must be eliminated or, at least, minimized, before approaching the patient.

A survey of the scene should also take into account subtle dangers to the patient, the members of the party, and you; dangers that will take longer to develop, e.g., cold, wind, rain, heat. These potential dangers should be attended to as soon as possible.

Mechanism Of Injury

With the safety of the scene established, or even during its establishment, and before the scene is cluttered with people wanting to help, further scene assessment includes assessing the *mechanism of injury* (MOI) the patient has undergone. MOI may be as important a consideration as the injury or injuries. As examples, consider: If the climber fell, what did he land on? Rocks? Compacted soil? Grass? In what position did you find him?

Much of the information concerning MOI may have to be gathered later through questioning the patient and/or eyewitnesses. As examples, consider: How far did the climber fall? What body part hit the ground first? Did a rope slow his descent? Was he wearing a helmet? Sometimes substantial forces can produce injuries that the patient will not be aware of early in your assessment. Knowledge of the MOI will help in your initial assessment and make you aware of possible changes in your patient later.

Body Substance Isolation

Communicable, or infectious, diseases must be considered a potential risk to rescuers. You should assume the possibility that every patient could spread germs that cause illness. You should also protect every patient from germs that you could be carrying (SEE CHAPTER 30: COMMUNICABLE DISEASES).

Use barrier devices to insure *body substance isolation*, to prevent your skin and mucous membranes from contacting the blood or other body fluids of a patient.

1. Keep protective disposable gloves available at all times, and wear them when there is the slightest chance you may contact a patient's blood, other body fluids, mucous membranes, or broken skin. Wear gloves when you may handle bandages, clothing, or other items contaminated with blood or other body fluids. When you no longer need them, pull the gloves off carefully from your wrist, leaving them inside out. Dispose of the gloves as soon as possible after use by sealing them in a plastic bag with other contaminated items and marking the

bag as contaminated material. Wash your hands as soon as possible after removing the gloves.

2. Wear protective glasses if the scene could involve the spraying of contaminated droplets, e.g., a coughing patient. Wear your sunglasses if nothing else is available.

3. Wear a protective mask over your nose and mouth if the scene could involve the spraying of contaminated droplets.

4. Use a rescue mask with a one-way valve, or a resuscitation device, if the patient requires artificial ventilations.

Number Of Patients

A final assessment of the scene should include scanning the area for other patients. One patient demanding attention, someone obviously afraid and/or in pain, can cause you to immediately focus on that patient. Meanwhile, sitting or lying quietly nearby, a second patient slowly dies from blood loss or loss of an airway. Make sure, as soon as possible, that you know how many patients are involved in the scene.

General Impression

What is your general impression of the patient? Hurt, or not hurt? Sick, or not sick?

If your impression is "This is a seriously hurt or seriously ill person," you should be preparing yourself for a rapid assessment, for rapid treatment, and for a rapid decision concerning transport of the patient from the wilderness. Keep in mind, however,

that "rapid" transport from the wilderness is most often a wishful thought rather than a reality.

Experience plays a role in helping you make a general impression, but examples of "serious" problems include 1) a patient unable to breathe, 2) a patient without a pulse, 3) a patient with pale, blue, or gray skin, 4) a patient with a decreased level of consciousness, 5) blood spurting into the air or pooling rapidly under the patient, 6) extremities with obvious deformities, and 7) extremities that are missing.

If your impression is "This person is not seriously hurt or seriously ill," then you can prepare yourself for a more relaxed assessment and treatment, and for a more relaxed decision concerning the need for transport.

Establish A Relationship

If the patient is conscious, there is an excellent chance she (or he) will be frightened, anxious, and in pain. If there are no obvious immediate threats to life (SEE BELOW INITIAL ASSESSMENT), take a minute to establish an open, clear, honest, effective relationship. Introduce yourself, if needed, and state your qualifications to provide care. Position yourself as close to eye-level as possible with the patient, and make eye contact. If you're wearing sunglasses, take them off. Speak reassuringly, quietly, but loud enough to be heard easily. If you don't know the patient, ask for her name . . . and use it. If the patient is older, it is usually best

to use the last name, e.g., "Ms. Smith." Maintain an open dialogue throughout your assessment and treatment of the patient, allowing time for questions about what you're going to do.

Touch is a universal way to show concern and provide comfort. Your hand on the patient's arm or shoulder, if you're comfortable doing it, can give valuable reassurance, but don't assume the patient wants you to touch her during your upcoming examination. Whenever possible, before touching in order to assess, be sure to ask permission. "I have to touch you in order to assess the extent of your injuries. I'll be as gentle as possible. OK?" If the patient says "OK," or nothing to indicate a lack of acceptance of your treatment, you have received consent to treat.

If the patient is unconscious and/or there are obvious immediate threats to life, relationship-building may have to wait. Remember, however, that the patient, even if unconscious, should still be treated with respect and compassion.

Compassion? You don't have to be compassionate. You can be effective by acting with competence and without showing an awareness of human distress and a desire to alleviate it. Arguably, however, compassionate care providers are better care providers. Few, if any, people would choose to be treated without compassion.

Stop! Survey The Patient For Immediate Threats To Life

Initial Assessment

The goal of the initial assessment is to find and treat any immediate threats to the patient's life. This is a Stop-and-Fix survey. If you find something that needs treatment during the initial assessment, you will immediately "stop and fix it." Although the initial assessment is presented here in a systematic manner--ABCDE--you may find what you actually do varies somewhat from alphabetical order. As you approach the patient, you should quickly scan for obvious threats. If your visual scan reveals blood squirting from an open artery, you might find yourself treating C (Circulation) a few moments prior to A (Airway). Still, the concept of ABCDE provides a sound basis from which to work.

Establish Responsiveness/ Control the Cervical Spine

The first step in the Initial Assessment is to determine the patient's ability to respond to stimuli, or, in other words, determine the patient's *level of consciousness* (SEE BELOW VITAL SIGNS, LEVEL OF CONSCIOUSNESS). This is the first step because a patient with a mental status altered from normal may need airway management or other early life-saving intervention.

If the MOI and/or the patient's mental status indicates the possibility of spine or head trauma, take immediate manual control of the patient's head and neck by placing one or both of your hands on the patient's head or by having an assistant rescuer take manual control of the patient's head and neck.

A is for Airway

Is the patient's airway open? If the patient speaks, the airway is at least temporarily open. If the patient is unconscious and/or if the patient's breathing sounds indicate difficulty moving air in and out, open the airway immediately with a *head-tilt/chin-lift*, if cervical spine damage is not suspected, or a *jaw thrust*, if cervical spine damage is suspected (SEE CHAPTER 4: AIRWAY AND BREATHING). Check the airway for blockages, e.g., blood, foreign bodies. Anything blocking the airway must be removed immediately. Ask a conscious patient to spit out anything in the mouth, e.g., gum, tobacco, anything that could later become an obstruction.

B is for Breathing

If the patient appears unconscious and/or does not speak, while maintaining manual stabilization of the patient's head and with the airway opened, place your ear against the patient's mouth in order to *look* across the chest and upper abdomen for movement, *listen* for the sound of breathing, and *feel* for the brush of moving air against your ear. If the patient is wearing bulky clothing, your second hand placed over the lower chest/ upper abdomen will allow you to feel for chest movement. Assess breathing for three to five seconds. Is the patient moving air in and out of the chest? If not, you will have to begin breathing for the patient (SEE CHAPTER 4: AIRWAY AND BREATHING).

You may find your patient in a position that makes it impossible to assess airway and breathing, or in a position that makes breathing for the patient impossible, e.g., face buried in snow. In these cases you will have to reposition the patient. Even though the possibility of spinal cord injury may exist, assurance of breathing takes precedence. Kneeling beside the patient, control the head and neck as best you can by cradling the head with one hand. Straighten out the legs. Roll the patient gently onto one side, and then into a supine (face up) position. This is easier and safer for the patient if two or more people are available to perform the roll. With two or more rescuers, the one controlling the head should be in charge of the movement (SEE CHAPTER 8: SPINE INJURIES).

C is for Circulation (and Bleeding)

With a conscious patient, check for a radial pulse, an indication of adequate circulation. With an unconscious patient, check for a carotid pulse on the side of the neck you are on. Do not reach across the trachea (windpipe) and do not try to check both carotid pulses at once. These maneuvers may partially block the trachea or reduce blood flow to the brain. If you find no pulse, you will have to start cardiopulmonary resuscitation (SEE CHAPTER 5: CARDIOPULMONARY RESUSCITATION).

If the patient's heart is beating, check for severe bleeding with more than a quick visual scan. Run your free hand, preferably a gloved hand, under the patient and inside of bulky clothing. Check your gloved hand for blood. If you see blood, check the wound. Bleeding can look deceptively serious and still be minor. Generally, only blood loss that is spurting or flowing heavily should be attended to in the initial assessment (SEE CHAPTER 6: BLEEDING).

D is for Disability

Since damage to the central nervous system--the brain and the spinal cord which runs down the neck and back--can cause permanent disability or death,

the patient should be kept immobile, preventing further damage, as long as there is a suspicion of spinal involvement. "D" reminds you to assume spinal cord injury until the pace of the emergency has slowed and sufficient information gathered to allow you to make a decision to treat or not treat the spine.

Early reasons for suspicion of spinal injury include 1) an unreliable patient, one with an altered level of consciousness, one not fully alert, 2) a positive MOI, e.g., a fall from a substantial height, 3) a patient complaining of neck

and/or back pain, 4) a patient complaining of an inability to move, and 5) a patient complaining of numbness or tingling in hands and/or feet. Keep the patient immobile until you have investigated further in the focused assessment (SEE BELOW).

Remember: You stop and fix threats to life, but discovered problems which do not threaten life are treated after the assessment is complete.

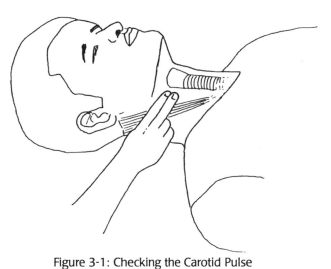

Figure 3-1: Checking the Carotid Pulse

E is for Expose, Environment

Clothing will often hide injuries you need to be managing. If, at this point, your initial assessment has revealed a serious injury, e.g., a bleeding site, consider cutting the patient's clothing to expose the injury for a better look. Keeping in mind that in a wilderness situation the patient may need those clothes later, remove no more clothing that you need to expose the injury. With a conscious patient, tell them exactly what you are

doing and why. Protect the patient's modesty as much as possible.

In extremes of cold, too much exposure of the patient can itself become a problem. Rely on your sense of touch through the clothing as much as possible. Look for convenient access points through winter clothing, e.g., zippers and velcro closures.

Cold, heat, wind, rain and other environmental conditions are almost always factors that require your consideration in the wilderness. Consider them early

and attend to them as soon as possible. The earth's surface, for instance, rarely rises to temperatures warmer than your patient's temperature, which means you'll want to get your patient on an insulating pad as soon as possible.

The initial assessment should take no more than 60 seconds if there are no immediate threats to life. However, you may be involved with the initial assessment for hours if there is an immediate threat to life.

Stop! Complete A Focused Assessment

Focused Assessment

When you have completed a thorough initial assessment, you have to make a decision about the further care of the patient. If the patient has any life-threatening problems that have not been managed in the field, or if the mechanism of injury suggests serious underlying problems, or if your intuition tells you more is going on than you are ready to handle, the patient should be on the way to the nearest hospital-- in an ideal world. The focused assessment could then be performed during transport. Rapid evacuation, however, is rarely possible in the wilderness, which means two things: 1) critical patients have a high mortality rate in the wilderness, and 2) you will usually have time to do a complete focused assessment. The focused assessment has three parts: 1) physical examination, 2) vital signs, and 3) relevant medical history. The order often varies. A patient, for instance, may calm down and reveal more in the physical exam if you take a history first. Treatment for discovered problems will wait until the assessment is complete.

Physical Examination

If you haven't asked yet, the physical examination should begin with the patient being asked for a *chief complaint*. This is done with a simple question, such as "Can you tell me what hurts" or "Can you tell me why you need help?" This is important because the patient may have an obvious and severely angulated fracture of the lower leg and respond to the question with: "I (gasp) can't (gurgle) breathe!" If the patient responds with two complaints ask which is the most bothersome. If the patient is unable to answer due to unconsciousness, "unconsciousness" may be recorded as the "chief complaint."

Knowing the chief complaint will give you another clue when you make your final assessment, as well as tell you what areas of the patient's body to be especially careful with during the exam.

The physical exam is a head-to-toe investigation during which you will Look for, Ask about, and Feel for (LAF), as well as Listen for and Smell for clues.

Look for bruises and other discolorations, bleeding, swelling and other deformities, or anything else out of the ordinary. Look for grimaces in response to pain from a patient with an altered level of consciousness.

Ask about pain (it hurts all the time), tenderness (it hurts only in response to being touched), or any unusual sensations.

Feel for unusual softness or hardness, rigidity, heat or cold, or anything out of the ordinary.

Listen for labored or unusual breathing sounds, grunts or groans from the patient when you touch a specific spot.

Smell for unusual body odors, breath odors, or odors from clothing or the environment.

The Head-To-Toe Examination

Position yourself at the patient's shoulder. If you have someone who can work with you, have that person hold manual stabilization of the patient's head during the exam if such immobilization is required. If you are alone, ask the conscious patient to refrain from moving his or her head. If you are alone with an unconscious patient, proceed with the examination, moving the patient as little as possible. Maintain a calm dialogue with patient, explaining what you are doing, asking for information. Even if the patient is unconscious, a calm, reassuring voice will often be of benefit. If the patient is seated, the same guidelines apply.

Head and Neck: Carefully remove a hat, cap or helmet. Run your fingers gently through the patient's hair. If hair is matted to the head, leave it in place but look closely for damage. If you discover a depression in the skull, be very careful not to move the bone fragments (SEE CHAPTER 9: HEAD INJURIES). Feel gently along the muscles and bones of the neck. Check for proper alignment of the trachea. Look for jugular vein distention (SEE CHAPTER 10: CHEST INJURIES) and Battle's sign (SEE CHAPTER 9: HEAD INJURIES). If at any time in your exploration of the neck, you find evidence of cervical spine (neck) injury, e.g., tenderness or deformation, place a cervical collar on the patient as soon as possible (SEE CHAPTER 8: SPINE INJURIES). Look for a medical identification tag at the neck, a tag that might relate important information such as allergies and pre-existing conditions.

Face: If the patient is wearing sunglasses, carefully remove them to assess the eyes, and replace them if the patient is more comfortable with the glasses on. Apply gentle pressure to the bony structures of the face and jaw. Without moving the head, check the eyes, ears, nose, and mouth for damage or unusual fluids. Ask the patient to follow your finger as you move it back and forth in front of the eyes. The eyes should move through a normal range of motion, and the pupils should be approximately equal in size and responsive to light (SEE BELOW PUPILS). Note any unusual breath odors, e.g., alcohol.

Chest: Spread your hands over the rib cage and check for instability of the ribs during respirations and asymmetry of respirations. Ask the patient to take a deep breath. A normal chest should rise and fall easily and equally on both sides without pain. Check high and low on the chest wall. Press gently on the sternum (breastbone). For more information SEE CHAPTER 10: CHEST INJURIES.

Abdomen: Press gently with one hand with the flat of your fingers, not your fingertips, on the four quadrants of the patient's abdomen. The four quadrants are the patient's Upper Right, Upper Left, Lower Right, and Lower Left with the navel as the central point. Do not press on obvious injuries. Check for pain, guarding (the patient protecting the abdomen from your palpations), rigidity in abdominal muscles, and distention of the abdomen. These are usual indicators of internal damage (SEE CHAPTER 11: ABDOMINAL INJURIES).

Pelvis and Lower Back: With your hands cupped over the iliac crests (pelvic crests), press gently downward, then inward. Without moving the patient, slide your hands underneath the lower back and check as much of the back and spine as you can reach.

Genitals: Unless damage is indicated, there is no need to check the genitals. If checking the genitals is required, state your reason for checking and ask permission first, if possible. Try to have a rescuer of the same gender and/or witnesses when checking genitals, especially with minors.

Note: If you need better access to a patient's back or buttocks in order to make an accurate assessment, gently lift the patient's arm, if the arm is unharmed, on the side you are assessing, place the arm across the patient's chest, and run your hand under the patient while moving the spine as little as possible. If a suspected back injury, e.g., a wound, requires taking a look, you may need to roll the patient to do so. Rolling a patient with a possible spinal injury requires great care (SEE CHAPTER 8: SPINE INJURIES).

Lower Extremities: Take a look at both legs for signs of injury, e.g., angulations, protruding bones, legs shortened and/or rotated abnormally at the hip. Check each leg, one at a time, from hip to foot. You will need to remove the shoes or boots and socks to inspect the feet of an unreliable patient, but you do not typically need to visually inspect the feet of a reliable patient who denies altered sensations in the feet. In a cold environment, however, visually check the feet for frostbite. Be prepared to protect the foot as soon as possible from cold. Check to see if the patient has sensation in the feet and the ability to wiggle the toes. Impairment of sensation and/or mobility may indicate spinal damage. In all patients suspected of spinal damage, compare the strength in each leg by asking the patient to push and pull her feet against the resistance of your hands.

Upper Extremities: Gently squeeze the shoulders, including the clavicle (collarbone) and scapula (shoulder blade). Check each arm separately. Check to see if the patient has sensation in the hands and the ability to wiggle the fingers. Impairment of sensation and/or mobility may indicate spinal damage. In all patients suspected of spinal damage, compare the strength in each arm by asking the patient to squeeze your hands.

Vital Signs

Vital signs relate how well the patient's basic life support systems--nervous system, circulatory system, respiratory system-- are doing their jobs. An accurate measurement of a body's vital functions do not tell you what is wrong with your patient, but they do relate how well your patient is doing. The second set of vital signs is more important than the first set. And the third more important than the second. Whatever the injury or illness, a stable patient's vital signs stay the same, an improving patient or a deteriorating patient will be indicated by changes in vital signs. Circumstances will dictate how often the signs are taken, but the change over time is the key to using vital signs in long-term patient care. A constant monitoring of your patient should be maintained until they are no longer in your care. And remember: Do not isolate on one vital sign, but take them as a whole picture.

The vital signs are 1) level of consciousness (LOC), 2) heart rate, or pulse (HR), 3) respiration rate, or breathing (RR), 4) skin color, temperature, and moisture (SCTM), 5) blood pressure (BP), 6) pupils (P), and 7) body core temperature (T). During a patient's progress through an injury or illness, the first four vital signs (LOC, HR, RR, SCTM) will change early and sometimes, if the patient is seriously in trouble, very fast. The last three vital signs (BP, P, T) will change late.

Since *when* vitals were measured and the *speed at which* vitals change are often critical factors in patient management, it is important, especially in the long-term care that a wilderness situation often demands, that you note and record the hour and minute you took a set of vital signs. "Time" may be considered almost a vital sign itself, a critical decision-making tool along with patient condition, distance from help, terrain, transportation options, strength of the group, etc.

Vital signs, including time, should be recorded as soon as possible after they are measured.

Early Changing Vital Signs

Level Of Consciousness (LOC)

The level of consciousness is a measure of a brain's ability to relate to the outside world. A normal level of consciousness allows your patient to answer intelligently in a way that tells you if he or she is oriented in person, place, time, and event (who, where, when, and what happened). LOC is the easiest sign to assess, and the first to change. It can be recorded simply by using the AVPU scale, which assigns the patient a letter grade from "alert" to "unresponsive."

Alert: The patient seems normal, and answers intelligently questions about person, place, time, and event: Who are you? Where are you? Approximately what time is it? What happened to you? A patient who responds appropriately to all four questions is fully alert and awarded an alert-and-oriented-times-four status: A+Ox4. A patient, however, may be awake but not fully alert.

LOC=A+Ox4: Patient knows person, place, time, and event.

LOC=A+Ox3: Patient only knows person, place, and time.

LOC=A+Ox2: Patient only knows person and place.

LOC=A+Ox1: Patient only knows who he or she is.

Verbal: Any patient with a level of consciousness below Alert is considered an "unconcious" patient. The "verbal" patient is not alert, but he or she does respond in some way when spoken to, e.g., a yell from the rescuer stimulates a grimace, grunt, or rolling away from the noise. The patient may even follow simple commands.

LOC=V.

Pain: The patient does not react to verbal stimuli, but he or she does react to being pinched or rubbed in sensitive areas, e.g., a pinch on the back of the arm, a knuckle rub on the sternum. Pulling away from a pinch or sternal rub or pushing away the hand that pinches or rubs are appropriate responses to pain. An inappropriate response to pain, such as curling toward a fetal position, indicates an even deeper level of unconsciousness.

LOC=P.

Unresponsive: The patient does not respond to stimuli.

LOC=U.

Heart Rate (HR)

Heart rate may be taken at any place where you can palpate a pulse. Pulse is a pressure wave created by the beating of the heart, a wave of expansion and contraction within an artery as blood rushes through. You can feel a pulse anywhere an artery passes over a bone or near the surface of the body. In the initial assessment you checked a pulse at the carotid artery, assuring yourself that your patient had blood being pumped to the brain. Now you are interested in the rate, rhythm, and quality of that pulse--in other words, how well the patient's heart is functioning. The *radial* pulse, inside the wrist, where the thumb side of the hand joins the arm, is usually the best place to check a pulse. Use the tips of two or three of your fingers. The radial pulse is easy to access. It's more reassuring to a conscious patient than having your fingers pressed into the carotid. It tells you, if you find an adequate radial pulse, that the patient's blood pressure is adequate (SEE BELOW BLOOD PRESSURE).

Rate: The quantity (number) of beats per minute. The normal range in an adult can vary greatly, as much as 50-100, although the range usually falls between 60 and 80. It will usually be higher in children, sometimes reaching a norm of 160 in an infant. Counting for one full minute is most accurate, but a count for 15 seconds and multiplying by 4 is acceptable and more often used. In the absence of a watch, take a pulse anyway. At least you can assess the rhythm and quality.

Rhythm: There will be either a clock-like regularity, or a sporadic irregularity.

Quality: This refers to the force exerted by the heart on each beat. The force will be best judged by its relation to previous pulse checks. A normal quality is "strong," a "thready" pulse is weak and an indication of inadequate circulation, and a "bounding" pulse is abnormally forceful.

Note: An absence of a radial pulse is cause for alarm, but delay panicking until you check the other arm. The cause might be an injury to the arm or shoulder.

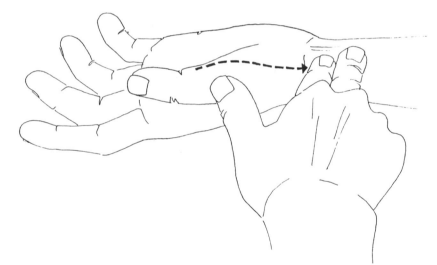

Figure 3-2: Checking the radial pulse

Respiration Rate (RR)

Breathe in and out once, and you've completed one *respiration*, or one breath. The rate, rhythm, and quality of respirations tell you how well a patient is moving life-sustaining air in and out. A patient alerted to the fact that you're checking respirations may voluntarily alter his breathing pattern. Keep your assessment a secret whenever possible by lightly placing one of your hands on the chest and/or upper abdomen and counting the movements without telling the patient you're counting.

Rate: The quantity (number) of breaths per minute. An adult normally breathes 12-20 times per minute. Children and infants breathe faster. Respiration rates are most accurate if taken for one full minute or, at least, for 30 seconds and multiplying by two.

Rhythm: Normally, breaths are even and regular, exhalations taking slightly longer than inhalations. Check for irregularities in the pattern, indications of a respiratory problem.

Quality: Normal breathing is quiet and effortless. Abnormal breathing might include unusual shallowness, unusual depth, labor, pain, noise (snores, wheezes, gurgles, gasps), and a flaring of the nostrils.

Skin Color, Temperature, Moisture (SCTM)

It's on the outside, away from the body's core where vital life processes are centered, but the skin gives pertinent information on the general well-being of your patient by giving evidence of changes in vital body processes.

Color: Pink is the normal color of skin in the non-pigmented areas of the body--the lining of the eye, inside the mouth, fingernail beds. It may be difficult to detect subtle changes in darker complexions, but the overall color of the skin is also an indicator. The size of the blood vessels near the skin, in most cases, determines skin color: Red, white, blue, or yellow. Vasodilation (widening vessels) produces a red, flushed color, and indicates problems such as fever or hyperthermia. Vasoconstriction (narrowing vessels) produces pale or blotchy skin, and may indicate shock or hypothermia. A blue hue, called *cyanosis*, shows a lack of oxygen in the blood. Yellowish skin, called *jaundice*, could indicate liver failure.

Temperature: Normal skin is relatively warm. Keep in mind that normal skin may feel cold on a cold day in the wilderness, and hot if the patient has been recently exercising. The temperature of the skin will not tell you anything exact about your patient's core temperature, but it will indicate whether or not the temperature is unusually high or low (SEE BELOW BODY CORE TEMPERATURE). You will get a more accurate check of skin tempera-

ture if you use the back of your hand instead of your palm or fingers.

Moisture: Normal skin is relatively dry. Wetness from excessive sweating may be evident, but if the skin is cool and moist, it may indicate shock. Hot, dry skin may indicate hyperthermia.

Late Changing Vital Signs

Blood Pressure (BP)

Blood pressure, the pressure of pulsing blood against arterial walls, is one of the most important vital signs, but one in which you will note changes *after* other vital signs have changed. You should know 1) how to get a BP with a sphygmomanometer and stethoscope, 2) how to get a BP with a sphygmomanometer only, 3) how to estimate a BP without instruments, and 4) what that information tells you about the patient.

A *sphygmomanometer*, or "cuff," is the instrument used to measure blood pressure. The cuff itself is a rubber bladder inside of a cover. The bladder has two tubes leaving its middle, one to a gauge, the other to the rubber bulb that inflates the bladder when squeezed. Bladder sizes vary and adults must have their pressure taken with an adult-sized cuff, children with children-sized cuffs, infants with baby cuffs, or else the readings will be inaccurate. The cuff is wrapped snugly around the patient's arm, about one inch above the elbow, with the two tubes centered over the *brachial* artery, the artery passing through the region of the elbow on the inside of the arm. Before taking the blood pressure, make sure

the patient's arm is relaxed and the cuff approximately on the same level as the patient's heart.

Attached to the cuff is an aneroid gauge or manometer. Mercury-gravity gauges, seen in hospitals, are more precise but impractical in the field. Inside the aneroid gauge is a metal bellows that expands or collapses with changes in pressure. Those changes are reflected on the dial of the gauge, calibrated into millimeters of mercury (mmHg) so everyone talks the same language. Advantages of the aneroid include portability, and disadvantages include susceptibility to inaccurate readings with major weather changes.

Most commonly, the cuff is used in conjunction with a stethoscope. Many stethoscopes have a two-sided patient end, one flat and called the diaphragm, one rounded and called the bell. Use the diaphragm side when taking a blood pressure, and, if there are two diaphragms, use the larger one. The bell is usually used for listening for specific respiratory or cardiac sounds.

With the gauge in view, the rescuer should palpate the radial artery, and then, with a finger on the radial, squeeze the bulb (with the other hand) and inflate the cuff until the radial pulse disappears plus about 20 mmHg more. Now the rescuer is ready to take a BP by *auscultation*, by listening. Place the diaphragm of the stethoscope over the brachial artery. Begin deflating the cuff at a rate of two-to-four mmHg per heartbeat. If you have taken a pulse first, it is easier to judge the rate of deflation. The needle on the dial should drop slowly. Sounds heard through the stethoscope, called Korotkoff sounds, relate the blood pressure. The needle will be pointing to the systolic pressure when the first sound is heard. *Systolic pressure* is the force exerted against the arterial walls by the blood when the heart's left ventricle contracts. A normal systolic is 100 plus the age of the patient up until 150 mmHg. Women's blood pressures are usually a little lower. Above 150 is often considered high blood pressure. When the last sound is heard, the diastolic is read. *Diastolic pressure* is the blood's pressure against the artery when the heart is at rest. A normal diastolic range is 60-90 mmHg, with anything above 90 generally considered hypertension, or high blood pressure. Blood pressure is recorded with the systolic over the diastolic: 120/

80. The difference between the systolic number and diastolic number is called the pulse pressure. Pulse pressures normally range between 35 and 50 mmHg, and are a measure of the pressure of the pulse wave.

Note: Although a blood pressure often measures a couple of mmHg's higher on the left arm, the difference between left and right arm is insignificant. Take a BP on the arm that's most available. If a second reading is necessary, wait at least 15 seconds before reinflating the cuff. Some patients will be in pain, or nervous, and their apprehensions will alter their pressure. The rescuer needs to be a calming influence.

Without a stethoscope but with a cuff, a systolic pressure

can still be obtained by *palpation*. The process is this: Palpate the radial pulse, inflate the cuff, maintain contact with the point of the radial pulse during deflation, note the position of the needle on the dial at the first palpable return of pulse, and that's the systolic. This offers a big advantage in a cold evironment since a relatively accurate BP can be obtained without removing clothing. You cannot obtain a diastolic pressure without a stethoscope. Systolic blood pressure by palpation is recorded as the number over P: 120/P.

Without a stethoscope or cuff, as often occurs in the wilderness, it is possible to guess blood pressures by palpating pulses. This may be called blood pressure by *estimation*. Here are suggested estimations:

Suggested estimations of blood pressure by palpating pulse

Carotid (neck) pulse present	Systolic BP is greater than 50mmHg
Femoral (groin) pulse present	Systolic BP is greater than 60mmHg
Brachial (arm) pulse present	Systolic BP is greater than 70mmHg
Radial (wrist) pulse present	Systolic BP is greater than 80mmHg
Pedal (foot) pulse present	Systolic BP is greater than 90mmHg

Typically, it is the falling blood pressure that most concerns us in the wild outdoors. When the BP drops below 70 mmHg, the kidneys lose their ability to remove waste products from the blood. As these waste products accumulate, the blood becomes toxic. When the BP drops below 50 mmHg, the other internal organs start to fail.

So, when your patient loses their brachial pulse, the BP is so low they're in trouble. When they

lose their carotid, they are in serious trouble . . . or dead.

Other indications of a dropping blood pressure include dizziness or lightheadedness if the patient sits up. Although often difficult to judge in the cold outdoors, the patient's skin will go pale, and eventually cyanotic.

Note: Since an adequate blood pressure in most patients is indicated by an alert level of consciousness, a strong radial pulse, and relatively normal skin color, temperature, and moisture, as a

general rule in wilderness medicine, LOC=A+Ox4 *plus* a strong radial pulse *plus* normal skin *equals* adequate BP.

Pupils (P)

Normal pupils are equal in size and round in shape, and they have a normal *pupillary response* to light: They *constrict*, or grow smaller, when exposed to light, and they *dilate*, or grow larger, when the light is reduced. You can check a patient's pupils by shining a light, e.g., flashlight, briefly into each eye, one at a time, and checking the response. In sunlight, you can cover an eye with your hand, wait a moment for the pupil to dilate, then uncover the eye and observe the response. Normal pupils may be recorded as pupils-equal-round-and-reactive-to-light: PERRL. Pupils that do not respond and pupils that respond unequally when one is compared to the other are significant discoveries.

Body Core Temperature (T)

The normal core temperature of a human runs around 98.6 degrees Fahrenheit (37 degrees Celsius). You can measure core temperature only with a thermometer, and even then you may get inaccurate results. In a patient suffering from the cold stress of hypothermia, for instance, oral thermometers sometimes register temperatures *lower* than the patient's core temperature, due to a cold mouth from breathing cold air. In a heat stressed patient who has been exercising vigorously, a rectal thermometer reading may be substantially *higher* than the core, due to the heat generated by muscular activity. Failure to properly use a thermometer, which is more likely in a wilderness environment, e.g., dark, wind, rain, can make it difficult even to monitor with relative accuracy the changes in temperature over time. Your best bet is to periodically check the reading until you find two consecutive readings of the same temperature.

Three areas of the body provide relatively convenient thermometer access: Mouth, armpit, and rectum.

Mouth: Oral thermometers provide the easiest access to an actual measurement. Your patient does not have to expose any body parts to the environment, and most patients are comfortable having the thermometer in place. Standard glass thermometers have found a home in many wilderness first aid kits, but they do break easily. Exposure to excesses of heat or cold can alter the accuracy of a standard glass thermometer, and cheap ones can lose their accuracy over time even under controlled conditions. Electronic thermometers are more durable and probably more accurate, but they only work as long as the battery does.

It is often suggested, sometimes strongly, that your thermometer should be one that reads low temperatures, sometimes called a "hypothermia" thermometer, because many standard instruments will not register in the hypothermia range. There are, however, many indications of hypothermia far easier to check and far more reliable than a temperature measurement (SEE CHAPTER 16: COLD-INDUCED EMERGENCIES). Thermometers are more trustworthy when used to check for rises in core temperature, e.g., fever.

The thermometer needs to be held in the mouth, under the tongue, for three to five minutes. The patient needs to remain still.

Armpit: The same glass thermometers used in the mouth can be used in the armpit, with the same pros and cons mentioned above. The thermometer may need to be left in place for up to 10 minutes. Axial (armpit) temperatures, in the wilderness especially, are at best a poor guess at "core" temperature, and are not recommended.

Rectum: Anywhere you can stick a regular glass thermometer, you can stick a "rectal" thermometer, and vice versa. Glass rectals are typically made, however, of thicker material, which means you'll have to leave it in a bit longer to get an accurate measurement. Digital thermometers with long flexible probes work well for taking a rectal temperature. Other than the heat-stressed patient mentioned earlier, you should get a fairly accurate estimate of "core" temperature with a rectal measurement. As you can easily imagine, a substantial amount of your patient will get exposed to the environment, and most patients will be made uncomfortable by the procedure. If you take a rectal measurement, the thermometer need only go in two to four inches.

Normal Vital Signs For An Adult

LOC	A+Ox4
HR	50-100, regular, strong
RR	12-20, regular, easy
SCTM	pink, warm, dry
BP	100-150/60-90
P	PERRL
T	98.6 F (37 C)

The Medical History

As you practice, you will gain pride in your ability to perform a patient exam and take a set of vital signs, but the tricky part of assessment, and probably 80 percent of your final verdict, will come from information gathered as you interview your patient. A wise old medical maxim states: It is more important to know what kind of patient has a disease than what kind of disease the patient has.

Approach the interview with a calm, confident, competent, compassionate attitude. An aura of calmness surrounding the scene will often do more for the sick and injured than all the splints and aspirin you can throw at patients. Quietly say, "Hi, I've been trained in wilderness medicine, and I can help you." Don't scream, "What happened? What happened?"

If you haven't already, establish a relationship with your patient. It is more effective to say sincerely, "I know you must be afraid and in pain, but we'll make you as comfortable as possible," as opposed to panting, "You'll be okay. You'll be fine."

Create a positive situation. Say: "Are you more comfortable sitting up or lying down?" Don't say: "Which hurts more?"

Be enthusiastic without being a cheerleader. Be kind without being nauseating. Be honest without saying everything you're thinking. Beware of the tone of your voice. Beware of your patient's tendency to take the slightest offhand comment as truth. Discuss with them the possible plans of action. They have a right to their say in what happens.

Effective communication with another person is exhibited by someone who:

1. Listens carefully.

2. Takes time to gather information before acting.

3. Gets specific details rather than general information.

4. Repeats what he or she has heard back to the other person to check for correctness of understanding.

5. Notices how the other person responds--verbally and non-verbally--and uses what has been noticed to improve communication.

6. Varies approaches to communication to meet the need of the specific situation.

7. Empathizes, demonstrates the ability to "step into someone else's shoes."

A helpful mnemonic for gathering information is SAMPLE:

Symptoms: "Describe what you're feeling. Pain? Headache? Dizziness? Nausea? Stomachache? Hot? Cold?" You need to know the sensations the patient is feeling.

Allergies: "Are you allergic to anything you know of? Foods? Drugs? Animals? Pollens?" You need to know if the patient contacted something that could cause an allergic reaction, and you need to prevent the patient from contacting something that could cause an allergic reaction.

Medications: "Taking anything currently? Over-the-counter drugs? Prescription drugs? Illegal drugs? Alcoholic beverages? Did you skip taking your medication? Did you take more than usual?" You need to know if medications are causing or could later cause a problem.

Past Relevant History: "Is there anything possibly relevant I should know about your health? Are you seeing a doctor for anything? Heart problems? Lung problems? Stomach problems? Seizures? Diabetes? Has anything like this ever happened before? You need to know a patient's medical conditions that could be causing or may later cause a problem.

Last Oral Intake: "When did you eat or drink last? What? How much?" You need to beware of what is currently in a patient's stomach, and you need to be aware of a patient's current and future needs for food and water.

Events: "What caused this illness (or injury)? Have you been feeling OK the last few days? Has anything unusual happened that could be related to this event?" And finally: "Is there anything else I should know?" You need to know if events leading to the problem are a part of the problem, and you need to leave no wilderness medicine stone of information unturned.

If the patient is in pain or discomfort, another mnemonic is OPQRST.

Onset: "What initiated the pain? Did it come on suddenly or gradually?"

Provokes, Palliates: "Does anything, such as changing position or taking a deep breath, make it better or worse?"

Quality: "Describe the pain or discomfort?" (e.g., sharp vs. dull, constant vs. erratic.)

Radiates, Refers, Region: "Does the pain radiate or refer from one part of the body to another? What is the region (location) of the pain?"

Severity: "How bad is the pain on a scale of one-to-ten with ten being the worst pain imaginable?"

Time: "How long has the pain or discomfort been going on? When did it start?"

If your patient is unconscious, you have to become even more of a Sherlock Holmes in your search for clues. Are they wearing medical alert tags on neck, wrists, ankles? Is there any information in their pockets? What can you learn from witnesses? Is there anyone around who knows the patient? What evidence does the scene hold for you? You need to figure out why the patient is unconscious (SEE CHAPTER 25: NEUROLOGICAL EMERGENCIES).

Stop! Complete Patient Care And Documentation

The SOAP Note

When time allows, or if there are spare hands at the scene, all the information gathered during assessment, and what was done for treatment, should be recorded on paper. You will never remember everything, vital signs slip away like autumn leaves in a high wind, and the patient deserves to have any physician who later takes over know the details of what happened and what was done. The note also becomes a legal record if a medical-legal question arises. Even if you're not sure what you're doing is absolutely correct, you want to record all your efforts on the patient's behalf. It shows you did your best, and it provides an essential element for others if you decide to send out for help.

The note can be divided into four sections for convenience of memory:

Subjective: : What happened (MOI) to who (include name, age, and sex), where and when? What is the chief complaint? OPQRST?

Objective: What did the physical exam reveal? What are the vital signs, and how did they change over time? What is the relevant medical history? SAMPLE? Are there pertinent negatives, e.g., "patient exam revealed no pain or tenderness."

Assessment: What are the possible problems?

Plan: What are you going to do? Do you have a plan for every assessment you've listed?

Sample Soap Note

Subjective	On 1 April 1997, John Doe, 22 year old, male, fell approximately 20 feet while rock climbing on Cannon Mountain, and pendulumed back first into rock wall. Patient was wearing no helmet. Patient denies loss of consciousness. Patient states: "My head hurts." Pain described as constant "5" on scale of 1-to-10.
Objective	Physical exam revealed pain on palpation in back of head, neck, and upper back of rib cage near the backbone. No bruising or deformities noticed. Good circulation, sensation, and motion noted in all four extremities. No other relevant findings.

TIME	6:05 pm
LOC	A+Ox4
HR	84,reg,str
RR	14,reg,easy
SCTM	pink/warm/wet
BP	str.radial pulse
P	PERRL
T	Did not check
SYMPTOMS	Pain described as dull ache "like a bad headache" with no radiation.
ALLERGIES	None known to patient
MEDICATIONS	Patient denies meds.
PAST RELEVANT HISTORY	Patient denies relevant medical history.
LAST ORAL INTAKE	Patient claims granola bar, cheese, one-half liter of water at noon approx.
EVENTS	Patient states "I slipped while climbing."

Assessment	Possible head and/or neck injury. Possible chest and/or spine injury. Possible loss of body temp.
Plan	Full manual head and spine immobilization on foamlite pad in sleeping bag. Monitor closely for changes. Send a team of "runners" with full documentation and location in order to get help.

Stop! Monitor

Patient assessment is an ongoing process. You will continue to monitor, to reassess, until the patient is no longer in your care.

Conclusion

You notice a backpack standing open near the patient sprawled on the banks of the Green River, and a pair of hiking boots near the pack. Your eyes leap to the young man's feet, feet wearing climbing shoes. The scene appears to be without immediate hazards. You dig your protective gloves out of your first aid kit.

As you approach the patient, he tries to sit up. You ask him to lay still, and you place a hand on his head. A few questions, and you learn his fall from the sandstone cliff was short, perhaps no more than six feet. His chief complaint is pain in his left ankle. He bit his lip, thus the smear of blood. The patient denies striking his head. Other than the left ankle and lip, your head-to-toe examination reveals nothing else. With support to the ankle, he will probably be able to walk out on his injury. Vital signs are all within normal limits. There is no medical history immediately relevant to this patient other than your discovery that he has had nothing to drink for several hours.

Despite the absence of Mr. Holmes, your Sherlockian approach to assessing the young man has allowed you to deduce that no serious injury has occurred. Indeed, by the time your assessment has ended, and he has downed a liter of water, he chats amiably about how fine most of this wilderness trip has been.

What if more serious problems had been discovered during your assessment? As you work your way through this book, you will gain knowledge and skills necessary to deal with specific emergencies. It will become, as Mr. Holmes would say, "Elementary, my dear Watson."

Chapter 4: Airway And Breathing

You should be able to:

1. *Describe the basic anatomy of the human airway.*

2. *Demonstrate ways to open an airway including head-tilt/ chin-lift, jaw-thrust, and tongue-jaw lift.*

3. *Demonstrate clearing an obstructed airway for an adult, a child, and an infant.*

4. *Demonstrate rescue breathing for an adult, a child, and an infant.*

It could happen to you

Few places on earth can compare to the beauty and peace of your campsite near Grave Lake in the Wind River Mountains of Wyoming. You've stepped away from the rest of the group, the group you've been hired to lead, to spend a few minutes alone near the water while dinner preparations near completion. You hear their laughter drifting from beneath the trees. Some of those guys are real jokesters. The faded yellow sun dissolves into rose and gray, and your contentment deepens... then a scream from camp sends the hairs up on the back of your neck.

Rushing to the campfire, you find a member of the group lying unconscious, not breathing.

You hear a voice sob, "He choked on something!"

Introduction

Nothing will strike more fear into a patient than the inability to breathe adequately. Nothing will strike more fear into you than a patient who is not breathing. Of all the skills performed by a First Responder, few, if any, will ever compare in importance to those involving a human's airway. If you can open an airway, clear an airway, maintain an airway, and breathe for someone not breathing, you possess skills that may make the difference between life and death.

Air moves in and out of an adult human body, a process called breathing or *respiration*, at an average rate of once every five seconds. The process has two parts: *Inspiration*, or inhaling, and *expiration*, or exhaling. Numerous incidents can cause *respiratory arrest*. To name the more common incidents: upper airway obstruction, drowning, electric shock, suffocation, heart failure, head injury, seizures, drug overdoses, and severe allergic reactions.

Take away the process of breathing a few minutes, and the heart begins to weaken. Without a return of breathing, the heart will sputter and stop, the moment of *cardiac arrest*, which is also the moment of *clinical death*. If the heart does not start again in an average of four to six minutes, irreversible brain damage occurs and the brain shuts down, the beginning of *biological death*. Although short time spans separate the cessation of breathing and cardiac arrest, and the moment of clinical death and biological death, these are the times when a First Responder must intervene.

Basic Anatomy Of The Airway

Air enters a human body either through the nose into the *nasopharynx*, the upper pharynx, or through the mouth into the *oropharynx*, the central portion of the pharynx. The *pharynx*, the air passageway from nose to *larynx*, or "voice box," at the top of the *trachea* (windpipe), also provides a passageway for food to the *esophagus*, or "food tube." The trachea, visible at the front of the neck, is held open by C-shaped cartilage "rings" with the "C" opening toward the back of the neck where the esophagus lies flat until something is swallowed. When something is swallowed, a flap of tissue called the epiglottis closes the opening to the trachea, the glottis, to prevent solid matter from descending the trachea. Behind the sternum (breastbone), the trachea splits into two bronchi, one going left and one going right. The bronchi split into bronchioles of ever decreasing size until each one comes to a dead end at a grape-like cluster of alveoli, the air cells of the lungs where oxygen from the air is exchanged for carbon dioxide from the blood. For an airway to be open, it must be open from the mouth and/or nose all the way down to the alveoli.

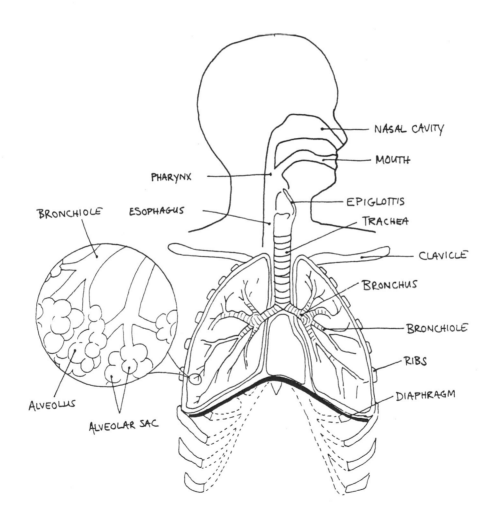

Figure 4-1: Anatomy of the airway

Opening An Airway

The scene is safe, and you have taken appropriate body substance isolation precautions. The patient appears unconscious. You are now at the A for Airway of the ABCDE of an initial assessment. Gently shake or simply tap the shoulder of the patient, and ask, Are you OK?, or something similar, in a loud voice. You are not after a specific answer per se, but after some response from the patient that gives you an immediate idea of his or her level of consciousness, a response such as a word, a groan, a movement, an opening of the eyes.

Remember, with any suspicion of head or spine injury, place your hand gently but firmly on the patient's head prior to asking for a response. *Do not shake a patient who may have a head or spine injury* (SEE CHAPTER 8: SPINE INJURIES). Unless otherwise indicated, the rest of this chapter assumes the patient has *no* head or spine injury.

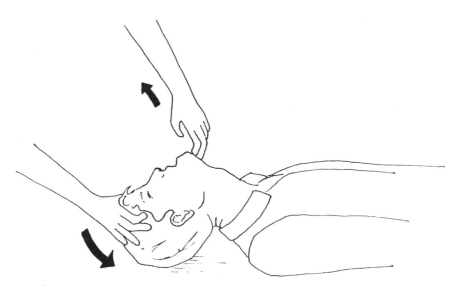

Figure 4-2: Head-Tilt / Chin-Lift Maneuver

Open the Airway

With any patient who may have a blocked airway, i.e., a patient who is not breathing or a patient with labored and/or noisy breathing, you must open the airway. Usually, this is best accomplished if the patient is in the *supine* position, on the back with face up and head in line with the back. A patient in a side position or in the *prone* (on the stomach) position who requires airway management will need to be rolled as a unit into the supine position. Rolling "as a unit" means to roll the patient's head, shoulders, and trunk simultaneously (SEE CHAPTER 8: SPINE INJURIES).

In an unconscious patient already on his or her back, the most common cause of airway blockage is the tongue. The tongue, a muscle, can relax and fall back far enough to prevent the passage of air. Sometimes simply and gently moving the head and neck into normal anatomical alignment will open the airway enough to save a life. Because the tongue is attached to the lower jaw, one of three maneuvers can be used to open an airway, three maneuvers that lift the lower jaw which in turn moves the tongue enough to allow air to pass.

Head-Tilt/Chin-Lift Maneuver

If you do *not* suspect head or neck injury, use the *head-tilt/chin-lift* to open an airway. Kneel beside the patient's head. With one hand on the patient's forehead, apply enough pressure to tilt the head back. At the same time lift the patient's chin with the fingers of your other hand. Be careful to not push in on the soft tissues under the chin which could further obstruct the airway. Continue to tilt and lift until the head is in an extended position, the chin pointed toward the sky. With a small child or infant, tilt the head only into a neutral position, the neck only slightly extended. Full extension could partially close the airway of a small child or infant.

Jaw Thrust Maneuver

If you do suspect head or neck injury, use the jaw thrust to open an airway. Kneel near the top of the patient's head, facing the patient's feet. With your elbows on the ground, place your hands on the sides of the patient's head, your thumbs on the cheek-

bones, two or three fingers of each hand at the corner of the patient's jaw where it angles between chin and ear. Lift the jaw with your fingers, using counter-pressure from your thumbs on the cheekbones.

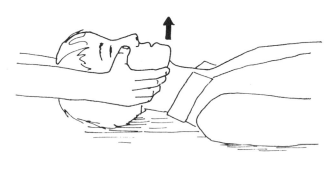

Figure 4-3: Jaw Thrust Maneuver

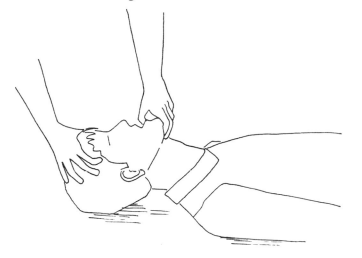

Figure 4-4: Tongue-Jaw Lift Maneuver

Tongue-Jaw Lift Maneuver

To open an airway in order to remove an object in the mouth, the tongue-jaw lift may be used. Grasping the tongue and lower jaw between your thumb and finger, lift the jaw up and out.

Assess Breathing

With the airway open, look, listen, and feel for air movement with your ear and cheek near the patient's mouth. Your head should be facing down the midline of the patient's body, allowing you to watch the chest for movement. Adequate breathing will be indicated by the rise and

fall of the chest and/or upper abdomen, the sound of air moving through the mouth, and the feeling of air from the mouth and nose blowing against your cheek. A breathless patient requires either removal of a foreign-body airway obstruction, or rescue breathing (SEE BELOW RESCUE BREATHING), or both.

Foreign-body Airway Obstruction: Conscious Adult

The most common cause of airway obstruction in a conscious patient is food. The obstructing object, whatever it is, usually lodges in the area of the glottis, and may form a partial or a complete obstruction.

A patient with a partial airway obstruction can get air past the obstruction and cough in attempts to clear the airway. This person requires no first aid and, indeed, should be allowed to cough his or her way to an open airway. This person, however, should not be left alone in case the obstruction shifts and becomes complete.

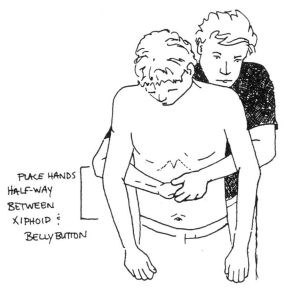

PLACE HANDS
HALF-WAY
BETWEEN
XIPHOID &
BELLY BUTTON

Figure 4-5: Heimlich Maneuver

A patient with a complete airway obstruction cannot get air past the obstruction, cannot speak or cough, cannot breathe. A patient with a complete obstruction may make weak breathing sounds and/or high pitched wheezing sounds but will not be able to adequately move life-sustaining air in and out. This person typically appears extremely panicked, and he or she may be grasping the throat, involuntarily displaying the "universal distress signal" of choking. This person requires immediate, life-saving help in the form of the Heimlich Maneuver, also known as abdominal thrusts.

Before beginning abdominal thrusts, quickly identify yourself to the patient as someone who can help. Then…

If the Patient is Standing or Sitting:
1. Stand behind the patient.
2. Wrap your arms around the waist of the patient, keeping your elbows out and away from the patient's ribs.
3. Make a fist and place it thumb in on the midline of the patient's abdomen, above the navel, well below the *xiphoid* process, the point of cartilage extending below the bottom of the sternum.
4. Grab your fist with your other hand.
5. Pull quickly in and upward with a powerful motion, a motion intended to force the object out of the airway.

6. Repeat the abdominal thrust until the airway clears or the patient goes unconscious.

If the Patient is Lying Down:
1. Place the patient in the supine position.
2. Kneel astride the patient's thighs.
3. Place the heel of one your hands on the midline of the patient's abdomen, above the navel, well below the xiphoid at the bottom of the sternum.
4. Place your second hand on top the first hand.
5. Press quickly in and upward with a powerful motion.
6. Repeat the abdominal thrust until the airway clears or the patient goes unconscious.

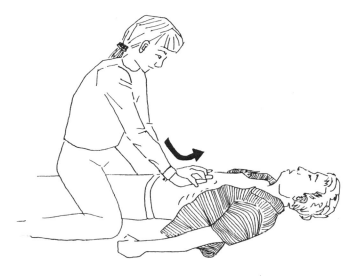

Figure 4-6: Abdominal Thrusts

If the Patient is Obese or Pregnant: For obese or pregnant choking persons, follow the above directions for the abdominal thrust with one important difference: Perform the thrust against the patient's chest with your hands on the *middle* of the sternum.

If You are Choking and Alone: If you suffer an upper airway obstruction while alone, perform the abdominal thrust on yourself. If this fails, press your upper abdomen against a firm object, e.g., backpack frame, log, and drop your weight against the object.

If the Patient goes Unconscious: If a patient goes unconscious during abdominal thrusts, place the patient on the ground in a supine position. This is easier said than done, especially if the patient is large and you aren't. Position yourself during abdominal thrusts in order to better control the patient's body weight should he or she lose consciousness.

1. Open the airway with a tongue-jaw lift and perform a finger sweep by running your index finger down the inside of one of the patient's cheeks, hooking your finger along the base of the tongue and back out in hopes of removing the obstructing object.

2. Perform a head-tilt/chin-lift and attempt to ventilate the patient by sealing your mouth over the patient's mouth, pinching the patient's nostrils firmly closed, and breathing in with enough force to cause the patient's chest to rise (SEE BELOW RESCUE BREATHING). If air doesn't go in, reposition the head and make a second attempt to ventilate.

3. If the airway remains blocked, straddle the patient's thighs and give up to five abdominal thrusts.

4. Repeat steps one through three until the airway has been successfully opened.

5. If the patient does not resume normal breathing, begin rescue breathing (SEE BELOW RESCUE BREATHING). If the patient does resume normal breathing, place the patient in the recovery position (SEE BELOW RECOVERY POSITION).

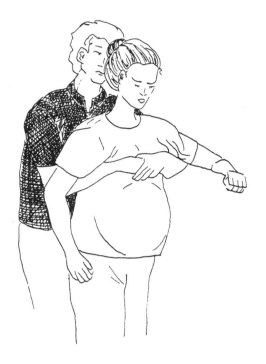

Figure 4-7: Chest thrust on pregnant patient

Foreign-body Airway Obstruction: Unconscious Adult

If the patient is found unconscious, immediately open the airway and look, listen and feel for breathing for three to five seconds. If the patient is not breathing:

1. Attempt to ventilate the patient. If air doesn't go in, reposition the head and make a second attempt to ventilate.

2. If the airway remains blocked, straddle the patient's thighs and give up to five abdominal thrusts.

3. Open the airway with a tongue-jaw lift and perform a finger sweep by running your index finger down the inside of one of the patient's cheeks, hooking your finger along the base of the tongue and back out in hopes of removing the obstructing object.

4. Repeat steps one through three until the airway has been successfully opened.

5. If the patient does not resume normal breathing, begin rescue breathing (SEE BELOW RESCUE BREATHING). If the patient does resume normal breathing, place the patient in the recovery position (see BELOW RECOVERY POSITION).

Note: The American Heart Association has established the following sequence for the rescue of an adult patient who is unresponsive:

1. Assess the patient to be sure he or she needs help.

2. Activate the Emergency Medical Services (EMS) system by dialing 911.

3. Begin resuscitation.

Obviously access to 911 will not be available in the wilderness. For that reason, the step of "activating the EMS system" is left out of sections of this chapter.

Foreign-body Airway Obstruction: Child

The American Heart Association defines someone between the ages of one and eight as a "child." An airway obstruction in a child is managed the same as in an adult with one exception: Tongue-jaw lifts are performed to open the airway, and if you *see* an object, you should remove it, but blind finger sweeps to remove unseen objects from the airway are *not* performed. A blind finger sweep could lodge the object deeper in a child's airway.

Note: The American Heart Association has established the following sequence for the rescue of a child or infant patient who is unresponsive:
1. Assess the patient to be sure he or she needs help.
2. If a second rescuer is available, send him or her to activate the Emergency Medical Services (EMS) system by dialing 911.
3. Begin resuscitation.
4. If alone and airway obstruction is not removed after one minute, activate the EMS system.

Obviously access to 911 will not be available in the wilderness. For that reason, the step of "activating the EMS system" is left out of sections of this chapter.

Foreign-body Airway Obstruction: Infant

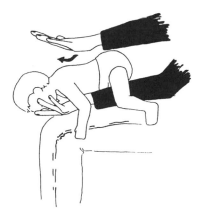

Figure 4-8: Back blows for choking infants

The American Heart Association defines someone less than one year in age as an "infant." Infants are not little adults, and management of an infant with a foreign-body airway obstruction differs from an adult's management.

If the infant is conscious:
1. Determine a serious breathing difficulty: lack of breathing, ineffective cough, weak cry.
2. Hold the infant face down on your forearm, supporting the head firmly with your hand. You may sit with your forearm on your thigh to increase support. The infant's head should be lower than his or her trunk.
3. With the heel of your other hand, deliver up to five forceful back blows between the infant's shoulder blades.
4. After the back blows, place your free hand on the infant's head, making a baby "sandwich" between your forearms and hands. Turn the infant carefully into a supine position with the head still lower than the trunk.
5. Deliver up to five quick chest thrusts with the fingers of your free hand on the lower half of the sternum, approximately one finger width below the infant's nipple line.
6. Repeat the back blows and chest thrusts until the airway is cleared or the infant goes unconscious.

If the infant goes unconscious:
1. Open the airway with a tongue-jaw lift, look for the obstruction, and, if you see it, remove it with your little finger. Do *not* perform a blind finger sweep.
2. Open the airway and attempt to ventilate by sealing your mouth over the infant's mouth and nose

and blowing in with only enough force to cause the infant's chest to rise. If the chest does not rise, reposition the infant's head and attempt a second ventilation.
3. If the airway remains blocked, give up to five back blows followed by five chest thrusts.
4. Repeat steps one through three until the airway is cleared.

If the infant is found unconscious:
1. Assess responsiveness, open the airway, and look, listen, and feel for breathing.
2. If the infant is not breathing, attempt to ventilate. If your air will not go in, reposition the infant's head and attempt a second ventilation.

3. If the airway remains blocked, give up to five back blows followed by five chest thrusts.
4. Open the airway with a tongue-jaw lift, look for the obstruction, and, if you see it, remove it with your little finger. Do *not* perform a blind finger sweep.
5. Repeat steps two through four until the airway is cleared.

Rescue Breathing

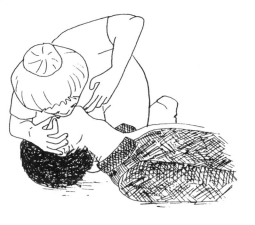

Figure 4-9: Mouth to mouth rescue breathing

The air you inhale contains approximately 21 percent oxygen, and the air you exhale approximately 16 percent oxygen. Only about five percent of the available oxygen is utilized by your body in each breath you take. So with rescue breathing you can provide adequate ventilation for a patient who is not breathing. Performed correctly, the First Responder may be able to save a life with rescue breathing.

Note: Use of a barrier device to prevent direct contact with a patient's mouth and body fluids is strongly recommended. Numerous commercial barrier devices

are available. Become familiar with the use of any device you carry *before* you need to use it. Most devices are used similar to the way mouth-to-mouth rescue breathing is delivered.

Mouth-to-Mouth Rescue Breathing:
After you have determined the patient is not breathing, use the thumb and first finger of your hand holding the patient's forehead to firmly pinch closed the patient's nostrils. If the nostrils are not pinched closed, the air you breath in will escape through the nose. Hold the mouth open with your other hand.
1. Take a deep breath. This will maximize the oxygen and mini-

mize the carbon dioxide in your lungs.
2. Open your mouth wide and seal it entirely over the patient's mouth. A poor seal is the single greatest cause of poor rescue breathing.
3. Deliver two initial *full, slow* breaths. Each of your ventilations should take one-and-a-half to two seconds. Blow only forcefully enough to fill the patient's lungs. *The rise of the patient's chest is the indicator you have delivered a full breath.* Too much air blown in too hard will force air into the patient's stomach causing gastric distention (SEE BELOW GASTRIC DISTENTION AND VOMIT).

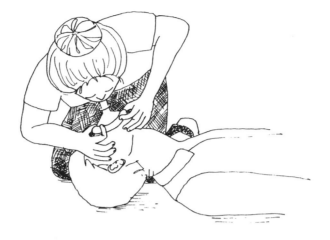

Figure 4-10: Mouth to mask rescue breathing

Note: If you're using the jaw-thrust maneuver to open the airway, you'll have to seal the patient's nose with your cheek, hold the patient's lower lip down with your thumbs and/or first fingers, and seal your mouth over the patient's mouth. Between breaths be sure to remove your mouth from the patient's mouth, and refill your lungs.

4. If your breath will not go in, reposition the patient's head and attempt to ventilate a second time. A second failed attempt indicates a foreign-body airway obstruction (see above).

5. Check for a carotid pulse. If the pulse is present, continue rescue breathing at the rate of approximately one breath every five seconds for an adult. This rate delivers approximately 12 breaths per minute. If the pulse is not present, initiate CPR (SEE CHAP-

TER 5: CARDIOPULMONARY RESUSCITATION).

Mouth-to-Nose Rescue Breathing: If the patient's mouth is injured or for some reason cannot be adequately opened, mouth-to-nose rescue breathing can provide adequate ventilation.

1. Perform the head-tilt/chin-lift maneuver, but hold the patient's lips closed.

2. Seal your mouth over the patient's nose.

3. Deliver two full, slow breaths, removing your mouth from the nose between breaths. If the patient does not exhale easily through the nose, you may open the mouth to let air escape the lungs.

4. Check for a carotid pulse. If the pulse is present, continue rescue breathing at the rate of approximately one breath every five seconds for an adult. This rate

delivers approximately 12 breaths per minute. If the pulse is not present, initiate CPR (SEE CHAPTER 5: CARDIOPULMONARY RESUSCITATION).

Mouth-to-Stoma Rescue Breathing:

You may have a patient who has had part or all of his or her larynx surgically removed. These people have a permanent opening inserted in the trachea, an opening called a *stoma*. Patients with a partial laryngectomy breathe through the stoma and through the nose and mouth. Patients with a full laryngectomy breathe entirely through the stoma.

Rescue breathing for patients with a stoma needs to be performed through the stoma. If the chest does not rise, suspect a partial laryngectomy, and use one of your hands to hold the patient's mouth and nose closed.

Rescue Breathing for Children and Infants

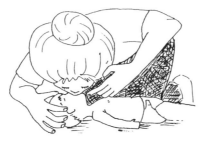

Figure 4-11: Rescue breathing for infants

Few differences distinguish rescue breathing for adults, children and infants. These differences may be summarized as:
1. Small children and infants should *not* have their heads fully extended to open an airway. Neutral or slightly extended is enough. Too much extension will close off a small airway.

2. For infants, seal off the mouth and nose with your mouth to perform mouth-to-mouth-and-nose rescue breathing.
3. Small lungs will take less time to fill with your breaths. Slow breaths on your part will help you control ventilation.
4. You may see the chests *and* abdomens of small children and infants rise when you ventilate.

5. For an infant, "puffs" of air from your mouth may adequately fill the lungs. Remember, the rise of the chest and abdomen are the indicators of a full breath.
6. The rate of breathing for small children and infants is approximately one breath every three seconds, or approximately 20 breaths per minute.

Gastric Distention and Vomit

Severe gastric distention (air inflating the stomach) during rescue breathing can cause vomiting and/or put enough pressure on the diaphragm to limit the air you can breathe into the lungs. Pressing on the stomach to release the trapped air is almost never recommended because it almost always causes vomiting. If, however, adequate rescue breathing is prevented, decompression may be the patient's only hope.

When the patient vomits, whether gastrically distended or not, immediately roll him or her into a side position to allow the vomit to flow out of the mouth instead of into the lungs where severe complications such as pneumonia may erupt. When the vomiting ends, wipe out the mouth—a T-shirt or bandanna will work for wiping— then roll the patient once again into a supine position, and continue resuscitation efforts.

Prevent gastric distention by:
1) maintaining an adequately open airway, 2) blowing air in slowly and with just enough force to see the chest rise, and 3) allowing adequate time for the patient to exhale between your rescue breaths.

Supplemental Oxygen

Rescue breathing will be more effective if supplemental oxygen, more often a wish than a fact in the wilderness, can be delivered. Several ways of delivering supplement oxygen exist

(SEE APPENDIX B: OXYGEN AND MECHANICAL AIDS TO BREATHING).

Recovery Position

Since every unconscious patient left on his or her back may lose an airway to a relaxed tongue and/or vomit, every unconscious patient should either 1) receive constant attention from a rescuer and/or 2) be rolled into the recovery position. Even one rescuer can move a patient with a suspected spine injury cautiously and successfully into the recovery position.

1. Kneel beside the patient at waist level.
2. Move the patient's arm on the same side of his or her body you're on until it is fully stretched out above the head, the reverse position to hanging straight down from the shoulder. The palm should be facing up.
3. Move the patient's arm on the side away from you across the patient's chest with the fingers pointing toward the opposite shoulder.
4. Flex the patient's knees and support them with your hand. If your strength does not allow you to flex and support the knees, cross the patient's legs with the away leg on top.
5. With your other hand support the patient's head and neck.
6. Roll the patient, as a unit, toward you by lowering the legs while assuring the patient's head stays in contact with the down arm. If you have crossed the legs instead of flexing the knees, roll the patient by grabbing firmly onto the hip.
7. Make sure the patient's nose points "downhill" to keep the airway open.
8. If the patient must be left alone, stabilize him or her in the recovery position with whatever is available, e.g., backpacks, rocks, logs.

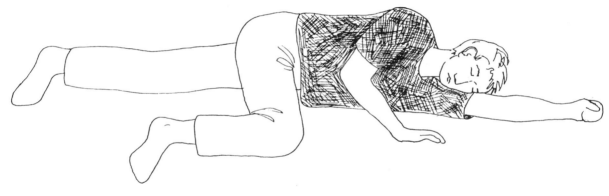

Figure 4-12: Recovery Position

Conclusion

Dropping to your knees beside your client in the Wind River Mountains, you attempt to get a response. Failing to establish responsiveness, you perform a head-tilt/chin-lift to open his airway. Looking, listening, and feeling for breathing, you detect none. Sealing your mouth over his, you pinch his nostrils closed and attempt a ventilation. It does not go in. Repositioning his head, you attempt a second ventilation without success. Leaping astride his thighs, you place the heel of one of your hands on his abdomen, well below the xiphoid, above the belly button, and your second hand on top of the first. With the fifth abdominal thrust, the client coughs out a chunk of canned meat. You open his airway and give two full breaths, watching as his chest rises and falls. He then spontaneously gasps out a few breaths before his respirations subside into a normal rhythm. The tension eases slightly between your shoulder blades.

Within a few minutes, his return to consciousness appears complete. Although you watch him carefully until fatigue sends everyone to their bags, you're able to fall asleep knowing you arrived in time.

Chapter 5: Cardiopulmonary Resuscitation

You should be able to:

1. Describe the basic anatomy of the heart.

2. Describe the signs of a patient in cardiac arrest.

3. Demonstrate cardiopulmonary resuscitation (CPR) on an adult, a child, and an infant.

4. Describe the complications that may occur during CPR.

5. List the criteria for stopping CPR.

6. Describe the special considerations concerning CPR in the wilderness.

It could happen to you

Colorado's San Isabel National Forest has attracted its usual large number of elk hunters, men and women from all over the United States who spend an October week in the Rockies. A few of those people will need help, and, as a volunteer on the local search and rescue team, you're ready to respond 24 hours a day. You're not surprised when a call comes during dinner.

This one is a little different: A man in his early fifties, not lost, but unable to walk the last half-mile to his car due to chest pain and the inability to catch his breath. His hunting partner hiked out and made the call.

You find the patient sitting against a tree beside a well-used trail, his orange jacket reflecting the beams of the headlamps of the rescue team. As you approach, he attempts to stand, and collapses face first to the ground.

Introduction

Cardiac arrest, the cessation of heart muscle activity, will end the lives of approximately one million humans suffering from heart disease in the United States over the next year (SEE CHAPTER 23: CARDIAC EMERGENCIES). Even with immediate cardiopulmonary resuscitation (CPR), most of these people will remain in cardiac arrest, but some can be saved by trained bystanders who witness the incident. Most of the patients who could have been saved, and most of the ones who are saved, receive not only immediate CPR but also more definitive medical treatment, such as defibrillation, administered by professional rescuers and hospital staff. In a wilderness environment, patients who go into cardiac arrest as a result of long-standing disease will rarely survive, even if your CPR skills are excellent.

Cardiac arrest, however, can be caused by other incidents, most commonly in the wilderness by lightning strikes, drownings, and burials by avalanche. In these cases, more often than not, you can save a life with CPR initiated without delay and performed correctly.

Basic Anatomy Of The Heart

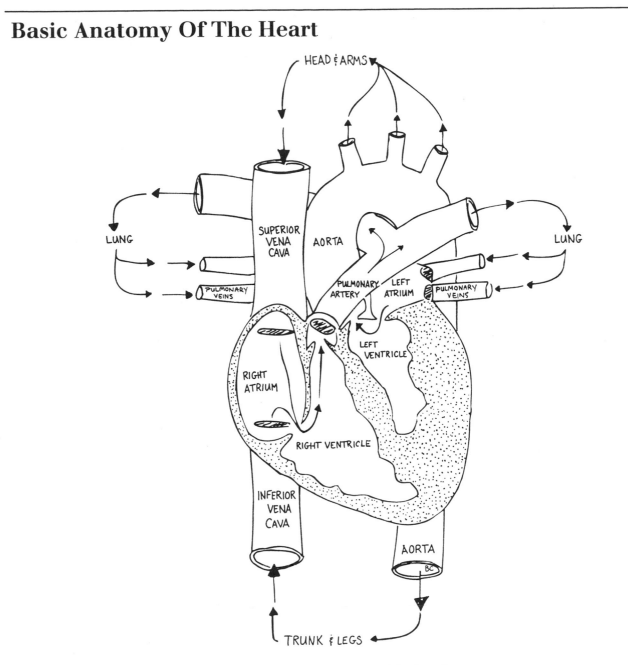

Figure 5-1: Basic anatomy of the heart

The heart is a muscular organ lying beneath the lower half of the sternum with the bottom "tipped" slightly to the left side of the body. Yours is approximately the size of your fist. Divided into four hollow chambers, the heart's two upper chambers, the right and left *atria*, are smaller than the two lower chambers, the right and left *ventricles*. These chambers are connected by one-way valves.

Blood from all over the body circulates into the right atrium via two large veins, the *inferior vena cava* and *superior vena cava*. Passing through the *tricuspid valve*, blood enters the right ventricle from where it is pumped through the *pulmonary valve* into the pulmonary artery and on to the five lobes of the lungs—three lobes on the right, two lobes on the left. From the pulmonary artery, blood squeezes through smaller and smaller arterioles until it enters capillaries that wrap around the alveolar sacs in the lungs. Alveolar sacs have microscopically thin walls, as do pulmonary capillaries. Here, on the alveolar level, gases are exchanged across the thin walls. After exchanging carbon dioxide for oxygen at the alveoli, blood travels through venules of increasing size until it reenters the heart at the left atrium via the pulmonary veins. It might be of interest to note that all veins in the body carry deoxygenated blood except the pulmonary veins, and all arteries carry oxygenated blood except the pulmonary arteries. All vessels carrying blood toward the heart are veins,

and all vessels carrying blood away from the heart are arteries. From the left atrium, blood passes through the *mitral valve* into the left ventricle. A hardy squeeze by the left ventricle sends blood through the aortic valve into the *aorta* and on to all parts of the body.

The pumping action of the heart keeps blood circulating under pressure, and each beat sends a pulse through the entire arterial system. Pulses are most easily palpated where large arteries run near the surface of the body. Two of those places are

the *carotid* pulse in the neck and the *radial* pulse at the wrist.

The heart and the lungs, the *cardiopulmonary system*, work together with the brain as an ultimate team, a perfect triumvirate, each precisely supporting the efforts of the other. If one of the team fails, the other two are soon to follow. Brain arrest, if you'll accept that term, is irreversible. Respiratory arrest (SEE CHAPTER 4: AIRWAY AND BREATHING) and cardiac arrest, however, may be reversed.

Cardiac Arrest & CPR

Respiratory arrest is the cessation of spontaneous breathing. Cardiac arrest is the cessation of heart function. A patient in respiratory *and* cardiac arrest is clinically dead: unresponsive, breathless, pulseless. Four to six minutes after cardiac arrest, the typical patient will have suffered irreparable brain cell death to the point where he or she is biologically dead. If CPR is initiated soon enough, done well enough, and

maintained long enough, the patient may eventually be resuscitated.

CPR consists of a rhythmic combination of rescue breathing and chest compressions. Rescue breathing keeps the patient's blood oxygenated. Chest compressions build up pressure in the chest cavity causing the blood to circulate with enough pressure to maintain life in the brain.

The basics of CPR may be summarized with the first three letters of the alphabet—ABC—the first three letters of the initial assessment.
A. Check for responsiveness. If unresponsive, open the AIRWAY.
B. Check for BREATHING. If breathless, give two full, slow breaths.
C. Check for a pulse. If pulseless, initiate CHEST compresssions.

Cardiopulmonary Resuscitation

The American Heart Association has established the following sequence for the rescue of an adult patient who is unresponsive:
1. Assess the patient to be sure he or she needs help.
2. Activate the Emergency Medical Services (EMS) system by dialing 911.
3. Begin resuscitation.
Obviously access to 911 will not be available in the wilder-

ness. For that reason, the step of "activating the EMS system" is left out of sections of this chapter.

Step One: Check Responsiveness

If the patient does not respond to an initial check for responsiveness, immediately open the airway with the head-tilt/chin-lift maneuver or the jaw-thrust maneuver (SEE CHAPTER 4: AIRWAY AND BREATHING)

Step Two: Check for Breathing

If a three to five second look, listen, and feel for breathing indicates the patient is breathless, give two full, slow breaths. If the patient's chest does not rise with your ventilations, reposition the patient's head and attempt to ventilate again (SEE CHAPTER 4: AIRWAY AND BREATHING).

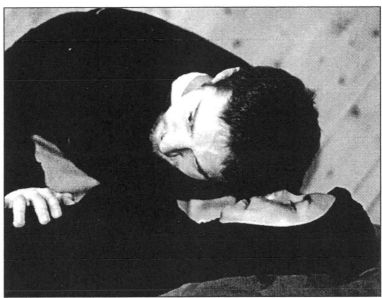

Figure 5-2: Checking for breathing: look, listen, and feel.

Step Three: Check for a Pulse

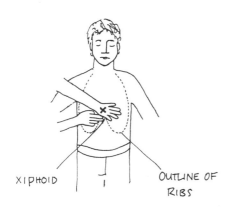

XIPHOID   OUTLINE OF
                              RIBS

Figure 5-3:
Hand placement for adult CPR

If you begin rescue breathing for someone who doesn't need it, you will do no harm. If you begin chest compressions on someone who doesn't need it, you could do harm. For that reason, your pulse check should be careful. Place two of your fingers on the patient's larynx (the "Adam's apple") and slide your fingers off to the side of the neck you are on. Do not reach across the trachea.

In the valley between the larynx and the large neck muscle you will find the carotid pulse. Check for at least five to 10 seconds before declaring pulselessness. If you find a pulse, continue rescue breathing. If you do not find a pulse, prepare to do chest compressions, but, before starting compressions:

1. Place the patient face up on a firm surface, e.g., the ground.
2. Expose the patient's chest. Time is of the essence: rip open or pull up shirts or blouses, cut off or slip up bras.
3. Kneel at the patient's shoulder with your knees approximately as far apart as your shoulders.
4. Find the xiphoid process (the point of cartilage extending below the lower end of the sternum) by running the fingers of your hand closest to the patient's feet up along the lower rib cage to the point where the ribs meet.
5. Mark two finger widths above the end of the sternum with your first hand, and place the heel of your second hand above the two fingers on the sternum. Place the heel of the hand that "land-marked" the xiphoid over the hand that's now on the lower half of the sternum. The lower half of the sternum is supported by carti-lege flexible enough to allow compressions. If you place your hands too high, you will fail to compress the chest enough. If you place your hands too low, you will soon break off the xiphoid, ribs, or even the sternum.
6. Straighten your arms and posi-tion your shoulders over the patient's chest.

Chest compressions should be fluid downward motions on the sternum followed by a release of pressure from the sternum which allows blood to flow back into the patient's heart and chest. Compression time and release time should be equal. Avoid jerky, jabbing motions. An adult patient's chest should be com-pressed one-and-a-half to two inches. Use the weight of your upper body instead of the strength of your arms and shoulders.

You will be performing 15 compressions to every two full breaths. The cycle ratio of 15:2 should be done in 15 seconds. Take nine to 11 seconds to do 15 compressions, which provides a rate of 80 to 100 compressions per minute. Take the remainder of the 15 seconds to give two breaths. In one minute you will have done 60 compressions and eight breaths. Counting softly out loud—"one, and two, and three"—will help you perfect your CPR compressions. *Practice, practice, practice.* Even the most excellent chest compressions will provide no more than one-third of the patient's normal circulation.

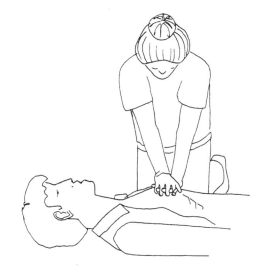

Figure 5-4: One rescuer chest compressions

Adult One-rescuer CPR

1. Check for responsiveness.
2. If unresponsive, open the airway and check for breathing for three to five seconds.
3. If breathless, deliver two slow, full breaths. Watch chest rise. Allow chest to deflate. Breathe between breaths.
4. Check carotid pulse for five to 10 seconds.
5. If pulseless, start cycles of 15 compressions to two breaths.
6. After four cycles of 15:2 (approximately one minute), recheck for a pulse. If still pulseless, continue cycles of 15:2 beginning with chest compressions.

Note: In case access to 911 is available, send someone to call immediately. If you are alone, you should run to call for help *before* initiating CPR.

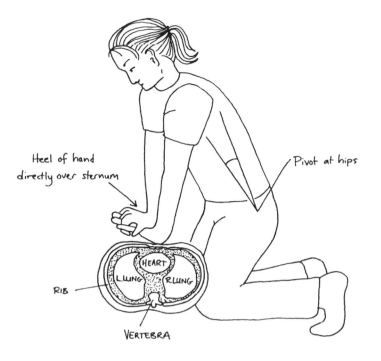

Figure 5-5: Cross section of chest during CPR

Adult Two-rescuer CPR

1. Check for responsiveness.
2. If unresponsive, Rescuer One opens the airway and checks for breathing for three to five seconds.
3. If breathless, Rescuer One delivers two slow, full breaths. Watch chest rise. Allow chest to deflate. Breathe between breaths.
4. Rescuer One checks carotid pulse for five to 10 seconds.
5. If pulseless, Rescuer Two, on the opposite side of the patient from Rescuer One, starts cycles of five compressions to one breath delivered by Rescuer One.
6. After approximately one minute of cycles of 5:1 (or approximately 20 cycles), recheck for a pulse. If still pulseless, continue cycles of 5:1 beginning with chest compressions.

If Rescuer Two arrives while CPR is in progress, Rescuer Two should state that he or she knows CPR. If Rescuer One is performing chest compressions, Rescuer Two should check for and find a weak carotid pulse, an indication that Rescuer One is delivering adequate compressions. Then Rescuer Two should prepare to do ventilations, and the ratio of 5:1 begins. If Rescuer One is doing ventilations, Rescuer Two should assume the position to do chest compressions. Rescuer One should finish his or her ventilations, check for a return of carotid pulse on the patient, and the ratio of 5:1 begins.

When a switch is needed, no exact sequence determines how the switch should be made. The compressor typically feels the greatest fatigue and may call for a "switch" on the first compression of a set of five. Following the five compressions, the ventilator gives a breath and moves to the chest while the compressor moves to the head and performs a five second check for a pulse. If no pulse is found, the new ventilator says, "No pulse, continue CPR." The new compressor begins compressions. Let it suffice to be said *you should reduce the amount of time the patient goes without CPR to a minimum.*

Child And Infant CPR

Cardiac arrest in children (one to eight years of age) and in infants (up to one year of age) rarely results from heart disease. The usual cause is an insufficiency of oxygen from suffocation, injuries, or illnesses. CPR in children and infants differs slightly from adult CPR.

Child CPR

1. Check for responsiveness.
2. If unresponsive, open the airway and check for breathing for three to five seconds.
3. If breathless, deliver two slow breaths. Watch chest rise. Allow chest to deflate. Breathe between breaths.
4. Check carotid pulse for five to 10 seconds.
5. If pulseless, start cycles of five compressions to one breath.

Compressions depress the chest one to one-and-a-half inches at a rate of approximately 100 compressions per minute. Most adults should be able to deliver the compressions with one hand while the other hand maintains the child's head and airway position.
6. After 20 cycles of 5:1 (approximately one minute), recheck for a pulse. If still pulseless, continue cycles of 5:1 beginning with chest compressions.

Note: In case access to 911 is available, send someone immediately to call. If you are alone, you should perform one full minute of CPR on a child *before* running to call for help.

Infant CPR

1. Check for responsiveness.
2. If unresponsive, open the airway and check for breathing for three to five seconds.
3. If breathless, deliver two slow breaths. Watch chest rise. Allow chest to deflate. Breathe between breaths.
4. Check brachial pulse for five to 10 seconds.
5. If pulseless, start cycles of five compressions to one breath. Compression site is approximately one finger width below an imaginary line between the infant's nipples. Use two of your fingers to perform the compressions. Compressions depress the chest one-half to one inch at a rate of at least 100 compressions per minute. The infant's head

should not be higher than the rest of the body.
6. After 20 cycles of 5:1 (approximately one minute), recheck for a pulse. If still pulseless, continue cycles of 5:1 beginning with chest compressions.

Note: In case access to 911 is available, send someone immediately to call. If you are alone, you should perform one full minute of CPR on a infant *before* running to call for help.

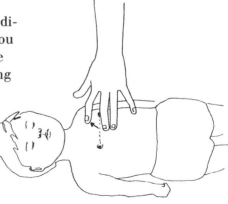

Figure 5-6:
Finger placement for infant CPR

Complications Caused By CPR

1. Even properly performed, CPR make break ribs and/or the sternum. If you feel a fracture occur, check your hand position and continue CPR.
2. The lungs may be bruised. Fractured ribs could cause lacerations of the lungs and the possibility of a pneumothorax and/or a hemothorax (SEE CHAPTER 10: CHEST INJURIES).
3. Lacerations to the liver may cause severe internal bleeding.
4. Patients, whether resuscitated or not, tend to vomit during CPR. In case of vomiting, immediately roll the patient into a side position and open the airway allowing the vomit to flow out of the mouth. When vomit has ceased to flow, wipe out the mouth—a T-shirt or bandanna will serve as a wipe—then roll the patient back into a supine position, and continue CPR.
5. Gastric distention may be caused by the rescue breathing phase of CPR (SEE CHAPTER 4: AIRWAY AND BREATHING).

Criteria For Stopping CPR

According to criteria established by the American Heart Association, CPR should be initiated as soon as possible after cardiac arrest and continued until:

1. You are exhausted and unable to continue.
2. You turn the patient over to rescuers or medical professionals of equal or higher training.
3. You resuscitate the patient.
4. The patient is declared dead by someone authorized to do so.
5. You find yourself in imminent danger.

Special Considerations For The Wilderness

Guidelines for the general use of CPR are well-defined, regularly updated, and widely distributed. Because the wilderness may impose circumstances which require special considerations in CPR, the following guidelines have been developed by the Wilderness Medical Society. Some of these guidelines will be relevant in urban situations as well.

A. Contraindications to CPR in the Wilderness: There is no reason to initiate CPR if you find 1) any sign of life in the patient, 2) danger to rescuers, 3) *dependent lividity* (discoloration of the skin, as from a bruise, where non-circulating blood has settled via gravity), 4) *rigor mortis* (stiffness occurring in dead bodies), 5) obvious lethal injury, e.g. decapitation, 6) a well-defined Do Not Resuscitate (DNR) status, 7) a patient who is rigid from a cold environment (but still may have an undetectable pulse).

B. Discontinuation of CPR in the Wilderness: Once initiated CPR should be continued until 1) resuscitation is successful, 2) rescuers are exhausted, 3) rescuers are placed in danger, 4) patient is turned over to more definitive care, 5) patient does not respond to prolonged resuscitative efforts (SEE BELOW SPECIFIC WILDERNESS SITUATIONS).

Specific Wilderness Situations

Hypothermia

A cold, rigid, apparently pulseless and breathless patient is not necessarily a dead patient. If you fail to find respirations, rescue breathing should be initiated immediately. The patient needs oxygen, and there is no danger to the patient from supplemental oxygen and/or rescue breathing. Failure to find a pulse in a cold patient should not necessarily lead to chest compressions. Apparent pulselessness may be due to hypothermia and the resulting tissue rigidity in combination with a very slow heart rate. Initiation of chest compressions 1) may cause a cold, slow beating heart to stop, and 2) will not be effective in someone dead from the cold. Chest compressions should *not* be initiated on the patient who is rigid from the cold. Rescue breathing, preferably with supplemental oxygen, and immediate gentle evacuation are indicated (SEE CHAPTER 16: COLD-INDUCED EMERGENCIES).

Avalanche Burial

Breathless and pulseless victims of avalanches are usually dead from suffocation and/or blunt trauma. Check for snow in the patient's airway which could block rescue breathing. Hypothermia is sometimes a confounding factor unless burial time is short. In case of hypothermia, guidelines for hypothermia (SEE ABOVE) should be followed.

Cold-Water Submersion

Near-drowning patients may be successfully resuscitated after prolonged (over one hour) submersion in cold water (70 degrees F or less). The younger the patient, the cleaner the water, the colder the water, and the shorter the duration of submersion, the greater the chance for success. CPR should be initiated immediately and continued, if possible, until definitive care is available (SEE CHAPTER 19: IMMERSION AND SUBMERSION INCIDENTS).

Lightning Strike

CPR should be initiated immediately on all pulseless, breathless victims of lightning strike. Following a severe electrical shock, respiratory paralysis may persist long after cardiac activity returns. Rescuers should be prepared to provide prolonged rescue breathing (SEE CHAPTER 20: LIGHTNING).

Evacuation Guidelines

Anyone who has been resuscitated via CPR should be evacuated to definitive medical care as soon as possible.

Conclusion

Kneeling beside the hunter in the San Isabel National Forest, you check for breathing and find none. You grab your pocket rescue mask from the outside pocket of your pack and give the patient two full breaths, watching the patient's chest rise and fall, rise and fall. A carotid check reveals no pulse. A fellow rescuer bares the chest of the patient and begins chest compressions. One, and two, and three, and four, and five compressions to your one breath. The routine continues.

Other rescuers assemble a break-apart litter the team carried in, preparing padding and straps for a carry. Tension stands thick in the dark forest. Beams from headlamps flicker back and forth. Orders are passed around in urgent whispers.

Gurgling in the patient's throat gives too short a warning of impending vomit, and stomach contents splatter the inside of your rescue mask. You are momentarily grateful for the one-way valve in the mask you've been blowing through. Quickly rolling the patient toward your partner, you remind him to open the airway. Vomits runs into the duff. You clean your mask with a wob of gauze someone stuffed in your hand. With the mouth wiped out by your partner, you roll the patient onto his back and continue Glancing at your fellow rescuer, you see a trickle of sweat beginning to run down his cheek, and you notice the dampness growing across your back beneath your heavy pile sweater. Suddenly, it all seems so hopeless, but you inhale to ventilate once more...

Chapter 6:   Bleeding

You should be able to:

1. *Describe the importance of blood and the dangers of bleeding.*

2. *Demonstrate how to control bleeding using direct pressure, elevation, pressure bandages, pressure points, and a tourniquet.*

It could happen to you

The knife slips out of a chunk of cheddar cheese and into her left hand. It's a Swiss Army Knife, new and razor-edged, the kind of blade that seems to first emerge from its red handle with a lust for blood. The cheese is cold and hard, her effort great, and the blade slices cleanly through her lower palm and deep into her upper wrist.

You, her backpacking companion, see little or no evidence of pain. There's a soft squeak of alarm, and a look of surprise on her face. But the knife has nicked her radial artery, and blood begins to spurt with each heart beat. Her look of surprise changes to anxiety and confusion. The pulse of escaping blood speeds up. Her skin color fades to pale. Her chest heaves in shallow gasps for breath. She stares at her wrist, and so do you, with a lack of comprehension. In moments blood has splattered "everywhere."

Introduction

The life of every cell in the human body depends on a continuous flow of oxygenated, nourishing blood. Blood is made up of red blood cells, white blood cells, platelets, and plasma. Red blood cells carry oxygen to body tissues and carbon dioxide away from body tissues; white blood cells attack invading microorganisms and produce antibodies in order to prevent infection; and platelets form clots which are essential if a wound is ever to stop bleeding. Plasma is the aqueous transportation medium for blood cells, platelets, and nutrients. This continuous flow of well oxygenated, nutrient-rich blood to cells, and the subsequent removal of waste products, is called *perfusion.*

Although amounts vary depending on body size, the average adult male has approximately 5.0 to 6.0 liters of blood (one liter is approximately two pints). The smaller the individual, the lower the blood volume. An adolescent of about 100 pounds body weight will have approximately 3.0 liters. Newborns usually have less than one-half liter of blood.

Blood is circulated throughout the body by the muscular pumping of the heart. The vessels that carry blood away from the heart are called arteries, in which the blood travels at the fastest speed under the greatest pressure. Arteries decrease in size to arterioles, then to microscopically-thin capillaries where the transfer of gases (oxygen into the cells, carbon dioxide out of the cells) takes place. From the capillaries, blood passes into venules, then to veins, which are vessels carrying blood to the heart.

An understanding of bleeding and, more importantly, how to control life-threatening bleeding in an injured patient, is one of the most critical intervention techniques the First Responder must learn. All bleeding stops—eventually—but you want to make sure it stops before the patient dies.

Types Of Bleeding

Hemorrhage is a word that means "bleeding from a wound." Hemorrhaging can be external or internal, and it can be further classified by the type of vessels that have been damaged. Capillary bleeding is slow, oozing from these small vessels, and usually bright red in color, although the blood from external wounds is often difficult to distinguish by color. Venous bleeding usually comes in a steady flow from these larger vessels, and it can be a heavy flow if the wound is significant. Venous blood tends to be a dark maroon color, due to its lack of oxygen. Arterial bleeding, under higher pressure, is usually rapid, often spurting each time the patient's heart beats. Arterial blood tends to be bright red, brighter than capillary blood.

Body Response To Bleeding

When blood vessels are damaged, the body almost immediately begins an involuntary process to stop the blood loss and start healing. The walls of the vessels constrict, helping to slow the flow of blood. Circulating platelets begin to stick to the tear in the vessel wall, and start forming a clot. A wide variety of "clotting factors"—some circulating in the blood, some released from platelets, some released from the damaged cells—interact at the site of the injury. A miraculous local actions of these factors is the formation of stable threads called fibrin that interweave to stabilize the clot and form a matrix which becomes the foundation over which new cells grow to create, eventually, new skin.

Most capillary and small venous hemorrhaging will form a clot and stop bleeding without your assistance, except in a few cases where disease conditions inhibit clotting. Although completely severed arteries will often constrict enough to seal off bleeding, arterial spurting and heavy venous bleeding will usually require outside control to stop the bleeding before serious harm is done.

Stages Of Bleeding

Although it is often difficult to judge the amount of blood an individual may have lost, it is important to make an estimate of the loss based on the signs and symptoms exhibited by the patient. This is especially true in the wilderness where fluid replacement may be limited or impossible, and rapid evacuation may be the determining factor in life or death. The stages of bleeding correspond to the stages of shock (SEE CHAPTER 7: SHOCK).

Stage 1: Compensatory Shock

When an adult donates blood, the amount taken is usually one unit (one-half liter, or about one pint), or roughly eight to 10 percent of the adult's total blood volume. Volume loss of up to 15 percent will usually be tolerated by the patient. As a crude estimate, this amount of blood will just about fill a one-liter water bottle, the size carried by most people on wilderness trips. Vital signs for this patient will remain within normal limits, and evacuation is typically not necessary, depending on the injury.

Loss of 15 to 30 percent of an individual's blood volume, however, may be considered serious. Peripheral vasoconstriction (constricting of the blood vessels on the periphery of the body) shunts blood away from the body's extremity and toward the vital organs. Vital signs usually show anxiety, confusion and/or restlessness, pale (often cool) skin, and increased pulse and respirations. The compensatory blood shunting usually maintains a normal, or even slightly elevated, blood pressure. Wilderness patients showing a decline in vital signs should be evacuated.

Stage 2: Decompensatory Shock

With a loss of 30 to 40 percent in blood volume, death may occur, especially if the loss is rapid. The patient's body can no longer compensate for the reduction in blood volume. Vital signs show what you would expect in shock: 1) anxiety, 2) rapid and weak pulse and respirations, 3) pale, cool, clammy skin, and 4) decreased blood pressure. But, even at this stage, the patient may be saved with rapid evacuation and aggressive treatment for shock (SEE CHAPTER 7: SHOCK).

Stage 3: Irreversible Shock

Loss of more than 40 percent of the blood volume, and the resulting inadequate perfusion, is often fatal. The patient becomes drowsy and lethargic, and eventually unresponsive. Vital signs continue to show increasing evidence of shock. Ultimately, irreversible brain damage occurs, and other vital organs start to fail. Only definitive medical intervention will preserve the life of this patient.

Control Of External Bleeding

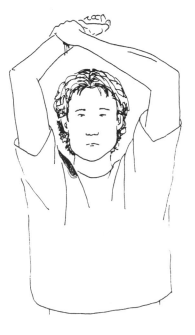

Figure 6-1: Direct pressure and elevation

The most immediate concern is not how much blood has been lost but how fast it is being lost. Severe blood loss must be stopped as soon as possible, taking precedence over almost everything else during the first few moments with a patient. The arrest of blood loss is known as *hemostasis*.

Despite the urgency of the situation, it is recommended that you first put on a pair of protective gloves, perhaps sunglasses if the blood is splashing, before touching blood or other body fluids. While locating your gloves, encourage a reliable, helpful patient to apply direct pressure to and elevate the wound, if possible, in order to facilitate control of the bleeding (SEE BELOW).

Direct Pressure

The first and best method for control of bleeding is direct pressure. Pressure should be applied directly to the wound with the heel of your gloved hand or, preferably, with a sterile absorbent dressing under your gloved hand. Without a sterile dressing, use the cleanest material available, e.g., shirt, bandanna. Most blood loss will slow appreciably or stop with 10 to 20 minutes of direct pressure.

In urban situations, if the absorbent dressing soaks through with blood, apply a second dressing and maintain pressure. In the wilderness, if the dressing soaks through, you may try a second dressing, or it may be preferable to remove the first dressing carefully, and start fresh with a second dressing, taking care to insure your pressure is exactly over the bleeding wound. Patience is almost always rewarded with success.

Huge wounds, in which your hands cannot cover the injury site, may require that you first pack the wound with absorbent material before applying pressure.

Highly vascular areas such as the scalp may require prolonged pressure with a bulky dressing. Scalp wounds should be assessed for stability of the skull before applying pressure.

Elevation

As soon as possible and whenever possible, the wound should be elevated above the patient's heart. This will further slow blood loss and encourage clotting. Elevation should be performed with extreme discretion if there is the possibility it will make the injury worse, such as wounds associated with severe fractures and dislocations.

Pressure Bandage

If bleeding persists after 20 minutes and/or if you need your hands free for another job, a pressure bandage should be applied. A pressure bandage is one that holds direct pressure on a wound. With a bulky dressing in place on the wound, conforming roller gauze, elastic wrap, or a clean strip of cloth is wrapped securely around the extremity and tied with the knot over the wound.

The pressure bandage should not be so tight that it causes a disruption in blood flow to the *distal* side of the bandage, the side farthest from the midline of the body. Distal blood flow should be assessed on a regular basis by checking distal pulses and sensation.

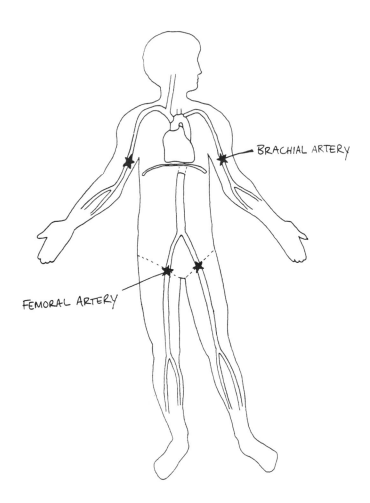

Figure 6-2: Pressure points

Pressure Points

A pressure point is a place where an artery lies close to a bone and simultaneously close to the surface of the body. By pressing with your fingers or hand on a pressure point, you can slow the flow of arterial blood. Pressure points should not be used in place of direct pressure but as an additional measure in stopping blood loss.

There are two pressure points immediately and easily available to the Wilderness First Responder: the brachial and the femoral.

The brachial artery lies on the inside of the upper arm between the armpit and the elbow. By holding the patient's arm with your thumb on the outside and your fingers over the artery, you can press the artery against the humerus (upper arm bone).

The femoral artery crosses the lower pelvis in the groin area. With the heel of your hand, you can press on the crease between pelvis and leg, reducing blood flow through that artery.

Tourniquet

Use of tourniquets in urban situations, where transport is imminent, remains controversial, seldom required, and recommended only as a last resort when the life of the patient is threatened. Using a tourniquet to control bleeding is extremely hazardous because it interrupts the blood supply and risks causing irreversible injury to the distal extremity due to lack of adequate perfusion.

In the wilderness tourniquets, though rarely necessary, may be of use more often than "on the streets." On upper arms and upper legs (the only places tourniquets should be used), they can be left in place for up to 45 minutes—less is better—before irreversible damage occurs. During that time the tourniquet may be useful in allowing you to stop blood flow long enough to find exactly where the torn vessels are located in order to increase the effectiveness of direct pressure, and useful in encouraging clot formation in severe wounds. If you apply a tourniquet and leave it applied, *you have determined to sacrifice the limb in order to save a life.*

Apply the tourniquet close to the *proximal* (closest to the midline of the body) side of the wound for upper arms or legs, or just above the elbow or knee for lower arm or leg wounds. Use a wide band and tie it just tight enough to prevent any leakage from the wound and no more. A loose "tourniquet," however, may actually increase bleeding by allowing arterial flow past the constriction but impeding venous return.

When you use a tourniquet, even for just a few minutes, always make note of that fact in your medical report. When you loosen a tourniquet, do it slowly to prevent the dislodging of any clots that have formed.

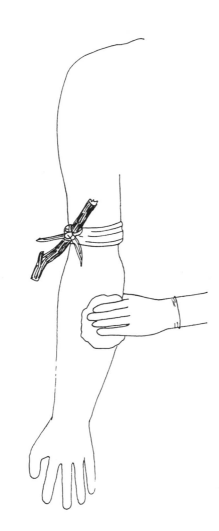

Figure 6-3: Tourniquet

Internal Bleeding

Internal bleeding can become life-threatening when it takes place inside a body cavity (chest, abdomen), if the pelvis is fractured, or if one or both femurs (upper leg bones) are fractured.

A threat to life may develop before you are even aware the patient is bleeding, and without a single drop of blood dripping onto the ground. Anticipate internal bleeding by careful assessment of the patient.

Given the mechanism of injury, for example a fall on or blow to the abdomen, the signs and symptoms of shock without another obvious cause are usually attributable to internal bleeding. Look for external bruising over a blood-rich internal organ. Watch for guarding, the patient's need to physically protect, in this case, the abdomen. Later signs of internal bleeding may be an increasingly rigid abdomen as the abdominal muscles spasm to protect the damaged area, and an extended abdomen as blood fills the cavity.

Unfortunately, there is little to be done by the Wilderness First Responder for internal bleeding other than stabilization of known injuries, treatment for shock, and rapid evacuation.

Evacuation Guidelines

Any patient who has bled enough to exhibit the signs and symptoms of compensatory shock and who does not improve rapidly with treatment, and any patient who has bled enough to exhibit the signs and symptoms of decompensatory shock should be evacuated. Any patient exhibiting the signs and symptoms of irreversible shock should be evacuated as soon as possible.

Conclusion

With sudden realization, you grab your bandanna from your pocket. Pressing it firmly over the gash in your friend's wrist, you squeeze down with enough force to stop the blood flow. Speaking quietly, your renewed calmness helps calm the patient. You lift her arm, elevating the injury above her heart level. A half hour later, when you gently remove the bandanna to check, the wound has ceased to bleed. Judging from her vital signs, you determine her blood loss is well within her physiological ability to compensate, and you begin preparations to treat the laceration.

Chapter 7:   Shock

You should be able to:

1. Describe the basic anatomy and physiology of the cardiovascular system.

2. Describe specific causes of shock.

3. Describe the stages and the accompanying signs and symptoms of shock.

4. Demonstrate the management of a patient in shock.

5. Describe the differences between managing shock in an urban environment and in the wilderness.

It could happen to you

Snow on the south slopes facing the midwinter sun has turned rock hard. The backcountry skiing, fast and furious, leaves the group exhilarated and exhausted, and the brown and gold tents of camp are a welcome sight. With dinner bubbling on stoves, you're surprised to see the look of concern on a young skier's face when she tells you her tent mate "seems really out of it."

Kneeling in the tent at the patient's side, you immediately notice her skin is pale, cool, and damp with sweat. Her breaths are rapid and shallow. A check of her pulse reveals to you a heart rate of 100, regular and strong.

You ask, "Can you tell me what's going on?"

She looks at you as if she didn't understand your question. Her face reveals a high level of anxiety. "I'm not sure," she finally answers, "I feel terrible."

Introduction

To function properly, the delicate and sensitive brain requires narrowly defined limits of sugar, temperature, oxygen, and blood pressure. When the body senses a drop in blood pressure, it initiates a series of coping mechanisms intended to supply an uninterrupted supply of oxygen-rich blood to the brain. These measures include complicated changes in blood chemistry, shifts in the location of body fluids, and other physiological adjustments. In response to minor problems, such as minor injuries, the system may maintain adequate blood circulation in the brain with little effort. Serious problems, such as injuries which involve major blood loss, require stronger compensatory actions. Attempts at regulation become increasingly more drastic until adequate pressure in the brain is restored, or until the brain dies from *hypoxia* (deficiency of oxygen). Sometimes, even if the person does not die from the initial injury or illness which caused the compensatory mechanisms to shift into high gear, the body is unable to recover as a result of the compensatory efforts themselves.

Perfusion is the constant bathing of cells with life-sustaining fluid under proper pressure. *Shock* is inadequate perfusion, a result of inadequate oxygen getting to the cells, and it can have numerous causes (SEE BELOW). Shock may be thought of as the "trigger" for the compensatory actions of the body.

As a WFR *you must vigilantly anticipate shock in all patients* because: 1) seemingly minor injuries and illnesses may trigger this life threatening condition, 2) by the time you notice the first signs, the downward spiral of shock may have already begun, 3) as shock progresses it becomes more difficult to treat, 4) you will not be able to predict how rapidly shock will progress, and 5) appropriate early interventions can save lives.

Anatomy And Physiology Of The Cardiovascular System

Your cardiovascular system (heart, vessels, and blood) is really two circulatory systems joined at the heart. The right side of the heart pumps blood to the lungs and back. The left side pushes oxygen-rich blood to all parts of the body and back. Both circuits work simultaneously. Cardiac output, the amount of blood pumped out by the heart every minute, is normally enough to meet the needs of all the cells of your body.

Blood leaves the heart through arteries, that branch and narrow to arterioles, that branch and narrow to capillaries. At the capillaries, the oxygen (and nutrients picked up from the digestive system) are diffused across cell walls, exchanged for carbon dioxide and the waste products of metabolism. The waste-carrying blood moves out the other end of the capillaries and into venules that come together to form veins. The veins return blood to the heart. Veins are more numerous than arteries, and can hold more of your blood. There is less pressure in the veins, and they have little one-way "doors" to keep the blood from backing up. All vessels can dilate or constrict to meet varying demands from the body.

Shock

The term "shock," once again, describes the body's condition and reactions when tissues are not being adequately perfused with oxygenated blood. Adequate perfusion requires a certain minimum blood pressure, approximately 90 mmHg, which is necessary for life-sustaining exchanges of oxygen and carbon dioxide to occur. The circulatory system's three main components—the heart, the blood, and the blood vessels—work in concert to maintain adequate pressure.

Heart: The heart must contract at a rate fast enough and strong enough to keep a steady stream of blood flowing through the system. Think of it as a water pump situated at the base of a hill below a cabin. If the pump does not supply water pressure great enough for the occupant of the cabin to take a shower, the occupant can build pressure by increasing the pump's rate, the number of strokes the pump makes per minute. Similarly, the body monitors blood pressure at sites called *baroreceptors* (nerve endings sensitive to pressure changes). When a baroreceptor detects low pressure, it sends a message which signals the pump, in this case the heart, to beat faster.

Blood: There must be enough blood in the system to keep the blood vessels filled. Using the cabin and water pump as a model, you can easily see that if there is not enough fluid in the system of pipes, no amount of rapid pumping will cause the water to rise all the way up to the cabin, and the occupant is left high and dry. Likewise, if the body is low on blood, through either dehydration or hemorrhage, the heart will not be able to work hard enough to maintain an adequate pressure. The only remedy to this problem is to add more blood to the system. The body will do this on its own, but the process requires time and raw materials: water and nutrients.

Vessels: The highly elastic arteries and veins form a container for the blood and must be precisely the proper size if the pressurized system is to function at its optimum. The occupant may determine that the only way to get suitable pressure in the cabin is to narrow the diameter of the pipes that lead there. You can see that given a certain volume, and a limited pumping capacity, forcing the same liquid through a smaller pipe will increase the pressure at the end of the run. The human body can narrow, or vasoconstrict, its "pipes" very efficiently.

A healthy body involuntarily makes minute adjustments in the functioning of the circulatory system that keep the body well pressurized. For example, when an adult male donates one-half liter of his approximately six liters of blood during the local blood drive, his vessels make up for the loss by constricting—shrinking the container, you might say—until his body is able to replenish the supply. Stress, trauma, and disease, however, are all capable of interfering with perfusion and initiating shock.

Causes Of Shock

All shock results from a failure of one or more of the major components of the cardiovascular system. With numerous specific causes, all shock is classified generally by the component of the cardiovascular system that is failing.

Cardiogenic Shock: The term *cardiogenic* describes shock stemming from failure of the heart. A heart attack, in which the muscle itself has sustained damage from *ischemia* (deficient blood supply), may result in cardiogenic shock. Trauma, too, may cause damage, such as a rupture of one or more of the heart's chambers, making it an ineffective pump.

Hypovolemic (Low Volume) Shock: The term *hypovolemic* describes shock that occurs from low fluid volume within the cardiovascular system. Severe bleeding secondary to trauma is a common cause of shock seen by WFRS. It will usually be easy to determine the relationship between large amounts of blood lost outside the body and the signs of shock in a trauma patient (SEE CHAPTER 6: BLEEDING). Always remember, however, that internal bleeding, whether caused by trauma or disease, can result in shock as well. Patients, for instance, can die from the amount of blood lost into the abdominal cavity. A ruptured spleen is one of the many causes of massive abdominal bleeding. As another example, a broken femur (upper leg bone), when it perforates the femoral artery, may cause serious internal loss of blood directly into the thigh.

Another common wilderness cause of hypovolemic shock is dehydration. Over-sweating, lack of adequate water intake, and gastrointestinal illnesses that result in diarrhea and/or vomiting are all culprits. When the general fluid level in the body drops, water is absorbed from the blood into other areas of the body to make up the deficit.

Burns are another major cause of hypovolemic shock. In addition to any blood loss associated with burns, the plasma that continues to leak from damaged tissue can account for significant fluid loss. The blisters that result from partial thickness burns serve as visible reminders that fluid is outside the body, rather than inside where it is needed. Usually much more serious, however, are full thickness burns which, having eliminated the protective barrier of skin, allow fluid to escape the body at a rapid rate.

Vasogenic (Low Resistance) Shock: The term *vasogenic* describes shock resulting from failure of the blood vessels to maintain sufficient resistance to blood flow. Spine injuries, for instance, may sever, pinch, or otherwise damage nerves that control muscles in the veins and arteries. When these muscles relax, the vessels dilate, and the container becomes too large for the amount of blood in the system, a condition sometimes called *neurogenic* shock. An overdose of some drugs that affect the nervous system may produce the same problem.

Septic shock, a form of low resistance shock, is the name given to shock stemming from infection. When a bacteria, virus, or some other agent proliferates rapidly in your system, the colony produces waste products. If these toxins are numerous enough, they damage your blood vessels, causing them to leak and to loose muscle tone. The resulting vascular dilation can initiate shock.

A severe reaction caused by over-sensitivity to an allergen is known as *anaphylactic* shock, another form of low resistance shock. Stings from honey bees and other *Hymenoptera* (wasps, hornets, etc.) and certain drugs, particularly penicillin-based antibiotics, are common culprits. This reaction causes the vessels to dilate and the pressure to drop, but patients will more likely die from airway obstruction caused by swelling of the airway (SEE CHAPTER 28: ALLERGIC REACTIONS AND ANAPHYLAXIS).

Because both septic and anaphylactic shock allow blood to leak into spaces between cells, called *interstitial spaces*, patients with either condition may look somewhat different than patients in other forms of shock. Their skin may be red or mottled and warm rather than the characteristic pale, cool, and clammy (SEE BELOW). Their bodies may be trying hard to get rid of the excess fluid, making them prone to vomiting and diarrhea.

Note: Sometimes fainting is referred to as *psychogenic shock*. In what is thought to be the mind's attempt to avoid an unpleasant situation, it will dilate the blood vessels, causing pressure in the brain to drop suddenly. Fortunately the condition is usually self-limiting because the skeletal muscles relax, too, and permit the body to drop into a horizontal position. Providing the person is not strapped into a seat and chest harness while dangling in a crevasse, or standing on a narrow rock ledge following a 5.9 lead, the body will slump to a level where the heart and brain are on the same plane, where blood can easily flow back into the brain and restore consciousness.

Stages Of Shock

Stage 1: Compensatory Shock

When blood pressure begins to drop, from blood loss, for example, the body will respond in ways that are intended to keep the pressure up. During this stage, the patient typically appears anxious and/or confused. Heart rate and respiratory rate increase. Skin typically grows pale or chalky white or ashen gray as peripheral blood vessels constrict to draw blood into the core. The patient usually begins to sweat. The redistribution of blood away from the abdomen may lead to nausea and vomiting, and the patient may be thirsty. If these actions maintain enough blood pressure to allow for adequate perfusion, and if, for example, no more blood is lost, this successful adjustment is called *compensatory shock*.

You may have experienced a temporary reaction very similar to compensated shock the last time a loud noise outside your tent startled you in the middle of the night or you suddenly realized a bear was following you down the trail. When the brain perceives some threat, it prepares the body for immediate action by directing the adrenal gland to release its hormones. This adrenaline rush, the "fight or flight" response, induces the same physiologic changes as those in compensated shock. This stimulation prepares you to make your best physical response to the situation. Once the threat subsides, a healthy body will return to a normal resting state. These "stress reactions" or "alert responses" to possible damage usually last no more than 10 to 20 minutes if no real damage to the patient has occurred.

Signs and Symptoms Compensatory Shock:

1. Anxiety, disorientation, confusion
2. Cool, clammy skin
3. Normal to pale or chalky white or ashen gray complexion
4. Thirst, nausea, vomiting
5. Shallow, rapid respirations
6. Dizziness, lightheadedness and/or weakness
7. Strong to weak rapid pulse
8. Blood pressure within normal limits
9. Pupils will be PERRL

Note: African-Americans and other people with dark skin are those most likely to appear ashen gray. One way to assess all patients for perfusion—and perhaps the best check for people of color—is to note the color of their mucus membranes. Pull down an eyelid or look at the inside of the lips. Reddish or bright pink is normal. Light pink or pale is a sign of diminished circulation.

If the injury or illness is severe enough, or if a seemingly minor problem is not managed properly, the patient progresses through compensated shock, on her or his way to the next, more serious stage.

Stage 2: Decompensatory Shock

Sometimes compensatory mechanisms are ineffective. Perhaps there is too much blood loss or other stressors are affecting the body, and blood pressure starts to drop. Now the body enters *decompensatory shock*, sometimes called progressive shock. The heart rate will continue to increase. There is a greater increase in the respiratory rate and a decrease in its depth—rapid, shallow respirations. The lesser amount of oxygen reaching the tissues changes the skin from pale to cyanotic (blue), evidence of lack of oxygen. *Diaphoresis* (profuse sweating) will begin and may soak the body. The patient may become obsessively anxious and spiral down through progressively deteriorating levels of consciousness.

> **Signs and Symptoms Decompensatory Shock:**
>
> 1. Altered level of consciousness
> 2. Cold clammy skin, diaphoresis
> 3. Very pale to cyanotic or mottled complexion
> 4. Rapid, shallow respirations
> 5. Weak and rapid pulse
> 6. Blood pressure dropping, with weak or absent radial pulse
> 7. Pupils sluggish to react

Stage 3: Irreversible Shock

Eventually the body runs out of options and begins to sink into *irreversible shock*. In this stage, hypoxia suffocates the brain, heart, liver, and other vital organs, and accumulating waste products poison the entire system. Blood pressure drops to the point of being undetectable, usually lower than 90 mmHg systolic. Respirations slow down and may become labored. The heart rate slows and weakens until it finally stops altogether. The skin grows cold and mottled. Most patients who enter this stage will die, and those who survive will probably suffer severe complications resulting from damage done to the vital organs by hypoxia.

Sometime during this final stage, the body releases an overwhelming surge of energy, a final all-out attempt to recover. This "bounce back," as it is sometimes called, may cause a return of blood pressure and consciousness. But, the effect is short-lived, and unfortunately so, usually, is the patient.

> **Signs and Symptoms Irreversible Shock:**
>
> 1. Unresponsive
> 2. Cold and damp, or cold and dry skin
> 3. Cyanotic or mottled appearance
> 4. Slow heart rate
> 5. Slow agonal respirations
> 6. Blood pressure undetectable, with no pulses palpable
> 7. Pupils very slow to react or fixed and dilated

Risk Factors

Bleeding and/or trauma are obvious conditions that predispose a patient to shock. Dehydration alone can lead to shock. The dehydrated person who is also a patient with trauma is doubly at risk. Children and young adolescents have dangerously deceptive reactions in shock. They compensate very well for a long period of time, often masking the severity of the condition. Then, with very little warning, they may decline through the progressive stage quite rapidly. The elderly and the chronically or acutely ill will often have weakened systems, impairing their ability to compensate. Pregnant women are supplying blood to two organisms, and, because the body diverts blood from the abdomen in shock, the fetus is placed in great jeopardy.

Management Of Shock

Because of the extended transport time associated with a wilderness environment, the downward spiral of shock must always be on the mind of the Wilderness First Responder. Anticipating shock in someone far from a hospital is so critical that the first act of management must occur while the group is still healthy. Proper hydration is the key. Be sure that all members of your party are maintaining an adequate water intake, generally indicated by clear and copious urine output. Then, whenever an injury or illness suggests, do not wait for the signs and symptoms of shock to appear in the patient. *Anticipate and treat for shock until you unequivocally rule it out.*

Early intervention will slow down the spiral and extend the amount of time a patient will remain viable. On the other hand, rough handling and anxious attention contribute to the general decline of the patient's condition. Handle her or him gently and speak in soothing, reassuring tones. Keep the patient informed of what you are doing and encourage a positive attitude. You will have comparatively long periods to spend with your patient. Use that time to attend rigorously to the details of patient care. Act deliberately and with confidence. Avoid panic or, at least, keep it to a quiet minimum. Move your patient only when necessary and strive to make her or him as comfortable as possible. Because of the significant role anxiety plays in exacerbating shock, *your calm attention may be all that keeps your patient alive.*

As a WFR, another priority will be to prevent further decline of the patient, and, therefore, whenever possible, it is important to treat the underlying cause of shock. During the initial survey on a trauma patient, for example, you should detect any gross venous and arterial bleeding, and stop this bleeding immediately (SEE CHAPTER 6: BLEEDING). Applying traction to a broken femur, as another example, will reduce pain and may tamponade, or slow down, hemorrhaging. In fact, splinting any fractures will lessen pain and anxiety associated with those injuries and should contribute to stabilizing your patient's condition (SEE CHAPTER 12: FRACTURES).

Remember, shock indicates that cells are not receiving an adequate supply of oxygen. Supplemental oxygen, although typically not available in the wilderness, may be of great benefit. High flow oxygen would best be administered via a non-rebreather mask (SEE APPENDIX B: OXYGEN AND MECHANICAL AIDS TO BREATHING).

You can further assist the body's compensatory efforts by placing the patient in a supine position (horizontal and face up) and raising the legs slightly, no more than 10 to 12 inches, a maneuver which allows whatever blood is circulating to flow more easily to the brain. You may hear this posture referred to as the *Trendelenburg position.* Some ambulance cots and most emergency room beds can be adjusted to the Trendelenburg position. You can position a shock patient in the wilderness by simply placing him or her on a gentle slope with the feet slightly higher than the head. Beware: Do not over-elevate the feet which puts pressure on the opening of the stomach and may encourage nausea and vomiting.

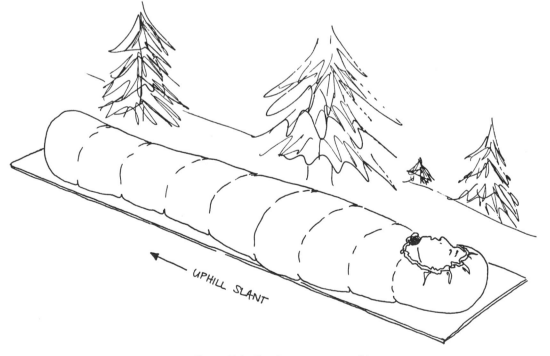

Figure 7-1: Shock treatment position

Note: Pregnant women do better in the *left lateral recumbent position* (on the left side with right knee drawn towards body and elevated on a pillow). In the supine position the heavy mass of the fetus may press on the inferior vena cava, reducing blood return to the heart.

The body's attempts at temperature regulation, a function normally carried out by the circulatory system, virtually cease during shock. Therefore, insulating your patient from the cold and preventing heat gain in an extremely hot environment may be important.

Monitor vital signs often, preferably every five minutes or so. Pay particular attention to the patient's level of consciousness. It will be your most useful indicator of how he or she is doing. An accurate chart of changing signs informs professional rescue and emergency room personnel how quickly they need to act and will assist them in making critical decisions in multiple casualty incidents.

"Nothing by mouth" is the standard of care for shock patients in the urban environment. You must be concerned with orally rehydrating the shock patient in the wilderness, as long as he or she is conscious, and can accept a container of water, and can swallow. You may administer liquids, preferably cool liquids in small amounts. Lightly salted water may be beneficial—the salt should not be detectable by taste—but avoid sweet drinks. Your goal is to speed absorption to the blood stream and anything too sweet will remain too long in the stomach, and may bring on nausea.

Note: Obvious abdominal trauma may eliminate your oral rehydration option (see CHAPTER 11: ABDOMINAL INJURIES).

Since definitively treating shock will often only be possible in a medical facility, a rapid evacuation must be considered.

General Shock Management:

1. Assess and monitor the ABCs
2. Keep the patient physically and emotionally calm
3. Treat any treatable causes, e.g., stop serious bleeding, splint fractures
4. Administer oxygen (high flow) if possible
5. Handle gently
6. Elevate legs
7. Maintain body temperature
8. Monitor vital signs
9. Orally rehydrate, when appropriate
10. Transport as rapidly as possible, when necessary

Evacuation Guidelines

Initiate a rapid evacuation of all patients who are decompensating. If the shock patient is not getting better, the shock patient should be getting out.

Conclusion

Although no cause is immediately evident, the skier-turned-patient shows signs of shock. So calmly and gently, you pad beneath her legs, raising them approximately 10 inches. You cover her with her tent mate's sleeping bag since she is already in her own.

Proceeding through a focused history and examination, you discover she took a hard fall on the last downhill run of the day. She landed, she says, on her left side. Your physical exam, performed reaching beneath the sleeping bags, elicits pain when you press on her left side, low on her rib cage. Taking a look, you see bruising approximately over the spleen. Ah ha, perhaps internal bleeding, a probable cause.

A second, and then a third, set of vital signs show increasing heart rate and increasing respiratory rate. More importantly, she shows an increasing level of anxiety.

Picking a team of your fastest skiers, you begin preparations to send out a request for a rapid evacuation.

Ken Thompson, WEMT, contributed his expertise to this chapter.

Chapter 8:   *Spine Injuries*

You should be able to:

1. *Describe the basic anatomy of the spinal column.*
2. *Describe the most common mechanisms of injury to the spine.*
3. *Demonstrate proper assessment for spine and spinal cord injury.*
4. *Demonstrate proper emergency care for the spine-injured patient.*
5. *Describe the special wilderness considerations for a spine-injured patient including the decision process for "clearing the spine."*

It could happen to you

April's sun-washed warmth only hints at the blast furnace heat of summer to come. Mountain biking the Kokopeli Trail, your group passed the Colorado border miles back. A lot of Utah stretches out dry and sandy ahead, and your party stretches out over a quarter mile. The silence breaks to a faint call of your name, drifting to you from somewhere behind. You stop and look back over the rough track you've just completed, a section that included a dicey piece of sloping sandstone. You see arms waving overhead in the distance. Nothing to do but retrace your hard-earned wheel turns.

You find Steve flat on his back in soft sand at the bottom of the sandstone slope, his bike approx-imately 10 feet away. The bike appears intact. His helmet is attached by its strap to the back of the bike. A nasty abrasion on your friend's forehead oozes blood. You hear him groan as you approach.

"He went over the handle-bars," someone says.

Introduction

Injuries to the spine rank among the most intricate and potentially devastating problems a Wilderness First Responder has to deal with. Spinal cord damage can produce paralysis or death as 1) a result of the initial mechanism or 2) as a result of mishandling by well-meaning rescuers. The problems of proper management are compounded by the lack of equipment and the remoteness of wilderness environments. Skilled handling and adequate equipment, some of which may need to be improvised, are keys to successful patient care.

Basic Anatomy Of The Spine

The spinal column is made up of 33 vertebrae. The top seven are called *cervical* vertebrae (C1-C7). They form the neck, the most flexible and least protected portion of the spine and, therefore, the portion most prone to serious injury. The topmost cervi-cal vertebra, C1, sometimes called the "atlas," supports the weight of the head as the mythi-cal Titan named Atlas supports the weight of the world on his shoulders. C2 is sometimes called the "axis," and most of the move-ment of the head on the spine occurs there. A small spike of bone, the *odontoid process*, rises from C2 into C1 forming a peg on which the head rotates. The 12 *thoracic* vertebrae (T1-T12) are attached to the ribs and protected by back muscles making them relatively rigid and secure. The lower back is composed of five *lumbar* vertebrae (L1-L5). They are large and strong, but the muscles supporting them are highly susceptible to injury and pain from improper lifting and moving techniques. The five sacral vertebrae are fused together to form the *sacrum* where the spine is attached to the pelvic girdle. The final four coccygeal vertebrae are fused together to form the *coccyx*, the lower tip of the vertebral column, the "tailbone."

The non-fused vertebrae of the neck and back are joined to each other by ligaments attached to their anterior (front), posterior (back), and lateral (side) surfaces. Between each of these vertebrae lies a disc of cartilage which allows some movement between bones and which serves as a shock absorber.

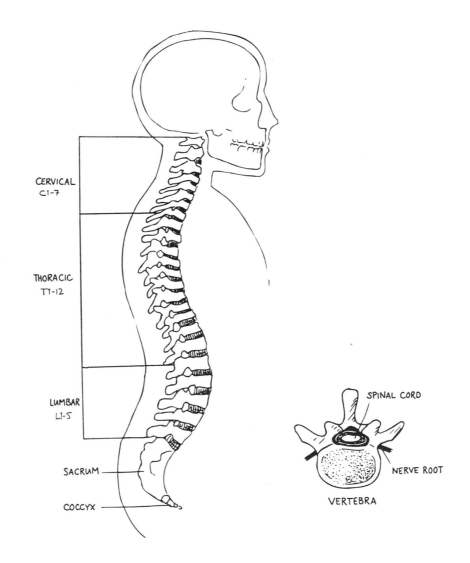

CERVICAL
C1-7

THORACIC
T1-12

LUMBAR
L1-5

SACRUM

COCCYX

SPINAL CORD

NERVE ROOT

VERTEBRA

Figure 8-1: Basic anatomy of the spine

Down through an opening in each of the vertebrae, an opening called the *vertebral foramen*, or spinal canal, passes the spinal cord. The spinal cord is a continuous bundle of nerves running from the brain to the juncture of L1 and L2 in the lumbar region, approximately the level of the "belly button." Below L1 the spinal cord branches into loose fibers called the *cauda equina* and resembling, somewhat, a "horse's tail." The spinal cord is protected by the bones of the spine, and by a continuation of the same meninges and cerebrospinal fluid that protect the brain (SEE CHAPTER 9: HEAD INJURIES). Spinal nerves branch out from the spinal cord between each of the vertebrae, sending countless peripheral nerves to the body. This is the connection of the brain to all parts of the body.

Mechanisms Of Injury

Most injuries to the spinal cord occur as a result of injury to the spinal vertebrae. Although spinal column injuries usually heal well, injuries to the nerve tissue of the cord are often irreparable. Spinal injury is produced by one or more of the following mechanisms:

1. Excessive flexion (chin forced toward chest, e.g., hiker tumbles backwards down hill. Flexion is especially dangerous when the head is axially loaded. e.g., diver hits bottom of shallow pond).
2. Excessive extension (head thrown backwards, e.g., driver thrown backwards when his vehicle is hit from behind by a second high speed four-wheel-drive vehicle).
3. Compression (vertebrae forcefully driven together, e.g., climber falls and lands sitting).
4. Distraction (vertebrae forcefully pulled apart, e.g., hanging).
5. Excessive rotation (vertebrae forcefully twisted, e.g., skier tumbles and skis fail to release).
6. Excessive lateral bending (vertebrae forced to one side or the other, e.g., standing skier hit from the side by high-speed skier).
7. Penetration injury (e.g., stabbing, gunshot wound).

Types Of Spinal Cord Injuries

Vertebral damage—breaks in the bones of the back—can occur without spinal cord damage, but the mechanism of injury can cause fragments of bone or disc to cut the cord. If the cord is cut on impact, the damage is almost immediately obvious. Spinal cord damage can also occur without significant damage to bones and discs due to swelling of the cord. An injury that causes swelling of the cord within the spinal canal can produce as serious an injury as a "broken back," injuries such as *paraplegia*, paralysis of the lower portion of the body, or *quadriplegia*, paralysis of all four extremities and almost always the trunk. Sometimes hours pass before obvious spinal cord damage from swelling shows up. Even though paralysis could occur hours later, some signs and symptoms of spinal damage will appear shortly after the injury.

Uninterrupted Spinal Cord

The spinal cord is intact despite the possibility of fractures and ligamental disruption. There are no changes in circulation, sensation, and motion (CSM) in the extremities: no decrease in strength of pulses, no loss of feeling, no loss of motor function, and no unusual weakness in the arms and/or legs. Proper care is critical to insure the spinal cord stays intact.

Partial Spinal Cord Injury

Normal blood flow to the spinal cord is interrupted with the possibility of damage to cord tissue. There are one or more changes in CSM, evidence of nerve injury: decreases in strength of pulses, loss of sensation, loss of normal motor function in the extremities, and possibly weakness in the arms and/or legs. Early recognition and stabilization in the field are critical in order to keep the patient's injury from getting worse.

Full Spinal Cord Injury

There is complete interruption of spinal cord function with obvious loss of CSM: decreases in strength of pulses, loss of sensation, loss of motor function, and perhaps paralysis. Early recognition and stabilization are critical in order to keep the patient alive.

Assessment

The first step in assessment of spinal injury is assessment of the scene. Attempt to determine, as accurately as possible, the mechanism of injury and the forces involved. Accidents that commonly include spinal injury are:

1. Sudden and forceful stops such as in motor vehicle accidents, falls from a height (especially if the height is as much or more than twice the patient's height), high speed skiing accidents, high speed bicycle accidents, and diving accidents (especially dives into shallow water and dives from a height).
2. Head injury, especially if the injury involves loss of consciousness.
3. Penetrating injury to the spinal region.

An adequate MOI is sufficient reason by itself to treat for spinal injury in an urban situation.

Assess the patient's level of consciousness. Any decrease in the level of consciousness following a blow to the head should raise the WFR's level of suspicion. Any unreliable patient due to the consumption of alcohol or any other mind altering substance should be treated for spine injury if sufficient MOI exists. *Treat all unconscious patients as if they have a spinal injury until it is proven otherwise*, preferably by physical examination in an emergency room.

Assess the patient for distracting injuries that may be making the spinal assessment less than accurate. Large wounds or obvious deformities to other body parts may distract the patient and make the spinal assessment questionable.

Assess for pain, and pain on palpation, along the spinal column. Pain and/or tenderness anywhere in the spinal column are indicators of possible spinal cord damage. The patient's back should be inspected visually, and palpated on the skin and not through thick clothing that could mask a proper assessment. In an urban environment, the clothes are typically cut away. In the wilderness, your wish to retain the integrity of the clothing—the patient may need them later—creates a situation requiring some thought. Removing clothing may cause too much movement of the patient. Clothing can usually be loosened, e.g., unzipped or unbuttoned, and pushed gently out of the way. A patient on his or her back may be safely log rolled in order to gain access to the back (SEE BELOW LIFTING AND MOVING A PATIENT).

Assess for neurological deficits in the extremities. With cord damage patients may complain of numbness or tingling in the hands and/or feet or unusual sensations of cold or heat in the extremities. Examination may disclose weakness or inability to move the extremities.

Assessment for Spinal Cord Damage:
1. Check the mechanism of injury
2. Check the patient's level of consciousness
3. Check for distracting injuries
4. Check for pain and/or tenderness in the spine
5. Check for neurological deficits (changes in CSM) in the extremities

Specific Signs And Symptoms Of Spinal Cord Injury

Injury to the spinal cord may produce one and usually more than one of the following signs and symptoms:

1. *Neurogenic shock* with loss of control over the dilation and constriction of blood vessels due to nerve damage. Although sometimes difficult to assess, the patient is often vasoconstricted (cool and pale) above the point of spinal cord injury and vasodilated (warm and flushed) below the point of injury.

2. *Difficulty breathing.* Nerve messages to the diaphragm come from between the upper cervical vertebrae, thus the old reminder: Above C4 they breathe no more! Damage between C4 and T1 often shows itself with "belly breathing" in a patient: the chest muscles are not working, so the patient's belly rises and falls, sometimes dramatically. This is sometimes called "diaphragm breathing" since the patient's diaphragm is doing all the work.

3. *Pain*, pain on movement, pain on palpation of any part of the spinal column. It is important to note that spine injured patients may initially move, even walk around, and still be seriously damaged. Base your assessment of the patient's pain on movement on questions you ask the patient, and *do not ask the patient*

to move his or her spine in order to confirm your assessment.
4. *Loss of consciousness* resulting from a blow to the head.
5. *Altered sensations* (e.g., numbness, tingling) in the arms and/or legs. It is important to note that other injuries (e.g., fractured bones) may cause altered sensa-tions when the spinal cord is per-fectly intact.
6. *Loss of strength* in the arms and/or legs.
7. *Loss of function* in the arms and/or legs.
8. *Loss of normal circulation* in the extremities causing sensa-tions of heat or cold.
9. *Obvious evidence of injury* to the spinal column (e.g., cuts, punctures, bruises).
10. *Incontinence* (loss of bladder and/or bowel control).
11. *Priapism* (a painful, constant, emotionally unprovoked erec-tion of the penis due to damage to nerves that control the genitals).

Emergency Care For Suspected Spinal Injury

In general, the immediate emergency care for a spinal injury is to immobilize the entire spinal column including the head and pelvis of the patient on a long backboard with a cervical collar in place, and transport the patient to a medical facility. The rule, in most cases, is to over treat rather than to under treat.

1. Manually (hands-on) stabilize the head and cervical spine, and assure an adequate airway, keep-ing the patient as still as possible. This may require gentle align-ment of the patient's cervical spine into a neutral position. Realignment should be slow and steady. *Do not attempt to realign the cervical spine if it requires force or causes pain*, in which case the patient must be immobi-lized as found. If the airway must be opened, use a jaw thrust (SEE CHAPTER 4: AIRWAY AND BREATH-ING). Ideally, maintain manual stabilization during the entire patient assessment and until mechanical stabilization is secured.

2. Check for adequate circulation, sensation, and motion in the extremities.

3. Apply a cervical collar. Com-mercial collars should be prop-erly sized for the patient and applied to the patient according to the manufacturer's instruc-tions. In the wilderness, cervical collars can be improvised (SEE BELOW SPECIAL CONSIDERATIONS FOR THE WILDERNESS). Collars do not adequately immobilize the cervical spine, but they will serve as an adjunct until full mechani-cal immobilization is estab-lished. Even after application of a cervical collar, commercial or improvised, manual stabilization should be maintained.

4. If supplemental oxygen is available, it should be started as soon as possible.

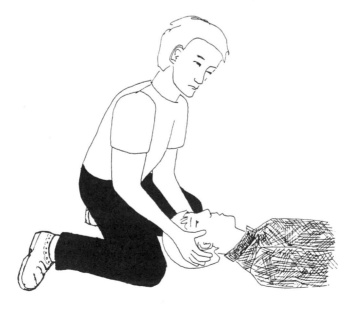

Figure 8-2: Manual stabilization of C-spine

5. Move the patient to a long backboard or a rigid litter (SEE BELOW LIFTING AND MOVING A PATIENT).

6. For comfort, pad the places where the patient will feel pressure, especially beneath the head. Use a thin pad beneath the head to prevent flexion of the cervical spine. *Avoid the voids*: Under the small of the back, beneath the knees and ankles.

7. Secure the patient to the long backboard or litter. Straps should be placed across bones: Upper chest and shoulders, pelvis, upper and lower legs. Conscious patients will prefer to have their arms free if the arms are undamaged. *Do not place the straps where they will interfere with breathing.* Pad the straps in places where they may cause the patient discomfort. Pad any spaces between the straps and patient to prevent shifting of the patient during carrying. *Secure the head last.* If the head is secured first, shifting of the cervical spine may occur during strapping. The patient should be completely immobile when you have finished.

8. Reassess the patient for adequate circulation and normal sensations in the extremities. Inadequate circulation may indicate you have strapped the patient too tight.

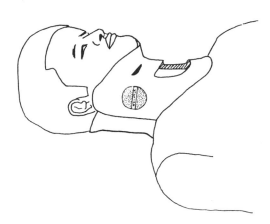

Figure 8-3: C-collar

Lifting And Moving A Patient

Although trepidation may surround movement of a patient with a suspected spinal injury, it must be done for one or more of several reasons, e.g., rolling the patient to assess the back, getting the patient off the cold ground, lifting the patient into a litter.

Log Rolling A Patient

Although one rescuer can successfully "log roll" a patient into a side position (SEE CHAPTER 4: AIRWAY AND BREATHING), three, or even four, rescuers make the process easier and safer for the patient.

1. One rescuer maintains manual stabilization of the patient's head and neck during the process. This "head" rescuer gives the movement commands.

2. Patient's arms are positioned along the sides of his or her body, if possible.

3. Additional rescuers position themselves on the same side of the patient, reaching across the patient at the shoulder, hip, thigh, and lower leg.

4. On command, rescuers roll the patient toward themselves and onto his or her side.

5. The back may now be assessed. Backboards, pads, sleeping bags, etc., may now be placed under the patient.

6. On command, rescuers roll the patient back into a supine position.

You may find you must log roll the patient onto a backboard. Place the board parallel to the patient and slightly off-center toward the patient's head. Place the patient's arms along the sides of the body (palms toward thighs), and log roll the patient as a unit, maintaining careful manual alignment of the head and spine. Slide the patient as a unit along the longitudinal axis of his or her body toward the head of the board in order to center the patient on the board. While the patient is in a side position, you can use the time to carefully check the back, again.

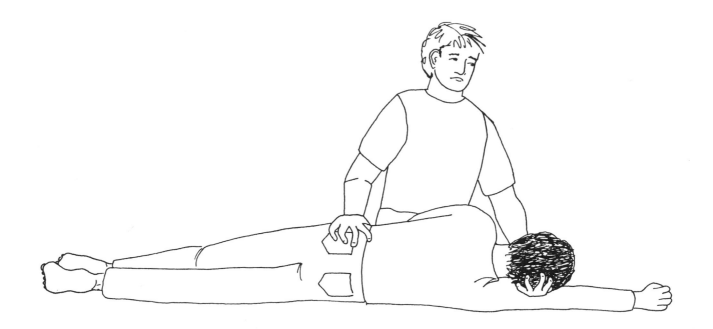

Figure 8-4: One rescuer log roll

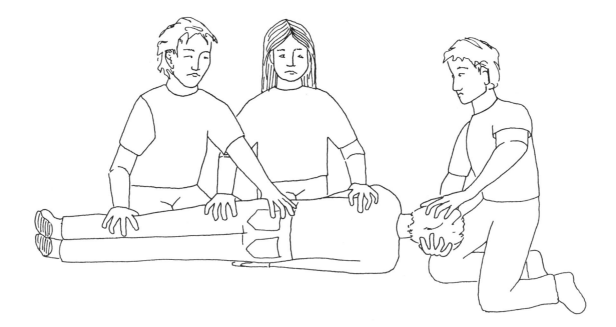

Figure 8-5: Three rescuer log roll

Lifting a Patient

It is better for the spine to lift the patient as a unit while maintaining careful alignment of the head and spine, slide the board or litter underneath, and lower the patient into position on the board or litter. This method requires an adequate number of people. Think of it as being "beamed aboard," a technique for moving people familiar to Star Trek fans. Think of BEAM as Body Elevation And Movement. With someone manually in control of the head and spine, five or six additional rescuers divide approximately according to strength to either side of the patient. Sliding their hands underneath the patient, the rescuers, using their legs not their backs, lift the patient on the command of the rescuer at the head, and lower the patient on the command of the rescuer at the head. Strong rescuers may even move patients short distances using this technique, e.g., out of the shallows of a lake onto shore. If you find yourself in charge of a group that has never "BEAMed" a patient before, since proper technique is critical, practice first, if time allows, on a healthy person.

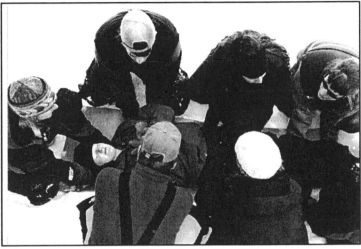

Figure 8-6: Preparing to BEAM against the patient's back and lower patient and device to the ground while maintaining careful manual stabilization of the head and spine.

Standing Take Down

If a patient who must be treated for spine injury is found standing, place the board or rigid litter

---

Special Considerations For The Wilderness

Patients suspected of having a spine injury should be rapidly evacuated from a remote environment with full immobilization. Swelling may be taking place, choking off the blood supply to the spinal cord, and rapid evacuation to definitive care may be beneficial. Intravenous drugs exist that could possibly, if administered soon enough, reduce or reverse the effects of some spinal cord injuries.

An improvised cervical collar should immobilize the cervical spine as much as possible. Some improvised collars will provide little immobilization, and some will provide a lot, but, the collar remains an important aspect of treatment. The fact that *something* is supporting a patient's neck reminds that person to refrain from moving.

While positioning a collar, the patient should be moved as little as possible, but a second rescuer may raise the head slightly to assist. What you use to improvise a collar should especially discourage flexion of the chin toward the chest. A few suggestions follow:

Packaging the Spine-Injured

In the wilderness, adequate packaging of the patient for a long evacuation is extremely important in order to reduce the chance of increasing the severity of the injury. It is difficult to improvise a safe, adequate "back-country backboard," especially one that must be carried over rugged terrain, but with attention to details it is possible to create a litter (SEE CHAPTER 36: WILDERNESS TRANSPORTATION OF THE SICK OR INJURED). *Improvised litters should be used to evacuate a spine-injured patient in only the most extreme circumstances*, e.g., there is no possibility that help will arrive with a commercial litter. Rigid litters, commercially available, provide adequate spine immobilization and are preferable for evacuating a spine-injured patient. During a wait for a litter, the patient should be moved onto a sleeping pad or similar protection from the ground. The patient should be collared, and the patient's head and neck should be kept manually stabilized or secured between padded rocks, logs, backpacks, etc.

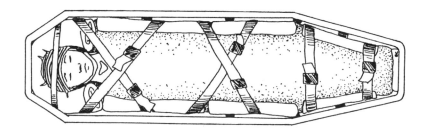

Figure 8-7: Patient secured in litter

When a litter is available, the patient should be packaged with attention and comfort. Padding should be placed under the entire patient, and extra padding should be placed at stress points created by being tied to a rack: behind the knees, in the small of the back, beneath the head and neck. All straps should be adequately padded for comfort. The patient is essentially made Free Of Any Movement (FOAM), but, while being carried, the straps can be tightened for steep terrain and loosened on flatter terrain for increased comfort. In addition, the patient usually requires insulation from the cold and protection from rain or snow.

1. A commercial product easily carried in wilderness first aid kits, the SAM Splint®, constructed from malleable aluminum, can be molded into a collar by wrapping one around the neck, flexing the front into a chin cup, and pinching the sides to add support. Mold the SAM first, put it in place, and fine tune it to the patient's anatomy.

2. Foamlite sleeping pads can be cut into the shape of a cervical collar and held in place with tape.

3. Sweaters or parkas can be rolled and placed around the patient's neck using the sleeves to secure the garment in place.

Remember: A collar is *not* a substitute for consistent hands-on stabilization of the head and neck.

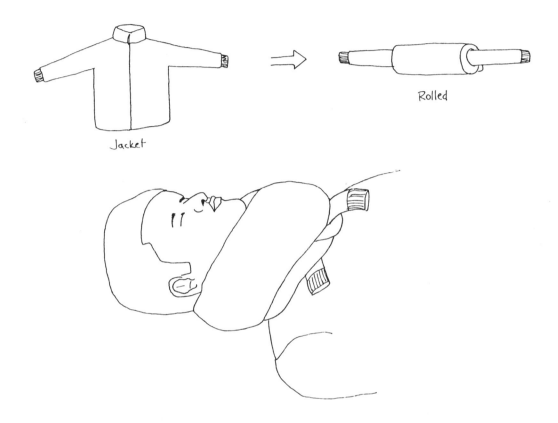

Jacket

Rolled

Figure 8-8: Improvised C-collar

Improvisation: Cervical Collar

An improvised cervical collar should immobilize the cervical spine as much as possible. Some improvised collars will provide little immobilization, and some will provide a lot, but, the collar remains an important aspect of treatment. The fact that something is supporting a patient's neck reminds that person to refrain from moving.

While positioning a collar, the patient should be moved as little as possible, but a second rescuer may raise the head slightly to assist. What you use to improvise a collar should especially discourage flexion of the chin toward the chest. A few suggestions follow:

1. A commercial product easily carried in wilderness first aid kits, the sam Splint®, constructed from malleable aluminum, can be molded into a collar by wrapping one around the neck, flexing the front into a chin cup, and pinching the sides to add support. Mold the sam first, put it in place, and fine tune it to the patient's anatomy.

2. Foamlite sleeping pads can be cut into the shape of a cervical collar and held in place with tape.

3. Sweaters or parkas can be rolled and placed around the patient's neck using the sleeves to secure the garment in place.

Remember: A collar is *not* a substitute for consistent hands-on stabilization of the head and neck.

Clearing the Spine

First, a disclaimer. There is always a slim chance you'll miss a spine injury and cause harm to the patient. If you always want to be certain, every patient with an MOI for spinal injury should be immobilized on a backboard or litter. Wilderness medical training offers a way to clear the spine, i.e., decide to not take spinal precautions, that is extremely accurate, approved by the Wilderness Medical Society (WMS), and adopted by the State of Maine for urban EMTS. It gives all those patients who don't have a spine injury freedom from hours or even days of spinal immobilization, and all those rescuers freedom from carrying a patient miles and miles to have him or her cleared five minutes after arrival at the hospital.

The patient should receive a full patient assessment with his or her spine manually immobilized prior to considering the patient as one who can have his or her spine cleared. Do not allow your wish to clear the spine interrupt the patient's need for a full assessment.

A decision to clear the spine should be made as a separate and distinct assessment, not as a part of the standard patient assessment.

The patient must be reliable: Alert, oriented, without drugs or alcohol on board. Does alert mean alert and oriented to person, place, time, and event, i.e., A+Ox4? That would be best, but if the patient is only A+Ox3 (with immediate loss of vivid memory as to the event), that person could still be considered for clearing if the rest of the criteria are met. A reliable patient is also *free of distracting injuries* that could block perception of spinal pain, injuries such as fractured femurs and dislocated shoulders. An unreliable patient with an MOI for spine injury must be treated for spine injury.

The patient must have no complaints of pain in the neck and back. Almost all patients with a spine injury will complain of pain, and those free of pain will almost always have some tenderness or guarding in the neck and/or back when palpated. A patient with an MOI for spine injury who has pain or tenderness in the neck and/or back must be treated for spine injury.

The patient must be free of altered sensations in the extremities, altered sensations such as numbness on palpation, weakness when checked for strength, pins and needles, inability to move, even temperature irregularities such as cold feet without another reason for cold feet. A patient with an MOI for spine injury who has altered sensations in the extremities must be treated for spine injury.

The patient should have palpable pulses in all four extremities. A patient with an MOI for spine injury who has no palpable pulses in the arms and/or legs must be treated for spine injury.

So far the patient has passed the test. Now, while supporting the head, ask the patient to gently flex the neck. If no pain occurs, then ask for rotation. If any pain on movement shows up, full spinal treatment follows. If the neck "locks" at one point, either to one side or the other, failing to move through a normal range of motion, full spinal treatment follows.

Now the patient may be allowed to move about freely but cautiously, if no other injuries, of course, would hamper moving about. If the patient experiences the onset of numbness or weakness later, or the onset of sharp pain later—not the tightness of muscle spasms—he or she gets the treatment later.

Note: In the past, wilderness medical training has suggested rescuers "wait two hours" after an MOI to clear a spine. This was based on clinical data which stated, and still states, that cord impingement will show up within two hours of the injury, a result of swelling. Some time should be allowed in order to let any adrenaline surge that might mask early pain to pass. There is, however, no need to wait beyond the time it takes to do a standard patient assessment: five to 10 minutes. If the spine is damaged, it will cause pain soon. Swelling, should it occur, will probably make the pain worse, but patients will experience some pain soon after the injury. To wait too long to clear the spine, even less than one hour, is to risk being fooled by the developing pain of muscular stiffness, a result of muscle strain and not an indication of spinal damage.

Process for Clearing the Spine

1. Is the mechanism of injury severe? Yes: treat. No: continue the process.

2. Have you completed a full patient assessment and found distracting injuries that could cloud a patient's reliability? Yes: treat. No: continue the process.

3. Is the patient unreliable due to decreased LOC, e.g., alcohol, drugs? Yes: treat. No: continue the process.

4. Does the patient complain of neck and/or back pain or tenderness, numbness, tingling? Yes: treat. No: continue the process.

5. Does the patient have altered sensations in the extremities? Yes: treat. No: continue the process.

6. Has the patient lost palpable pulses in the extremities? Yes: treat. No: continue the process.

7. With the head supported, does the patient complain of pain when you gently move the head and neck? Yes: treat. No: continue the process.

8. Does the neck "lock" at some point, failing to go through a normal range of motion? Yes: treat. No: continue the process.

9. Does the patient complain of sharp neck and/or back pain after being allowed to move about? Yes: treat. No: clear the spine.

Evacuation Guidelines

Initiate an immediate evacuation for anyone treated for a suspected spine injury.

Conclusion

Back in the sand of Utah, Steve moans and tries to sit up. You discourage any movement, placing your hands on his head, lowering him once again to the ground.

A full assessment reveals no injuries other than mild abrasions to the forehead and right forearm. Approximately 20 minutes have now passed since you heard the call for help. Taking a deep breath, you methodically check off the points that must be covered before the spine can be cleared: no loss of reliability, no pain or tenderness in the neck and/or back, no altered sensations in the extremities including no loss of ability to move, no loss of circulation in the extremities, no pain on gentle movement.

The wounds are cleaned and dressed. Reminding your friend to immediately let you know if his condition changes, specifically changes in neck or back pain, the trip continues.

Chapter 9: Head Injuries

You should be able to:

1. Describe the basic anatomy of the head.

2. Describe the signs and symptoms of the types of injuries to the head including scalp damage, closed head injury, and open head injury.

3. Describe and demonstrate, where applicable, treatment for the types of injuries to the head.

4. Describe when a patient with a head injury needs to be evacuated from the wilderness.

It could happen to you

Ice formed overnight on the rocky slope called Central Gully at the head of Huntington Ravine. It happens that way sometimes in October on New Hampshire's Mount Washington. Two 20-year-old hikers, one male, one female, move off the trail seeking surer footing. She doesn't find it. Slipping on a more technical section of the ravine, she tumbles about 100 feet. Somewhere on the way down her head strikes forcefully against a stone.

Her boyfriend descends carefully to find her sitting up, bleeding heavily from the nose, a nose that has already begun to puff up alarmingly. He has had enough first aid training to assess the young woman for spine damage. He decides her spine has not been involved. They choose to hike out.

Within a half hour, the young man notices his girlfriend beginning to act "weird." She grows increasingly irritable and confused. She can't remember if this is the right trail. Before long she asks, "What happened to me?"

He tells her, but five minutes later she asks the same question again.

Within an hour, she sits down beside the trail, refusing to walk further. When he tries to help her to her feet, she slaps his hands away and angrily uses words he has seldom heard her utter. As he sighs deeply in frustration, she collapses. He is unable to get any response from her other than moans.

Introduction

Head injuries range from simple scalp damage to severe brain damage. Serious, potentially life-threatening injury is usually a result of the uncompromising structure of the *cranium* (skull)—if the brain starts to swell, it is squashed because there's no room up there for the swelling to take place. Head injuries that involve the brain are a major source of disability and death in the wilderness because there is little the Wilderness First Responder can do other than recognize the risk to the patient, offer what small aid is available, and arrange an evacuation as soon as possible. Knowing when and how fast to work toward an evacuation of a head injured patient is a critical skill for the WFR.

Basic Anatomy

The bulk of the brain is the *cerebrum*, the gray matter, the center of higher functions like thought and emotion. In the back of the head, beneath the cerebrum, is the *cerebellum*, where equilibrium and coordination are controlled. The *brain stem* grows out of the base of the brain and is responsible for vital vegetative functions, including circulation and respiration. Enclosing the brain, and the spinal cord, are three blood-rich layers of tissue called, collectively, the *meninges*. Their names, from the brain outward, are the *pia mater, arachnoid,* and *dura mater. Cerebrospinal fluid*, a clear liquid manufactured at a constant rate in cavities in the brain called ventricles, continually circulates through the *subarachnoid space*, the space between the arachnoid and the pia mater.

The brain sits about one millimeter from the inside of the cranium, well protected by hair (on many people), the scalp, the thick skull, and the shock absorbency of tissues and the cerebrospinal fluid surrounding the brain. The brain maintains control of almost everything that goes on within the human body as long as levels of oxygen, temperature, blood sugar, and pressure stay adequate and balanced within the head. When brain tissue is damaged, however, it does not repair itself like other tissues in the body. Loss of brain cells is permanent. Loss of too many brain cells adds up to the death of the patient.

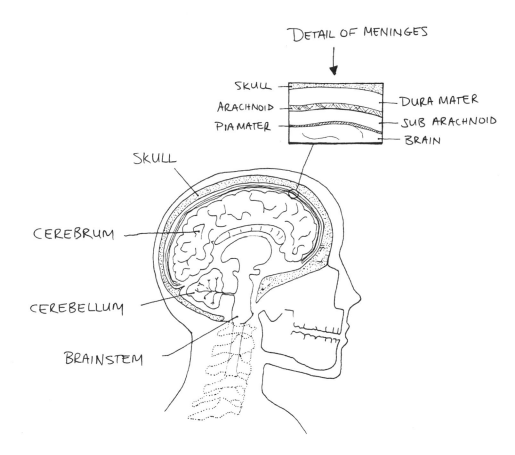

Figure 9-1: Basic anatomy of the head

Types Of Head Injuries

Injuries to the head may or may not involve scalp damage requiring medical attention. Injuries to the head that involve the brain may be closed (the integrity of the skull remains intact) or open (the skull is fractured and/or an object penetrated the skull). All injuries that may involve the brain require immediate attention.

The single most important sign indicating the possibility of brain damage is a change in patient's level of consciousness. A normal level of consciousness—alert and oriented to person, place, time, and event—will deteriorate and typically involve alterations in personality as the pressure from swelling increases on a damaged brain.

Scalp Damage

Lacerations and avulsions of the scalp have a habit of bleeding profusely due 1) to the blood-rich nature of the scalp and 2) to the fact that blood vessels in the scalp do not constrict rapidly after injury to help slow bleeding. Scalp tears, also, tend to reveal the skull, which tends to make rescuers nervous. Fortunately, for rescuers and patients, scalp damage is seldom a serious injury, and shock rarely results from scalp bleeding alone except in small children.

To encourage the bleeding to stop, apply direct pressure with a bulky dressing. The recommendation of a bulky dressing is based on consideration of the integrity of the skull beneath the wound. If the blow to the head was forceful enough to fracture the skull, too much direct pressure could press bone fragments into the brain with devastating results. A bulky dressing disperses the pressure. Blood loss can be further discouraged by pulling the edges of the wound together, perhaps with wound closure strips, although it may be difficult to get the strips to stick to a bloody scalp.

Once bleeding has stopped, the wound should be cleaned and dressed (SEE CHAPTER 15: SOFT TISSUE INJURIES). Hair may be clipped to make wound management easier, but do not shave the scalp. Shaving increases the risk of infection.

There may also be a rather large "goose egg" developing rapidly on the head of the patient after an impact injury to the skull. Types of helmets worn, for instance, by rock climbers or mountain bikers may prevent the "goose egg" but do not necessarily prevent a brain injury, even though helmets typically lessen the severity of the impact. The "goose egg" may be treated with the application of cold and, by itself, is not a cause for concern. The amount of brain damage, which may be cause for great concern, is usually relative to the forces involved.

Closed Head Injury

A *closed head injury* involves an immediate and often transient loss of normal brain function—a period of unconsciousness—following a violent impact to the head. No matter how minor the severity of the closed head injury there will always be some damage to brain cells. Two immediate factors will help you decide how severe the trauma to the patient's brain has been: 1) the duration of unconsciousness, and 2) the duration of *amnesia* (loss of memory) following the return of consciousness.

In the urban environment, any blow to the head resulting in loss of consciousness and/or any post-trauma amnesia lasting more than 30 minutes should send the patient to a hospital for evaluation. In the wilderness environment, the decision-making process leading to the evacuation of someone knocked unconscious may be plagued with doubt. If you evacuate anyone knocked unconscious, you will be acting responsibly, but if the loss of consciousness lasts momentarily, and if the patient remains without symptoms of brain injury after regaining consciousness, you may sometimes choose to let the patient remain in the wilderness (SEE BELOW). Keep in mind that many outdoor organizations have a standing protocol to evacuate anyone who has been knocked unconscious. Such a protocol eases the burden of decision on the WFR.

Note: Successive closed head injuries, even minor ones, may cause cumulative brain damage and increase the risk to the patient. Therefore, if the patient reveals that this is the second or third time, etc., he or she has been knocked unconscious, your eagerness to have the patient evaluated in a hospital should increase.

A serious injury to the brain may or may not be associated with any obvious signs of damage to the head or face. There does need to be sufficient force to slam the brain around inside the skull. What may happen inside the patient's head is this: Blood flows out of broken blood vessels and, sometimes, blood serum starts to leak out of the damaged area of the brain. Swelling results. As the size of the brain increases, there is less and less room for the flow of life-sustaining blood. *Intracranial pressure* (ICP), the normal pressure inside the skull, starts to rise, and, as a result, the brain may sustain permanent damage or death.

Brain injuries may be categorized into one of several types that include: 1) A contusion (bruise) to the brain that may lead to cerebral edema (swelling) that could cause an increase in intracranial pressure. 2) An *epidural hematoma* (bleeding above the dura) which is almost exclusively arterial bleeding and typically causes a rapid rise in intracranial pressure and a quick death. 3) A *subdural hematoma* which involves bleeding between the dura and the arachnoid and/or bleeding between the arachnoid and the cerebrum. Bleeding between the arachnoid and the cerebrum may be called a *subarachnoid hematoma*. Subdural bleeding is almost exclusively venous bleeding which causes a slow rise in intracranial pressure and may lead to death hours or even days after the accident.

Although the progress of increasing intracranial pressure is not absolutely predictable, certain changes in the patient will probably occur, sometimes fast, sometimes slow. Once regaining consciousness, she or he will become increasingly disoriented and irritable, and, perhaps, combative. These changes in level of consciousness are a result of pressure on the cerebrum. *Remember: Level of consciousness changes are the first and foremost signs of brain damage.* Breathing will tend to be erratic early, rapid and deep later. Heart beats will slow down and begin to bound. Blood pressure will rise. Heart rate and blood pressure changes are serious, and both are caused by pressure on the brain stem that is being crushed against the floor of the skull. Skin may appear flushed, especially in the face. Later indications of increasing ICP may include pupils that become distinctly unequal, and unusual, rigid body postures.

Note: Signs of increasing intracranial pressure should not be mistaken for signs of shock. The triad of changes indicating a rise in ICP are 1) erratic respiratory rate growing rapid and deep, 2) heart rate slowing and bounding, 2) blood pressure rising. The triad of changes indicating shock are 1) respiratory rate rapid and shallow, 2) heart rate increasing and weakening, and 3) blood pressure dropping. Although a patient may have sustained injuries that could cause increasing ICP and shock, the signs and symptoms tell which problem should be treated. In other words, vital signs showing increasing ICP mean treat for increasing ICP, and vital signs showing shock mean treat for shock (SEE CHAPTER 7: SHOCK).

Serious brain damage may be detectable by other signs and symptoms that include:
1) prolonged unconsciousness, 2) a headache that increases in intensity, 3) complaints of blurred vision or other visual disturbances extending over one hour, 4) excessive or unusual tiredness or sleepiness, 5) protracted nausea and vomiting, 6) seizures, and 7) ataxia (unusual loss of balance).

Without definitive treatment for increasing intracranial pressure, the patient's brain may rupture through the floor of the skull, the only point with any give to it. Death immediately follows. Even if the brain manages to gain control of the swelling, the loss of circulation often results in permanent loss of the brain's normal function.

**Signs and Symptoms
Increasing Intracranial Pressure:**

1. Distinct changes in mental status often described as disoriented to irritable to combative to coma
2. Slowing and bounding heart rate
3. Erratic respiratory rate later becoming rapid and deep
4. Rise in blood pressure,
5. Flushed skin
6. Intense headache
7. Disturbances in vision
8. Excessive Sleepiness
9. Protracted nausea
10. Vomiting
11. Ataxia
12. Seizures
13. Unequal pupils
14. Rigid body postures.

Open Head Injury

A skull fracture is an *open head injury*, an injury accompanied by a break in the integrity of skull, as opposed to a closed head injury. A fracture of the skull may be indicated by obvious signs that include

1) fracture lines visible beneath a tear in the scalp,

2) deformity, often a depression, at the injury site,

3) *raccoon eyes* (black-and-blue discoloration around swollen eyes),

4) *Battle's sign* (black-and-blue discoloration behind and below the ears),

5) seizures, and

6) cerebrospinal fluid or blood mixed with CSF leaking from the nose and/or ears. A patient with a fractured skull should be evacuated as soon as possible.

Note: You should not attempt to stop the flow of cerebrospinal fluid resulting from a head injury. The patient may be relieving some increasing intracranial pressure. If you're unsure whether or not CSF is mixed with blood, catch some of the blood on a piece of sterile gauze. CSF will spread out farther than the blood on the gauze forming a halo around the blood spot. The haloed blood spot appears somewhat like a target, giving this test for CSF the nickname "target test."

**Signs and Symptoms
Skull Fracture:**
1. Visible fracture line
2. Depression in the skull
3. Raccoon eyes
4. Battle's sign
5. Seizures,
6. Cerebrospinal fluid or blood mixed with CSF from the nose and/or ears.

When an object penetrates the skull, an object such as a ice axe, knife, or bullet, permanent brain damage almost always results. The wound should be covered with bulky sterile dressings. Often the object lodges in the brain, sticking out of the skull. Impaled objects should be stabilized in place with large bulky dressings, not removed. Bleeding should be allowed to continue, not stopped with direct pressure, in hopes some of the pressure within the cranium will self-release. Any penetrating wound to the head requires an immediate evacuation of the patient.

Levels Of Head Injury

For quick reference, all head injuries can be loosely divided into three levels:

1) *No loss of consciousness* means only an extremely rare chance of serious problems, despite the fact heavy external bleeding and a huge "goose egg" sized bump may accompany the injury. In the wilderness, monitor the patient for about 24 hours, watching primarily for changes in level of consciousness, and evacuate if the signs and symptoms of serious brain damage develop.

2) *Momentary loss of consciousness* tells that the patient's brain underwent some transient loss of function and, therefore, some brain cell damage. Keep in mind the patient may not be aware they have been unconscious. Ask witnesses, if possible. People knocked unconscious only momentarily are often okay, but they may only appear okay initially, and then start to deteriorate. Either evacuate the patient as soon as possible, or monitor closely for 24 hours, awakening the patient several times during the first night—every two to three hours—to evaluate the LOC. Evacuate if the signs and symptoms of serious brain damage develop.

3) *Long-term loss of consciousness* and/or other warning signs and symptoms indicating the brain has been seriously damaged warrant an immediate evacuation.

Treatment For Serious Head Injury

Any force severe enough to cause unconsciousness may have caused damage to the cervical spine. If the patient regains consciousness and reliability, you may proceed with your assessment with the possibility of clearing the spine (SEE CHAPTER 8: SPINE INJURIES). Any patient who remains unreliable must, of course, be treated for spine injury as well as brain injury.

If the spine is cleared, and the patient is capable and free of signs and symptoms of brain damage, you may decide to start walking the patient out as a means of evacuation. A patient incapable of walking and/or a patient with obvious signs and symptoms of increasing ICP and/or a skull fracture or penetrating head wound should be evacuated as soon as possible by whatever other means are available.

If the patient must be left alone for any reason, roll her or him carefully into a stable side position, the recovery position, to ensure an airway.

Elevation of the patient's head to decrease increasing intracranial pressure is controversial. Some experts believe it reduces ICP, a "good" thing. Some experts say it reduces cerebral perfusion, a "bad" thing. If local protocols exist, you will follow those protocols. Without protocols, since patients with a serious head injury are almost always being treated for spine injury as well, stabilization of the patient supine with the head in a neutral position is a priority, and keeping the patient flat is recommended.

Since oxygen deprivation is the immediate threat to life, supplemental oxygen, when available, would be of great benefit. In the wilderness with a patient in the later stages of brain injury, artificial respirations—mouth-to-mouth/mouth-to-mask—*may* help keep the patient adequately oxygenated. Breath for any head injured patient who has inadequate respirations, e.g., less than the normal rate, at a rate of approximately 18 to 20 breaths per minute.

Do *not* give pain killing medications to head injured patients with signs and symptoms of brain damage or during an evaluation period while you're waiting to see if signs and symptoms appear. These medications may mask the signs and symptoms you are trying to monitor. Some medications, such as aspirin and ibuprofen, may increase the rate of bleeding in the brain.

Once in a hospital, even the seriously head injured patient has a chance of survival. Oxygen therapy, drug therapy, and surgical intervention are available. That's why they keep the patient awake, or arouse them regularly. If arousal is impossible, the hospital staff knows it's time for radical procedures. In a wilderness situation, you'll wake the patient periodically to assess the level of consciousness and, thus, the level of brain damage. In sleep, however, the brain will have the best chance of controlling its own swelling. Once you have decided to evacuate the patient for treatment for serious brain damage, you may let them sleep.

Evacuation Guidelines

Immediate evacuation is a necessity for any patient with signs and symptoms of increasing intracranial pressure and/or a skull fracture or penetrating head wound. You may decide prior to the start of a wilderness trip to evacuate any patient forcefully knocked unconscious.

Conclusion

Fortunately for the young woman lying unconscious in New Hampshire, her boyfriend remembers to leave her in the recovery position—to maintain her airway—while he hurries on for help. He leaves his parka covering her as much as possible.

The rescue team arrives to find the ground around her face splattered with vomit. Her respirations are deep and sighing, her heart beats slow and hard, her face appears deeply flushed. She does not respond to any stimulus. Supplemental oxygen is started at a high flow. She is loaded into a litter with her head and shoulders elevated approximately 30 degrees for the carry to the nearest road.

Long after dark, she lifts off for a quick helicopter flight to Boston. After extensive surgery she is able to return finally to a full and healthy life.

Chapter 10:   Chest Injuries

You should be able to:

1. *Describe the basic anatomy of the chest and normal breathing.*

2. *Define and describe the signs and symptoms of the most common chest injuries including fractured ribs, pneumothorax, hemothorax, flail chest, pericardial tamponade, and traumatic asphyxia.*

3. *Describe the treatment for the most common chest injuries.*

It could happen to you

Posted at the trailhead, a small sign read "Beware of Bears," which explained why Dave straddled a limb high in the ponderosa pine tying off a bag of food. The knot held, but Dave didn't. Smashing into several branches on the way down, his rush to the ground ended with a gut-wrenching thud and an ooooff of forcefully expelled air.

Kneeling close to the baghanger-turned-patient, your first words are "Don't move." To your assessing eye, clues begin to appear: scrapes on bare legs and arms—ugly but not serious; respiratory effort—shallow and labored, an immediate concern; a ragged tear on the upper left side of Dave's T-shirt reddening with seeping blood.

Dave, fully alert, denies pain in his head or spine, but you opt on the side of caution, asking another member of your party to maintain manual control of his head and neck. His heart beats fast but strong and regular. You lift his shirt to take a close look at his chest. Any injury to the chest may lead to severe respiratory difficulty and a critical patient. If there's a chest injury, you want to know as much about it as possible... as soon as possible.

Introduction

Few traumatic injuries offer Wilderness First Responders as great an opportunity to watch a patient die as a serious chest injury. Although well protected by the construction of the chest, the organs within the chest cavity—lungs, heart, great blood vessels—once damaged, can quickly develop into a threat to life. For that reason, *any injury to the chest should be considered an immediate life threat until proven otherwise.*

Basic Anatomy And Normal Breathing

Ribs form a bony cage that surrounds the *thorax* (chest cavity). Each of the 12 pairs of ribs attach to a thoracic vertebrae. The top 10 pairs attach to the sternum by way of cartilage. The last two pairs of ribs are shorter and "float" free with no anterior attachment. Beneath each rib runs an intercostal nerve, artery, and vein.

Lungs fill both sides of the thorax which is lined with a tough membrane called the *parietal pleura*. The lungs are covered with a membrane called the *visceral pleura*. Between the two pleuras exists a potential space, the pleural space.

Between the lungs, beneath the lower half of the sternum, lies the heart, surrounded by its own membrane of fibrous connective tissue called the *pericardial sac*. The central area of the thorax also houses the great vessels—aorta and vena cava—carrying blood from and to the heart respectively.

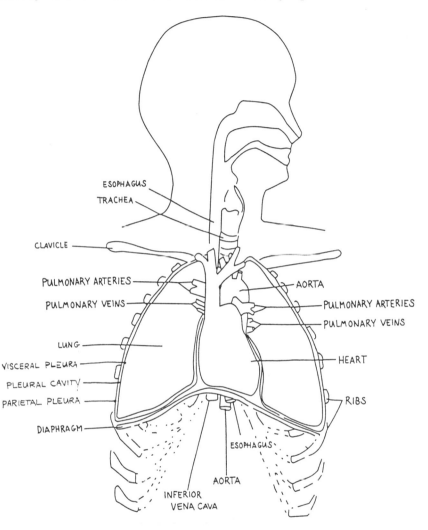

ESOPHAGUS
TRACHEA
CLAVICLE
PULMONARY ARTERIES
PULMONARY VEINS
LUNG
VISCERAL PLEURA
PLEURAL CAVITY
PARIETAL PLEURA
DIAPHRAGM
AORTA
PULMONARY ARTERIES
PULMONARY VEINS
HEART
RIBS
ESOPHAGUS
AORTA
INFERIOR VENA CAVA

Figure 10-1: Anatomy of the Chest

Being spongy and relatively flaccid, the five lobes of the lungs (three on the right side, two on the left) depend on nearby muscles in order to function. A domed shelf of muscle, the *diaphragm*, relaxes between the chest and abdominal cavities when not in use. Every few seconds it contracts and flattens downward, enlarging the chest cavity. Secondary to the diaphragm, *inter-costal muscles*, the ones that lie between the ribs, contract to lift the rib cage and expand the chest cavity. Lungs slide along the chest wall as it moves up and down, slipping easily on a lubricating layer of synovial fluid. But, since the fluid keeps the lungs stuck to the chest wall, they are pulled open as the chest expands. On inhalation, air rushes in to fill the void created by the expansion of the chest cavity: the active phase of breathing. As tension releases from the diaphragm and intercostal muscles, air leaves the lungs: the passive phase of breathing. The breathing process, all things considered, resembles very much the action of bellows that once hung beside just about every fireplace in the world.

Types Of Chest Injuries

Injuries to the chest may be closed (the skin of the chest is unbroken) or open (an object penetrates the chest wall). These injuries may result from blunt trauma, penetrating trauma, or compression trauma.

Two important signs indicate the possibility of a serious chest injury: changes in respiratory rate and changes in respiratory patterns. Normal breathing at 12 to 20 breaths per minute is effortless and painless. A patient with rapid breathing, painful breathing, and/or difficult breathing should send you into quick response mode.

Fractured Ribs

**Signs and Symptoms
Fractured Rib:**
1. Pain at the fracture site
2. Point tenderness at the fracture site
3. Pain on movement
4. Pain on coughing
5. Pain on deep breathing
6. Shallow breathing
7. Guarding the fracture site
8. Bruising

Broken ribs account, by far, for most chest injuries. And cracked ribs, although painful, rarely create a serious patient. Pain explodes in the damaged area whenever the patient inhales, when the active phase of breathing causes contraction of the muscles around the broken bone. The patient will take shallow breaths to ease the pain. Typically, the patient also presses a hand over or squeezes an arm against the fracture site to help stabilize the broken bone or bones, another pain reducer.

Supplemental oxygen, if available, will ease the pain and anxiety. As long as spinal precautions need not be taken, aid the patient in assuming a semi-reclining position which should make it easier to breathe. You can help the patient by doing more than he or she is doing to stabilize the fracture. The simplest and most effective treatment involves suspending the arm on the damaged side of the chest in a sling. The arm then hangs protectively over the fracture in a position similar to the one the patient was probably already holding the arm. Secure the arm in place by tying strips of cloth around the chest and the slung arm, or by putting the patient's sweater or jacket on over the arm. If your first aid kit does not contain sling material, you can improvise with relative ease using extra clothing, or even by folding the shirt the patient is wearing up over the arm and safety-pinning it in place.

The sling-and-swathe technique leaves one arm virtually useless, sometimes a disadvantage on the trail. Less protective but functional, you can help stabilize the fracture by padding the site with a folded cloth, say a T-shirt, and securing it with an elastic wrap that encircles the chest. Tape can be used, too, but the strips of tape should not wrap completely around the chest, a technique that may make it even more difficult for the patient to breath.

Anti-pain, anti-inflammatory drugs such as ibuprofen may be given, but avoid pain medications that depress the patient's respiratory drive.

Patients with minor fractures to the ribs may need nothing done for them. His or her ability to deal with the discomfort will be your best guide. But all people suspected of having a broken rib should be watched over the next day or two. Any marked increase in a patient's respiratory effort indicates a need for rapid evacuation. Since patient comfort is also a factor, you may decide to evacuate someone with a suspected fracture to the ribs simply because he or she is not able to enjoy the wilderness experience.

Pneumothorax

**Signs and Symptoms
Pneumothorax:**
1. Sharp chest pain
2. Increasing difficulty breathing
3. Increasing anxiety
4. Rapid pulse
5. Diminished breath sounds on the affected side
6. Bruising
7. Pale, cool, clammy skin.

A simple fractured rib may not be so simple if a bone fragment stabs inward to puncture a lung. Air escaping the lung on inhalation and collecting in the chest outside the lung in the pleural space creates a condition called a *closed pneumothorax*. Over a period of time determined by the extent of the injury, the "dead air" in the chest cavity grows in size. The patient will experience increasing difficulty breathing, especially difficulty taking a deep breath, and a rising level of anxiety as the trapped air takes up more and more breathing room. With a stethoscope, you may hear diminished breath sounds on the affected side, beginning in the upper chest. If your hearing is acute, you may be able to hear diminished breath sounds on the affected side by pressing your ear against the patient's chest

Treat the patient as you would a patient with a fractured rib: supplemental oxygen, semi-reclining position, stabilization of the fracture site. More often than not, a pneumothorax reaches a point where it gets no worse. But it can worsen until the patient is unable to breath adequately, a condition known as a *tension pneumothorax*, one of the most life-threatening chest injuries. In a tension pneumothorax, air keeps leaking from the damaged lung, collecting in the pleural space until the lung on the affected side compresses to the size of a tennis ball. Air continues to leak out, compressing the heart, the great vessels, even the other lung. Neck veins may bulge, sometimes called *jugular vein distention* or JVD, and the trachea may deviate toward the uninjured side. With a stethoscope, you may hear diminished breath sounds or fail to hear breath sounds on the affected side. When the pressure of trapped air inside the chest reaches maximum tension, breathing stops.

Signs and Symptoms Tension Pneumothorax:
1. Sharp chest pain
2. Increasing difficulty breathing
3. Decreasing level of consciousness
4. Rapid pulse
5. Distended neck veins
6. Tracheal deviation
7. Falling blood pressure
8. Pale, cool, clammy skin.

Medics with advanced training are often able to puncture the chest with a small hole that lets the trapped air out. Since most of us can't do that, and since you never know whether a pneumothorax will go to tension or not, *suspicion of any pneumothorax calls for an immediate and rapid evacuation.* Although circumstances could demand otherwise, it's best for the patient to be carried, preventing an increased work load on an already damaged lung. While waiting for transport or even while being carried, remember to aid the patient to sit in a semi-reclining position which makes breathing easier.

Of value to note, a pneumothorax can occur spontaneously, without an injury to the chest. Seldom life-threatening, a *spontaneous pneumothorax* results when a weak spot on a lung ruptures. The patient—often a tall, thin, male, adolescent who recently experienced a growth spurt—is usually involved in some activity when sudden chest pain and difficulty breathing strike. Treatment is the same as for any pneumothorax.

With a chest injury that tears a lung or a bronchial tube, little bubbles of air may move into subcutaneous tissue and appear on the skin of the chest, neck, or face. Termed *subcutaneous emphysema*, the bubbles move around and may make a crackling sound when you push on them. Not a problem itself, subcutaneous emphysema is another indication of a serious chest injury, most often a pneumothorax.

Hemothorax

Signs and Symptoms Hemothorax:
1. Sharp chest pain
2. Increasing difficulty breathing
3. Increasing anxiety
4. rapid pulse
5. Decreased breath sounds on the affected side
6. The possibility of hemoptysis
7. Pale, cool, clammy skin

Broken ribs can tear into blood vessels causing enough damage to allow an accumulation of blood in the pleural space, a condition known as a *hemothorax*. A small hemothorax can create no signs and symptoms, but blood may accumulate to the point, as air may accumulate in a pneumothorax, where the lungs cannot expand and breathing ceases to be possible. With a stethoscope, you may hear diminished breath sounds or fail to hear any breath sounds on the affected side, usually at the base of the lungs. If the hemothorax is extensive, you may see *hemoptysis* (blood coughed up). A hemothorax and pneumothorax can occur simultaneously.

Shock is possible, and treatment for shock, if it develops, would be appropriate, except the patient will probably breathe much easier sitting up instead of lying down. Otherwise, the patient with a hemothorax receives the same treatment as a patient with a pneumothorax.

Sucking Chest Wound Open Pneumothorax

If the chest has been opened by a penetrating object (if Dave, for instance, fell on a sharp stick), the resulting hole may bubble and make noise when the patient breathes. When the chest moves, air flows in and sometimes out through the wound as well as through the mouth and nose. This is appropriately called a *sucking chest wound*, and the air being sucked in through the wound does nothing to sustain life.

Signs and Symptoms Sucking Chest Wound:
1. Difficulty breathing
2. A moist sucking sound and/or bubbling from an open wound
3. Increasing anxiety
4. Rapid pulse
5. Pale, cool, clammy skin

Immediate action is required. Plug the hole. Your hand, preferably gloved, will work fine, and quick action could prove life saving. Continue treatment by covering the wound with an occlusive dressing—something that lets no air or water pass through. Clean plastic will work. Tape this dressing in place leaving one side, or at least one corner, free in hopes air collecting under tension in the chest will self-release. If collecting air doesn't release, an *open pneumothorax* may develop, and may progress to life-threatening tension.

If the patient's pneumothorax goes to full tension, he won't be able to breathe. Death is imminent. You can try pushing your little finger, or some dull-ended object, gently into the hole in an attempt to release the trapped air. Not fun or advisable in most situations, this may your only chance to save the patient.

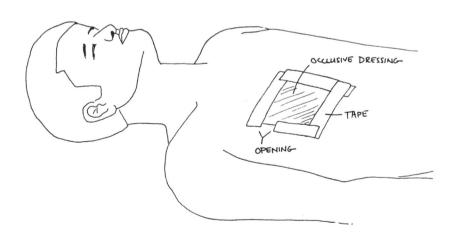

Figure 10-2: Bandaging of open chest wound

Impaled Object

When you inspect the chest and find an object still wedged in a wound, don't attempt to remove it. Removal has an excellent chance of making the injury worse by encouraging serious bleeding or creating a sucking chest wound. Pad well around the impaled object with the padding rising at least as high as the object, and tape the padding in place to stabilize the object. Evacuation of the patient, of course, should be high on your list of priorities.

The Wilderness First Responder

Flail Chest

Signs and Symptoms Flail Chest:
1. Chest pain
2. Difficulty breathing
3. Paradoxical respiration
4. Deformity at the fracture site
5. Bruising
6. Decreased level of consciousness
7. Pale, cool, clammy skin

If several ribs are broken in several places and/or the sternum has broken loose (if, for instance, Dave fell on a large rock instead of a sharp stick), a free-floating section of chest wall, called a *flail*, sometimes results. A minor flail is often a subtle injury, never assessed until the patient is x-rayed. A major flail, however, is a major threat to life. You may see the flail move in opposition to the rest of the chest wall during breathing, a condition known as *paradoxical respiration*. Paradoxical movement is easiest to see when the patient lies on his or her back. A severe flail makes it extremely difficult for the patient to adequately breathe. A pneumothorax and/or a hemothorax may develop as well.

Taping a bulky dressing securely over the flail to stabilize the fracture site often allows the patient to inhale a little more easily. If the tape runs from midline to midline, halfway around the patient's body, the stabilization is usually improved. If, however, the patient gets worse with the flail secured, remove the tape and dressing. Evacuation of the patient on his or her side, injured side down, sometimes aids breathing, but the patient, other injuries allowing, may prefer to assume a semi-reclining position. Supplemental oxygen at a high flow would be of great benefit. In addition, with severe cases (profound respiratory distress, cyanosis, mental status changes) you need to provide positive pressure ventilations for the patient. These ventilations are somewhat tricky since you need to synchronize your breaths with the patient's efforts to breathe. In other words, when he or she attempts to inhale, you assist by blowing in air and/or supplemental oxygen.

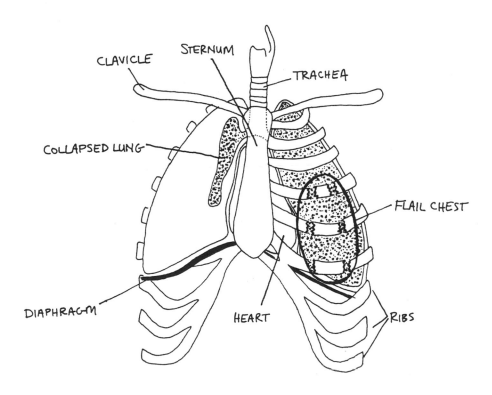

Figure 10-3: Anatomy of collapsed lung and flail chest

Pericardial Tamponade

Blunt trauma to the chest wall may cause *pulmonary contusions* and/or *myocardial contusions*, producing shortness of breath or chest pain respectively. These contusions may, of course, be small or large. But, in addition, chest trauma, blunt or penetrating, may cause blood or other fluids to leak from the myocardium (heart) itself into the pericardial sac. The sac will not stretch, so the heart is squeezed by the increasing pressure, a condition known as *pericardial tamponade*, an immediate threat to life. As the heart beats with less and less efficiency, the pulse pressure, the difference between the systolic and diastolic blood pressure, narrows. In other words, the two numbers grow closer and closer to the same number. You should see the pulse growing weaker and shortness of breath increasing. You may see distended neck veins. Shock results. Death is imminent.

There's little to be done in the field other than early recognition, supplemental oxygen, if available, and the most rapid evacuation possible.

Traumatic Asphyxia

A sudden and violent compression of the chest wall can force blood out of the heart the wrong way, into the veins instead of into the arteries, especially the veins of the shoulders and head, causing an immediate threat to life known as *traumatic asphyxia*. Head, neck, and shoulders appear swollen. Neck veins distend. Eyes bulge. A blue tongue protrudes from blue lips. Hemoptysis and/or *hematemesis* (vomiting blood) may occur. Shock develops. Death is imminent.

There's little to be done in the field other than early recognition, supplemental oxygen, if available, and the most rapid evacuation possible.

Tearing the Great Vessels

A sudden and violent deceleration, once rare, now common with modern high-speed vehicles, can tear one of the great vessels in the chest. Massive bleeding results in an instant threat to life. Fiery pain burns through the chest and/or back. Blood pressure plummets, although it can be high in the arms and low in the legs. Death is very imminent. Only surgery can save the patient.

General Treatment Guidelines

1. Maintain an adequate airway
2. Give supplemental oxygen, if available
3. Inspect the bare chest: look, ask, feel
4. Treat any injury you find: stabilize fractures, close open wounds, stabilize impaled objects
5. When no other injuries prevent movement, allow the patient to assume a position that provides the most comfort
6. Avoid pain medications that depress respiratory drive
7. Plan an evacuation (except for simple fractured rib)

Evacuation Guidelines

Any patient with increasing difficulty breathing and increasing anxiety following an injury to the chest and/or any patient treated for a serious chest injury should be evacuated as soon as safely possible. Decreasing level of consciousness, increasing respiratory rate, and diminishing breath sounds on the affected sides are further indications of the need for a rapid evacuation.

Conclusion

Beneath the tear in Dave's shirt you find a superficial abrasion, the source of the blood. His breathing remains labored, but he appears to be getting no worse. His chest expands equally on both sides when he inhales. A complete examination reveals no serious problem, and you decide, after a second and closer look for signs and symptoms of spine damage, to clear his spine. Sitting up, Dave is able to breathe easier.

Your careful palpation of the ribs below the abrasion elicit a pain response at a specific point. With encouragement because it hurts, Dave is able to take a deep breath. Your assessment: a cracked rib.

For the next day the group remains camped at this spot, and Dave wears a sling supporting the arm on his injured side. He reports sleeping "fairly well" through the night. Although extensive bruising appears on his injured side, his ability to breathe without pain increases.

You keep a watchful eye on his condition, but he is able to finish the trip with the rest of the group.

Chapter II: Abdominal Injuries

You should be able to:

1. *Describe the basic anatomy of the abdomen.*

2. *Describe the general signs and symptoms of abdominal injuries.*

3. *Describe the general treatment for abdominal injuries.*

4. *Demonstrate specific treatment for blunt abdominal trauma and penetrating abdominal trauma.*

It could happen to you

As a novice wrangler, you're happy to have gotten a job with a small company that leads horse-packing trips in the Wenaha-Tucannon Wilderness, a vast area shared by Washington and Oregon. One of the reasons you got this job is your medical skills. None of the other wranglers on this 10-day ride have more training than an urban-oriented basic first aid course. It's the evening of the fourth day before your skills are needed.

The dinner bell rings the call to grub, but one of the clients is a no-show. Another client says the missing rider was complaining of a stomachache. He says he saw him lying down by the river after the horses were unsaddled and hobbled for the night. You go to investigate, and most of the group follows.

You find the man on his side with his legs drawn up in a fetal position, his arms crossed over his abdomen to guard his abdominal area. He moans softly. His skin appears pale, cool, and clammy. His breathing is rapid and shallow.

"Anybody got an idea about what happened," you ask.

"Well," offers one of the other wranglers, "he got kicked in the gut by that ol' pack mule at lunch break, but he jumped right up and seemed OK."

Introduction

Abdominal injuries, trauma to internal structures of the body between the diaphragm and the lower end of the pelvis, may be generally classified in two categories: 1) *blunt trauma*, a closed abdominal injury caused by a forceful blow to the abdomen, and 2) *penetrating trauma*, an open abdominal injury caused by an object being forced into the abdomen. The extent of injury is often difficult to assess in the wilderness—or anywhere, for that matter. No other region of the human body has more potential to conceal serious blood loss. The mechanism of injury may seem trivial, and the patient may initially present with signs and symptoms that appear relatively normal before indications of serious injury seem to suddenly manifest themselves.

Serious abdominal trauma in the wilderness carries a high risk for mortality due to two factors: 1) several body systems may be involved in the injury, and 2) several hours to days may lapse before definitive care can be reached, and there's little treatment that can be provided in the field. The chance of saving a patient with serious abdominal injury depends largely on the First Responder's ability to make an early accurate assessment and provide rapid evacuation.

Basic Anatomy

The abdominal cavity extends from the vertebral column in back to the abdominal muscles in front, from the diaphragm on top to the pelvis on the bottom. It is important to remember that the diaphragm may rise as high as the fourth rib on exhalation, and injury below that point may involve the abdomen.

The abdominal cavity is divided into four quadrants for assessment purposes by drawing an imaginary vertical line and horizontal line through the *umbilicus* (belly button). The quadrants are named "right" and "left" in reference to the patient's body, not the rescuer's body. The contents of each quadrant are:

Right Upper Quadrant (RUQ): the right and largest section of the liver, gallbladder, part of the transverse colon, right kidney, and duodenum (first section of the small intestine).

Left Upper Quadrant (LUQ): the left and smaller section of the liver, stomach, transverse colon, spleen, left kidney, and pancreas.

Right Lower Quadrant (RLQ): part of the small intestine, ascending colon, appendix, right ureter, bladder if it is distended, and, in females, right ovary, right fallopian tube, and uterus if it is enlarged.

Left Lower Quadrant (LLQ): part of the small intestine, descending colon, sigmoid colon, left ureter, bladder if it is distended, and, in females, left ovary, left fallopian tube, and uterus if it is enlarged.

Some of the abdominal organs are solid—pancreas, liver, kidneys, spleen—and mostly tucked under the rib cage for more protection. Some are hollow—stomach, intestines, gallbladder, urinary bladder, female reproductive organs. Solid organs can be damaged by penetrating trauma, but they can also rupture from blunt trauma. Blood loss from solid organs can be life-threatening, especially from the liver, which receives about 30 percent of heart's output every minute, and the spleen, which receives about 10 percent of the heart's output every minute. Hollow organs are more likely to be damaged by penetrating trauma, but they also can rupture from blunt trauma, especially if they happen to be full of a transient substance on impact, e.g., a full bladder, a full stomach.

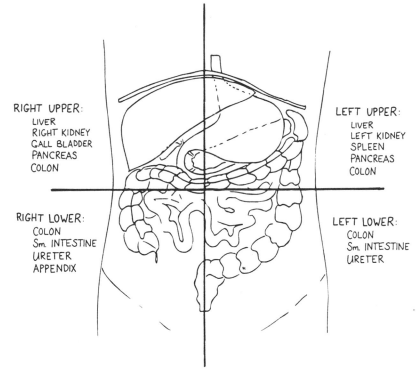

RIGHT UPPER:
LIVER
RIGHT KIDNEY
GALL BLADDER
PANCREAS
COLON

LEFT UPPER:
LIVER
LEFT KIDNEY
SPLEEN
PANCREAS
COLON

RIGHT LOWER:
COLON
Sm. INTESTINE
URETER
APPENDIX

LEFT LOWER:
COLON
Sm. INTESTINE
URETER

Figure 11-1: Anatomy of the abdomen showing quadrants

General Abdominal Trauma Assessment

1. Determine the mechanism of injury, and assess if it is indicative of abdominal trauma.

2. Observe the patient's body position. Although pain is not always a reliable indicator of the seriousness of the injury, a patient who lies still with legs drawn up into a fetal position is often assuming a posture that minimizes serious pain.

3. Look at the abdomen with the patient lying down. A normal abdomen is gently rounded and symmetrical. Look for distention and/or an irregularly shaped abdomen, both of which indicate a serious injury. Look for bruises, penetrating wounds, or obvious injuries, and don't forget to check the flanks where damage to the kidneys might be indicated. Find out as much as you can about any object that has penetrated the abdomen. If you see a gunshot entrance wound, check as soon as possible for an exit wound.

4. Feel the abdomen with flat fingers. Press gently in all four quadrants of the abdomen. Watch for a pain response. Normal abdomens are soft and not tender to palpation. Feel for rigid muscles, lumps, and pain specific to a local spot, all of which may be signs of injury.

5. Ask the patient about his or her condition. Has this ever happened before? The OPQRST questions will be very helpful:

O-Onset: Did the pain come on suddenly or gradually?

P-Provokes, Palliates: Does anything make the pain worse or better?

Q-Quality: How does the patient describe the pain? Sharp? Dull?

R-Radiate, Refers, Region: Where is the pain, and does it radiate or refer to another region?

T-Time: How long has the pain been there?

6. Listen with an ear or stethoscope pressed against each of the four quadrants. This takes time. In two or three minutes, within each quadrant, bowel sounds (gurgling noises) should be heard. Absence of noise means something is not working right.

7. Monitor the vital signs for indications of shock.

8. Ask about blood which may appear in the urine, stool, or vomit.

Blunt Trauma Assessment & Treatment

A patient suffering a severe blow to the abdomen needs to have an adequate history taken since damage on the inside is often not very obvious from the outside. What hit the patient? How fast was it going?

When you look at the abdomen, you may see bruising. When you press gently on the abdomen during your examination, the patient may reflexively "guard"—a sign of a serious abdominal problem. When you palpate the abdomen, you may feel unusual lumps.

Hollow organs, when ruptured, may release substances into the abdomen such as stomach acid, digested food, or bacteria. Hollow organs contents are highly irritating. *Peritonitis*, an inflammatory reaction in the abdominal cavity, will probably develop with pain—described as sharp, stabbing, or burning—increasing and spreading throughout the abdomen. Pulse and respiration quicken. The muscles of the abdomen become increasingly rigid and distended. Your ear placed against the patient's abdomen, periodically, reveals a decrease in the gurgles and rumbles of normal bowel activity as the intestines become paralyzed. The patient will lie very still on her or his back or side but demand flexion of the knees to take pressure off the abdominal muscles. Pain is provoked by movement and any attempt to straighten the legs.

Since solid organs bleed when ruptured, and since blood is less irritating than hollow organ contents, the signs and symptoms of peritonitis may not appear. The signs and symptoms of shock may appear. You should also see increasing rigidity, distention, and possibly the loss of bowel sounds. Pain may increase. Pain from a damaged liver may refer to the right shoulder, and pain from a damaged spleen may refer to the left shoulder. Threat to life may be immediate.

With any abdominal injury anticipate nausea and vomiting. Over time, blood may appear in the vomit (often looking like "coffee grounds"), in the urine (often appearing pale pink), or in the stool (often described as "black and tarry"), depending on where the damage occurred. Over time, a fever may develop.

As with all patients, treatment should involve maintenance of the airway. Stay alert to the possibility of vomiting. Generally, treat for shock. Patients suffering blunt trauma should be kept in the position of comfort they choose—if no other injuries prevent this—and kept warm. If you are involved in their evacuation, comfort and warmth should be extended to them during the carry. In general, nothing should be given to them by mouth, but on an extended evacuation sips of water, preferably cool, may be necessary to prevent dehydration.

Penetrating Trauma Assessment And Treatment

The immediate seriousness of any penetrating abdominal injury, as with blunt trauma, is determined by what got damaged inside and how bad it's bleeding. With severe bleeding, shock is imminent, and immediate evacuation the only chance of salvation. Over time the risk of infection is very high. General assessment of the patient is the same as with a closed injury. General treatment of the patient is the same as for a patient suffering blunt abdominal trauma. Specific treatment will vary somewhat depending on the soft tissue involvement. External bleeding should be controlled. Wounds should be cleaned and bandaged (SEE CHAPTER 15: SOFT TISSUE INJURIES). Impaled objects, in almost all cases, should be stabilized in place.

An *evisceration* is a specific type of penetrating injury that opens the abdomen and lets intestines protrude. In short term care, cover the exposed bowels with sterile dressings soaked in disinfected water to prevent drying out. Check the dressings every two hours to make sure they stay moist. Cover the moist dressings with thick, dry dressings, and rapidly evacuate the patient. In long-term care, over several hours, the exposed intestines will do better if they are flushed clean with disinfected water and "teased" back inside by gently pulling the wound open. If teasing doesn't work, you may have to gently push the exposed loops of intestine back inside the abdominal cavity. Then clean and bandage the wound.

**Signs and Symptoms
Serious Abdominal Trauma:**

1. Obviously serious abdominal injury, e.g., impaled object, evisceration
2. Signs and symptoms of shock
3. Blood in the vomit, feces, or urine
4. Pain in the abdomen persisting for more than 12 to 24 hours
5. Localized abdominal pain, especially with guarding, tenderness, rigidity, palpable lumps, distention and/or asymmetry
6. Fever above 102 DEGREES F (38 DEGREES C)

Evacuation Guidelines

All patients with serious abdominal injuries require rapid evacuation. The evacuation should be as gentle as possible. Often surgical intervention is all that will eventually prevent their death.

Conclusion

Exposing the abdomen of your horsepacking client, you notice substantial bruising over the left upper quadrant. In response to your questions he says, yes, that's right where the mule kicked him. When you press on the left upper quadrant, the patient groans, flexing his abdominal muscles to guard the area. Palpation of the other three quadrants produces unremark-able results. He refuses to roll onto his back. He says when he's curled up on his side the pain eases a little. A first set of vital signs shows a heart rate of 110, strong and regular; a respiratory rate of 20, shallow and slightly labored.

Organizing members of the party, you lead a carry of the patient to his tent where he is bedded down as comfortably as possible. A second set of vitals shows a marked increase in the numbers.

You begin immediate preparations to send for help. The trail in was easy, and a group of competent riders, led by one of the other wranglers, will travel through the night, carrying full documentation and location information.

Chapter 12: *Fractures*

You should be able to:

1. *Describe the basic anatomy of the musculoskeletal system.*

2. *Describe the signs and symptoms of upper and lower body fractures.*

3. *Demonstrate how to treat simple upper and lower body fractures.*

4. *Demonstrate how to treat complex upper and lower body fractures including femur fractures, angulated fractures, and open fractures.*

It could happen to you

You've set a camp near Minnesota's Blue Mounds because it's a pleasant spot and one of the few places in the Land of 10,000 Lakes where you can rock climb. Early summer mosquitoes and ticks make you glad you brought the tent. To the west the first hint of color announces the beginning of the end of the day, but the routes here are short. You and your partner agree there's ample light for an hour or so of climbing.

Half way up a straightforward 30 foot crack, you've broken a mild sweat. Safely belayed by your partner, you ease off a moment and look to your left. A solo climber has started up an open face about 50 feet away. He's only, maybe, eight feet off the ground. As you watch, he reaches high and both his feet come off their precarious steps. He drops to the broken rock at the foot of the face, landing on his feet.

It doesn't look like much of a fall, and you return your attention to the route you're on when the solo climber's scream of pain jerks your head back in his direction. Even from up here you can now see the weird angle at which his lower right leg lies.

Introduction

Injuries to muscles, bones, tendons, and ligaments—the musculoskeletal system—are, undoubtedly, among the most common emergencies dealt with by the Wilderness First Responder. Your quick and adequate response will prevent further injury, reduce pain, and, sometimes, make the difference between discomfort and permanent disability.

Basic Anatomy

The two principle parts of the musculoskeletal system are muscles and bones. Muscles are specialized tissues that contract, or shorten, when stimulated, providing power and motion. Bones—the skeletal system—give muscles attachment points in order for locomotion (movement from one place to another) to occur. Muscles and bones also provide support and protection for vital organs. The rest of the musculoskeletal story includes *tendons*, connective tissues holding muscles to bones; *ligaments*, connective tissues holding bones to bones; and *cartilage*, which is tough, elastic tissue forming protective pads where bone meets bone.

Types Of Fractures

Any break in the normal continuity of a bone is a *fracture.* These breaks can be caused by force being applied directly to a bone, such as a skier's leg striking a tree, or they can be caused by indirect force, such as falling on an outstretched hand and breaking the collarbone or the larger lower arm bone near the elbow. Fractures may be closed, when the skin is intact, or open, when the skin is broken over the site of the fracture. Bone does not have to be visible through the opening in the skin for the fracture to be called "open."

Wilderness Assessment

In addition to strong assessment skills, managing fractures in remote environments requires common sense and sensitivity to the needs of the patient. For example, in a badly sprained ankle, where a fracture is a possibility, you would ideally immobilize the part and put the patient at rest with instructions for elevation and ice. In the wilderness, however, you must weigh other factors: the desire of the patient to ambulate on a suspicious ankle injury; the availability of people to transport the patient; the type of terrain involved in transport; the severity of the environment; and the patient's need or desire to continue the trip. Even though the best medical judgment would preclude using the injury, the best decision in a remote environment might be, if the patient can use the injury, to immobilize the ankle in a splint that allows the patient to hobble along on his good ankle using an ice axe, ski pole, or wooden stick as a crutch. This could be the safest and most reasonable decision based on the situation.

General Assessment

> ### Signs and Symptoms
> ### Fracture:
> 1. Pain specific to the injury site
> 2. Swelling and/or bruising
> 3. Deformity
> 4. Tenderness or point tenderness
> 5. Sounds, e.g., snaps, pops, crepitus
> 6. Loss of circulation, sensation, and/or motion (CSM)
> 7. Wounds at the site with or without protruding bone

The general principles of any assessment involve Looking, Asking, and Feeling (LAF).

Looking requires careful removal or cutting away of the patient's clothing. In cold environments, perform the examination, as much as possible, by reaching beneath clothing that is left in place. Much can be gained by comparing the injured and uninjured sides. Look for bruising, bleeding, deformity, and symmetry. Look for guarding: over-protectiveness of the injury site by the patient.

Asking starts with finding out what happened and what forces were involved. The greater the forces involved, the greater the chance of a significant injury. Ask about pain—where, how much. Ask about sounds—snaps or pops heard when the injury occurred.

Feeling means palpating the injury site for signs of a fracture. Do you feel muscles spasming around the injury? Does it feel unstable? Do you feel (or hear) crepitus, the grating of bone against bone? Is there "point tenderness," a certain spot that hurts when you touch it? Is there adequate circulation (pulses), sensation (feeling), and motion (the ability to move distal to the injury site)?

In most cases, fractures are determined by x-rays, not by field assessments, unless there are obvious signs such as gross deformity—two knees, as it were, on the same leg. You are looking, asking, and feeling for signs and symptoms of a fracture, but, in the end, a great deal of your wilderness assessment of a possible fracture will include the willingness of the patient to use the injury. If you and the patient decide the injury is not usable, you will, in most cases, splint the injury as if it were a fracture and arrange an evacuation.

General Treatment Principles

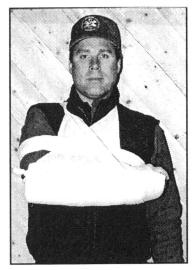

Figure 12-1: Sling and swathe

The basic treatment for all suspected fractures is the same: a splint. A patient with a bone that might be broken should have circulation, sensation, and motion assessed beyond the injury before and after splinting. CSM should be regularly monitored as long as the patient is in your care. Any loss of CSM should be immediately investigated, in case you can do something to reestablish healthy blood flow, e.g., loosening the splint.

Suspected fractures, in most cases, should be splinted in position of function which means arms flexed at approximately 90 degrees at the elbow, hands slightly curled, legs flexed at approximately five to 10 degrees at the knee, feet approximately perpendicular to legs.

A splint should involve plenty of padding for support and comfort, and it should incorporate something rigid for additional support. Sufficient padding can almost always be found in the wilderness in the form of extra clothing. The padding should be thick enough to provide comfort and arranged in a manner that eliminates voids within the completed splint. Voids allow the possibility of painful shifting. Avoid the voids! Rigid splinting materials also typically abound in the form of stays from packs, Crazy Creek Chairs®, sticks, sleeping pads, etc. Therm-A-Rest® pads offer an advantage: They can be deflated, secured in place, then inflated for additional rigidity. Commercial splints of practical value for some broken bones in wilderness situations include the SAM Splint® and foldable wire splints.

A splint should immobilize the joints above and below a long bone injury or the bones above and below a joint injury. Remember: There should be adequate circulation, sensation, and motion before *and* after a splint is applied.

Most upper extremity fractures can be adequately immobilized with a *sling and swathe.* Both sling and swathe may be created from triangular bandages, but many improvisational techniques can also be used successfully. A long-sleeved shirt, for instance, can be formed into a sling using the arms of the shirt to go around the patient's neck. Cut a few strips from the bottom of a T-shirt to use as swathes.

After you've cut a few swathes from the bottom of a T-shirt, the rest of the shirt can be used as a sling by putting the patient's head through the head-hole on the shirt and using the arm-holes to hold the patient's arm. As a minimal sling and swathe, you can fold up the bottom of the shirt the patient is wearing and safety pin it in place for a sling, and zip a jacket closed over the torso as a swathe.

Most lower extremity fractures can be immobilized with sleeping pads held firmly in place with any material that can be wrapped around the splint and secured in place, e.g., elastic wraps, triangular bandages, belts, rope, strips of cloth. In the absence of sleeping pads, lower extremities can be splinted with paddles, ski poles, ice axes, sticks, etc., and adequate padding.

It is important to give reliable patients the responsibility of notifying you of any changes in circulation, sensation, and motion, changes such as pain, numbness, and tingling.

Almost all patients with a fracture will benefit from RICE: Rest, Ice, Compression, Elevation (SEE CHAPTER 14: ATHLETIC INJURIES). If your protocols allow, give medications for pain and inflammation, medications such as ibuprofen or another non-steroidal anti-inflammatory drug. If your protocols allow, severe pain from a fracture may be treated with stronger pain medications.

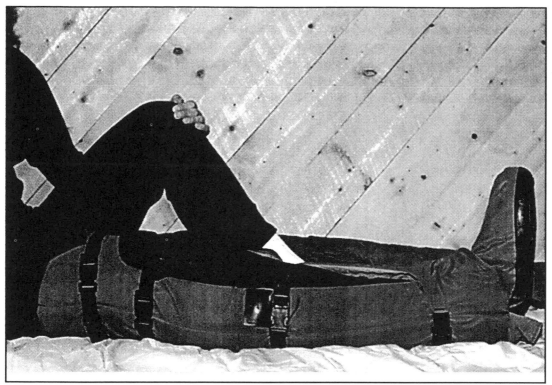

Figure 12-2: Leg splinted with Crazy Creek Chair

Treatment For Upper Body Fractures

The Mandible (Jaw)

Secure the jaw in place with a wide wrap that goes around the head. Be sure to provide for an adequate airway, and a way for the patient to quickly remove the wrap should they feel like vomiting (which they often do after a severe blow to the jaw)

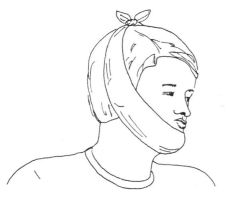

Figure 12-3: Stabilized Jaw

The Scapula (Shoulder Blade)

Fractures of the *scapula* are quite often stable and require nothing more than sling and swathe immobilization. Immobilizing the arm against the body wall is nature's best splint, and many upper extremity injuries can be very adequately padded and immobilized in this manner with a sling and swathe. With any sling and swathe, the hand and wrist should be accessible so that pulses may be monitored.

The Clavicle (Collarbone)

The *clavicle* is a small bone, easily fractured by a direct blow, by falling on the shoulder, or by falling on an outstretched arm where the force is transmitted up to the clavicle. Patients with a fractured clavicle often support the weight of the arm on the affected side with their opposite hand. A fracture of the clavicle may be treated with a sling and swathe which should support the weight of the arm, taking pressure off the clavicle. Monitor the patient for increasing difficulty breathing, an indication of lung involvement (SEE CHAPTER 10: CHEST INJURIES).

The Humerus (Upper Arm)

It is worth noting that the humeral shaft may be palpable on the medial (inner) side throughout its entire length. Therefore, when a fracture of the *humerus* is suspected, beginning either proximal or distal to the patient's area of complaint, palpate the entire shaft. In this way, very small, non-displaced fractures may be identified. Checking radial nerve function is important in humeral fractures and is done by asking the patient to extend his wrist, digits, and thumb. Document the presence or absence of radial nerve function for future reference. A fractured humerus may be immobilized with a sling and swathe. It may be beneficial to place a pad over the outside of the humerus to protect the fracture. With an unstable humerus, if the patient will be walking, the elbow may be left free of the sling, allowing it to hang free, thereby letting gravity pull gentle traction on the fracture, which may increase patient comfort.

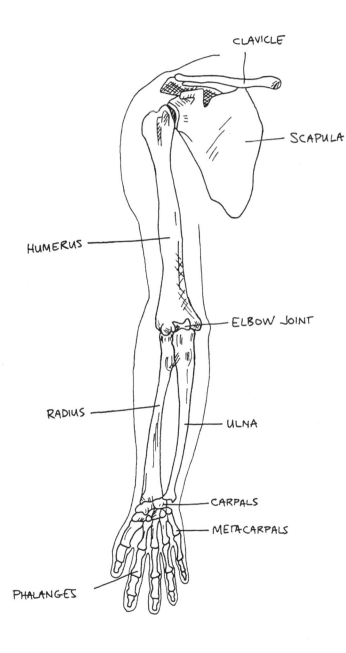

Figure 12-4: Bones of shoulder and arm

port. Place the hand in a position of function with a rolled up glove, sock, or other soft material tucked in the palm. Then immobilize the hand, wrist, and forearm in a splint

functional position with a rolled elastic bandage or a suitable similar sized material in the palm of the hand, and then wrapping the entire hand with an elastic wrap or roller gauze dressing. Torn strips of clothing can be used for an improvised hand splint. Phalangeal fractures should be splinted in a position of function, not in an extended (straight) position. The use of adjacent digits for splinting may be appropriate at times, depending of the severity of the injury.

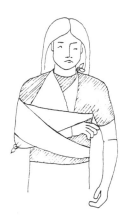

Figure 12-5: Sling and swathe

The Lower Arm

Fractures in the region of the elbow, the *radius* (large lower arm bone), *ulna* (small lower arm bone), and wrist should be adequately splinted, incorporating the joints above and below. If at all possible, splint the elbow at approximately 90 degrees of flexion to elevate the forearm and hand and, thus, reduce swelling. The stability provided by a solid splint is worth the effort, especially in a long and difficult trans-

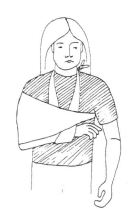

Figure 12-6:
Sling and swathe with elbow free.

The Hand

Fractures of the hand are fairly common and often related to fractures of the *phalanges*, the finger bones. When splinting the entire hand is advisable, a suitable splint may be made by placing the entire hand in a

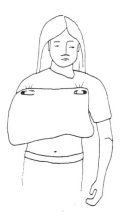

Figure 12-7:
Improvised sling from a shirt

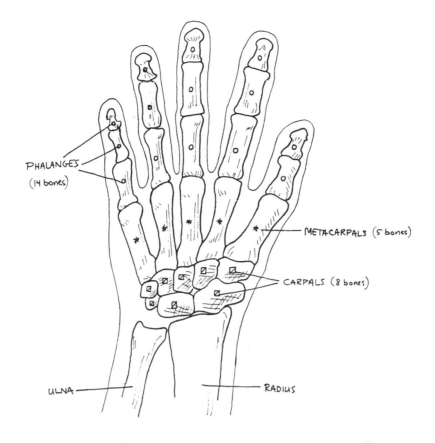

PHALANGES
(14 bones)

METACARPALS (5 bones)

CARPALS (8 bones)

ULNA

RADIUS

Figure 12-8: Bones of the hand

Treatment For Lower Body Fractures

Fractures of the hip, pelvis, and femoral shaft present major problems in wilderness medicine, due foremost to the potential for shock, the forces involved which create a possibility of spinal involvement, and the inevitable transport problem and, in the case of a femoral shaft fracture, the necessity of maintaining adequate traction for extended periods of time.

The Hip

First of all, in fractures of the hip, the typical position of external rotation and shortening may or may not be present. The fracture may be an impacted femoral neck type or an *acetabular* fracture (a fracture of the socket portion of the hip). Making the assessment might be difficult. As a general guideline, if a patient has sustained significant trauma and has painful motion in the region of the hip, plus pain with weight bearing, anticipate carrying him or her out well-padded and secure on a litter, sled, or backboard. The patient should be carefully assessed for the possibility of spine involvement. It is usually beneficial to pad between the patient's legs and to secure the legs together. Suspected fractures about the hip should not be placed in traction, an unnecessary technique that could reduce healthy blood flow to the joint.

The Pelvis

In suspected fractures of the pelvis, it is imperative that the patient be observed for progressive shock due to the significant blood loss often associated with these fractures. Because of the possibility of bladder trauma, check the patient for *hematuria* (blood in the urine). The patient should be carefully evaluated for the possibility of spine involvement, and transported in a well-padded litter during evacuation. Securing the pelvis by carefully wrapping a sleeping pad around the pelvic region and tying the pad snugly in place may provide some relief for the patient. Inflatable sleeping pads may be secured around the pelvis prior to being inflated, and then inflated for additional support.

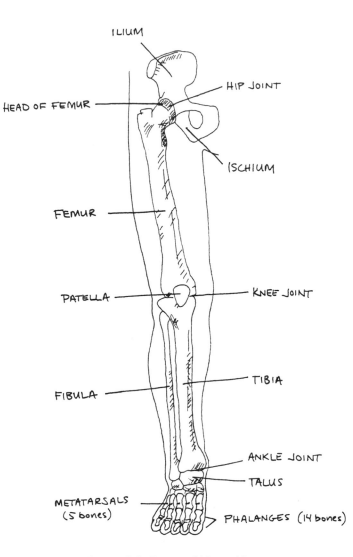

Figure 12-9: Bones of hip and leg

The Femur (Thigh Bone)

Fractures of the femoral shaft require traction, except for fractures of the upper end (hip region) and lower end (knee region) of the femur. Although upper and lower end femur fractures are technically femur fractures, it is *not* recommended to place such fractures in traction. In a major expedition or in an extended trek in remote regions, the Wilderness First Responder in charge should plan ahead for the type of traction that will be utilized if a femoral shaft fracture

should occur. There are commercial traction devices available which are lightweight, easy to apply, and fairly efficient, such as the Kendrick Traction Device® or KTD. Improvising femoral traction can be satisfactory, but should definitely be practiced prior to the actual event so that everyone understands and is familiar with the plan.

The fracture of the femoral shaft must be treated in traction for many important reasons. The most important is that traction reestablishes normal length and

conformity of the musculature and this tends to slow the bleeding which occurs in the thigh. A patient with a femoral shaft fracture can easily lose more than a liter of blood and, if the fracture is movable and the thigh unstable, this bleeding can continue. With bilateral fractured femurs, bleeding may constitute a threat to life. In addition to that the fracture fragments may cause further vascular damage. The additional reasons for femoral traction include the relief of pain, stability of the fracture fragments, prevention of converting a closed fracture to an open one, and reduction of further soft tissue damage.

Once a fractured femur has been assessed, someone should be assigned to apply manual traction to the extremity with the patient protected against the environment until the mechanical traction device is in place. *Once initiated, at no time prior to full mechanical traction should manual traction be released.* A general rule of how much traction to apply is 10 percent of the patient's body weight or until the pain is relieved.

Many improvisation techniques have been devised for creating a femur traction splint. More wait to invented. Here is one that has proven successful:

1. Secure a fixation splint, e.g., sleeping pad, firmly to the injured leg. This will provide support of the fracture, and

patient comfort, while the traction device is being improvised, and after the device is in place. Extend the fixation splint beyond the knee and place padding behind the knee to create five to 10 percent of knee flexion because this will make the extremity much more comfortable than if the knee is fully extended into traction.

2. Create an anchor at the sole of the foot, a point from which traction will be mechanically applied. This is often referred to as an *ankle hitch*. An ankle hitch can be made from rope, webbing, belts, cloth, duct tape, etc. Numerous techniques can be used to create an ankle hitch. A few ankle hitches include: 1) With a single piece of material, form a "Z" over the patient's lower leg. Run the tips of the material under the leg and back through the loops of the "Z." Tighten the system around the

patient's leg, and make an anchor at the sole of the foot by tying the ends together. 2) With two pieces of material, place a loop of one over the patient's leg, and a loop of the second piece under the patient's leg. Pass the ends back through the loops. Tie the ends together to form an anchor at the sole of the foot. 3) Remove the boot from the injured leg. Cut holes in both sides of the boot near the sole in line with the ankle bones. Run a piece of material through the holes and tie the ends below the boot. Replace the boot and secure it to the patient's foot. 4) Remove the boot from the injured leg. Place a piece of material inside the boot under the arch, a piece of material long enough to allow it to be tied under the boot after replacing the boot on the patient.

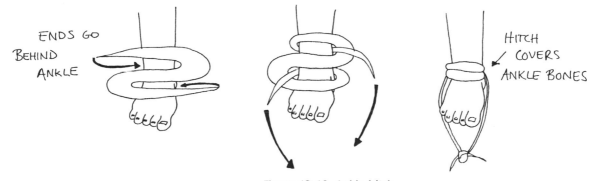

ENDS GO BEHIND ANKLE

HITCH COVERS ANKLE BONES

Figure 12-10: Ankle hitch

Is the patient better off with boot left on or the boot taken off? The boot and sock provide padding for the ankle hitch. If you do leave the boot and sock off, you'll need to pad well beneath the ankle hitch. With the boot on, the dorsalis pedis pulse (located on top of the foot near the bend of

the ankle) can be palpated within the sock and, also, a gross determination of sensation and skin warmth can be made by palpation. The patient can relate the sensation of numbness or tingling in the toes, if this should occur. In cold weather, however, the patient may not be able to

maintain adequate foot warmth with the boot on, depending on the type of boot. Foot warmth may be easier to maintain with the boot off and adequate insulation added to the foot. The determination to remove footwear should be left to the person in charge and should be based on consideration of all pertinent factors.

3. A shaft approximately 18 inches longer than the injured leg—measured from the groin or the hip—needs to be found. This can be a stick, a ski pole, a tent pole, a paddle, etc.

4. One end of the shaft should be securely attached to the patient's upper thigh on the injured side.

5. A piece of rope, cord, or strong cloth is needed to make a trucker's hitch. Traction by the trucker's hitch is pulled from the loops at the sole of the foot and the end of the shaft until the trac-

tion of the device is equal or greater than the manual traction. The best judge of the amount of traction is the patient. They usually offer this judgment without your asking for it.

6. When mechanical traction is stable, use wraps of cloth, elastic bandages, etc., to secure the shaft firmly in place. The "bad" leg can be secured to the "good" leg for additional support.

If you find yourself alone with a patient suffering a fractured femur, you'll have to forego manual traction, gather the materials, and carefully apply mechanical traction when everything is in

place. A rigid litter is usually required to get the patient out of the backcountry. The patient needs a hospital as soon as possible to guarantee prevention of permanent loss of function or loss of leg.

An extended transport over uneven terrain is extremely difficult, entailing risk of injury to the carriers and risk of further injury to the patient. Therefore, if there is a reasonable alternative, including helicopter evacuation, it should be strongly considered.

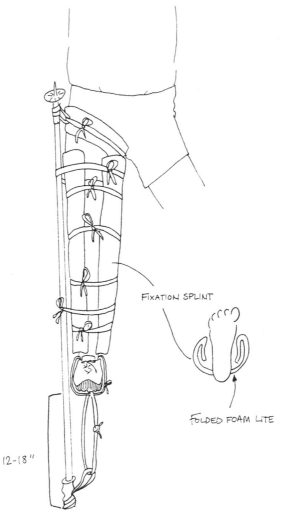

FIXATION SPLINT

FOLDED FOAM LITE

12-18"

Figure 12-11: Improvised traction splint

The Patella (Kneecap)

Fractures of the *patella* may result from a fall directly on the knee and may be difficult to differentiate from a severe contusion unless there is an obvious deformity. Therefore, a patient with such an injury should be immobilized in a splint that extends from well above the knee to well below the knee, and may be permitted to walk with assistance if terrain and other factors dictate that this is the best course of action. A sleeping pad rolled up from both ends simultaneously and secured around the knee, leaving the kneecap free, works well to immobilize injuries about the knee.

Tibia/Fibula (Lower Leg)

Fractures of the *tibia* (large lower leg bone) and *fibula* (small lower leg bone) require adequate fixation splinting: The knee, ankle, and both lower leg bones are stabilized. Remember: Pad behind the knee to keep the knee comfortably flexed at about 10 degrees, secure the ankle at 90 degrees to the lower leg, avoid the voids, check CSM before and after splinting.

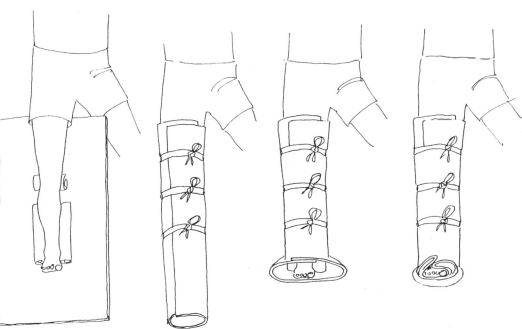

Figure 12-12: Splinting of lower leg

The Ankle

Fractures of the ankle may be difficult to assess. Early examination and treatment, prior to gross swelling, are important. Take all steps possible to rest the injury, then elevate and apply ice, cold water, or snow to the injured extremity to prevent excessive swelling. A well-wrapped compression dressing is also quite helpful. In fracture-dislocations of the ankle, early gentle reduction of the deformity is extremely important and most often quite easy to do. Simply holding the foot and applying gentle traction can greatly improve the deformity. The sooner this is done, the better. Basically, the damage has already been done by the fracture-dislocation and, therefore, any attempt at improving the position will have a beneficial effect on circulation (SEE CHAPTER 13: DISLOCATIONS). This also makes splinting more stable and comfortable. Ankle splints need to hold the foot approximately perpendicular to the leg.

The Foot

Fractures of the foot may be splinted similarly to fractures of the ankle. Fractures of the phalanges (toes) seldom require anything more than walking carefully and swallowing pain killers. Additional support for the toe may be gained by padding between the fractured toe and neighboring toes, and "buddy splinting" the injured toe to an uninjured toe.

Complicated Fractures

Angulated Fractures

In deformed fractures, when angles exist in bones where no angle should exist, gentle traction to obtain better alignment for stable splinting is the appropriate and preferred treatment. Generally, no harm will be done by gently realigning a long bone fracture to a more anatomically aligned position. Applying a splint to a badly angulated fracture is difficult and, most often, unstable. Gentle traction with an assistant applying counter-traction to the extremity results in an overall improvement in pain, circulation, and splint stability with a negligible risk of creating further vascular or neurologic damage.

Few protocols require that you realign an angulated fracture except when the angulation is severe enough to reduce normal circulation distal to the injury. If circulation, sensation, and/or motion has been impaired by the fracture, an attempt to return the injury to normal anatomical alignment is strongly recommended.

Traction should first be applied in line—in the direction the bone presents. Then, when the patient has relaxed, movement toward normal alignment should progress slowly. Patient relaxation is often signaled by a significant reduction in pain after traction-in-line is applied. Two signals will indicate that you should stop your attempt to reposition the fracture: 1) a need to use force indicating, possibly, the bone ends are somehow trapped out of alignment, and 2) a marked increase in pain indicating, possibly, nerves and/or blood vessels are caught at the fracture site. *Do not use force. Do not cause patient a marked increase in pain.* Once the bone has been returned to normal anatomical alignment, splinting may proceed without any need to maintain traction except in the case of a fractured femur (SEE ABOVE). Remember: Check CSM before and after traction.

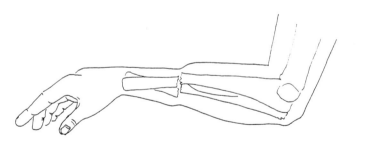

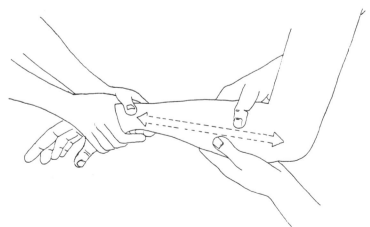

Figure 12-13: Reduction of angulated fracture

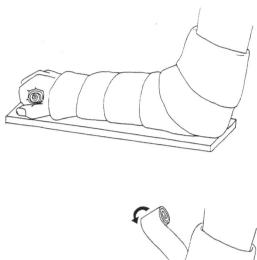

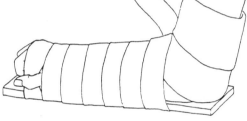

Figure 12-14: Lower arm splint prior to sling and swathe

Open Fractures

In an open fracture without visible bone ends, the wound should be thoroughly cleaned and bandaged prior to splinting (SEE CHAPTER 15: SOFT TISSUE INJURIES). The rigid part of the splint should not press on the wound.

In case of an open fracture with visible bone ends, the best approach is to gently cleanse the protruding bone ends with any cleaning agent available or even plain soap and water. Bone ends should be irrigated and/or flushed and not scrubbed. In a wilderness environment, gentle traction-in-line should be applied, a technique that almost always results in the bones ends slipping back under the skin. A sterile bandage or the cleanest available material should be placed over the wound, and the fracture then splinted. The rigid part of the splint should not press on the wound. Broad spectrum antibiotic therapy is indicated, if available. It is recommended that a physician be consulted well in advance concerning the wilderness use of antibiotics. The point here is that correction of gross angular deformity and adequate splint immobilization takes precedence over concern regarding protruding bone ends. The fact that bone ends slide back under the skin during realignment should not be a major concern during treatment of an open wilderness fracture. If, however, the bone ends fail to slip back under the skin, they should be covered with a moist sterile dressing prior to splinting.

Evacuation Guidelines

Almost all suspected fractures, especially those that are unstable, should be evacuated to definitive medical care. There is no great rush except in the case of open fractures, fractures with decreased CSM distal to the injury, and fractures of the femur and/or pelvis.

Conclusion

After a careful, belayed descent, you hurry to the side of the injured climber. His face a grimace of pain, he breathes between clinched teeth. Your initial assessment reveals no immediate threat to the patient's life, and your focused assessment uncovers no injuries other than an angulated fracture not far above the right ankle.

With your climbing partner holding counter-traction well above the injury site, you take careful hold of the patient's foot and pull traction-in-line. After a moment of increased pain, the patient remarks that it "feels better now, please don't stop pulling." Under traction, you slowly return the leg to normal anatomical alignment.

Releasing traction but holding the leg firmly in position, you ask your partner to return to your tent for a sleeping pad and the first aid kit. When he returns, you create a well-padded and rigid splint that encloses the lower leg, stabilizing the knee and ankle. With the injury splinted, you and your partner lift and carry the patient to a relatively comfortable nearby spot. You intend to stay with him while your partner goes for help.

Chapter 13: Dislocations

You should be able to:

1. *Describe the difference between long-term (wilderness) care and short-term (urban) care of dislocations.*

2. *Describe the signs and symptoms of upper and lower extremity dislocations.*

3. *Demonstrate how to treat upper and lower extremity dislocations.*

It could happen to you

A period of melt-and-freeze temperatures in the Old Cascades region of Oregon has left the snowy surface hard, but not hard enough—just enough of a crust to hold weight a teasing moment before dropping snowshoers through into softer underlying whiteness. For additional support, everyone in the group you're leading is using two ski poles. It could have been frustrating, but the day's weather is pleasant, the group congenial, and spirits are high. The walk up the ridge goes quickly.

On the descent, the trip goes even quicker for Deborah. Her lighter weight kept her from crunching through on an especially dense crust in an opening on the steep forested hillside. She "skies" away from the group on her snowshoes. Planting a pole instinctively to brake herself, she slips to the end of her arm's reach, and levers her right shoulder out of joint. Deborah plops into a sitting position with a look of surprise that alters rapidly into one of intense pain. She sits huddled in the snow with her right arm cradled in her left.

Introduction

Any joint of the body can come out of joint, out of its normal bone to bone relationship. The definition of a *dislocation* is a complete or partial disruption of the normal relationship of a joint. The mechanism of injury can be *indirect*, e.g., the stuck ski pole levers out a shoulder, the high brace of the kayaker pries out a shoulder, or *direct*, e.g., a fall on a shoulder forcefully knocks it out. Direct mechanisms tend to cause more damage to the joint because of the forces involved.

Dislocations are sometimes associated with fractures, the probability being higher if the forces involved were direct.

Our concern is primarily with the more obvious complete dislocations of joints. These are more easily identified and more incapacitating to the patient. In an urban situation, the treatment for a dislocation rates as relatively simple: The injury should be stabilized—splinted—in the position found, and the patient should be expeditiously transported to a medical facility. In the unique situation of a wilderness accident, however, it is extremely important to be able to make an accurate assessment and attempt a *reduction*—a return to a normal bone to bone relationship—of a dislocation as quickly as possible after it occurs. Discretion must obviously be used when evacuation to a nearby medical facility can be easily accomplished, when the patient is approximately an hour or less from definitive medical care.

Reduction

Some of the major advantages in early reduction of dislocations are:

1. Reduction is easier immediately after injury, before swelling and muscle spasm have developed.

2. Transport of the patient is easier after reduction.

3. Reduction most often results in dramatic relief of pain.

4. Immobilization of the injured joint is easier to accomplish and more stable after reduction.

5. The safety of the entire party may be jeopardized during the evacuation of a patient with an unreduced major joint dislocation.

6. Early reduction reduces the circulatory and neurological risks to the extremity.

General Assessment And Treatment

As with any musculoskeletal injury, have a good LAF—Look, Ask, Feel—at the patient (SEE CHAPTER 12: FRACTURES). There are many signs which may be helpful in identifying a dislocation. Remember that when a joint is dislocated, there is nearly always restriction of motion through its normal range. There is often obvious deformity in comparison with the uninvolved side. Crepitus or grating of bone on bone is almost always absent. There is very often a typical, identifiable posture of the dislocated joint, which the patient will maintain to minimize the pain. Obtaining a history of the mechanism of injury can also be helpful and will be discussed below for individual joints.

Assess for normal CSM—circulation, sensation, motion—distal to the injured joint. Any vascular or neurological deficits distal to the injury 1) should be noted, and 2) should initiate an immediate attempt to reduce the dislocation in order to prevent permanent disability.

A note of assurance: Do not be concerned about causing additional damage to any fracture associated with a dislocation. These fractures will most often be improved in alignment with the reduction of the joint. The same is true of vessel or nerve impairment associated with a dislocation—reduction will reduce the impingement to these structures, as well.

When a major long bone fracture, such as femur or humerus, accompanies a dislocation at the hip or shoulder respectively, the dislocation may not even be assessed in view of the more apparent major fracture. In these cases, splinting of the fracture is the main concern. The dislocation, for all practical purposes, is a secondary issue and usually not amenable to reduction by ordinary means.

When reducing dislocations, try to have as many factors in your favor as possible. Utilize other party members where necessary; communicate with the patient very openly about what you are going to do; be very positive and deliberate in your approach. There is nothing magic about reducing a dislocated joint and, in fact, if it's any consolation, not too many years ago, reduction of dislocations was done by laypersons, not physicians. The use, however, of intramuscular or intravenous drugs can make the job much easier, should they and a person

licensed to use them be available. Gentle, but steady, and persistent traction is the rule rather than forceful jerking or ballistic maneuvers to reduce the joint. Remember: You and the patient have much to gain.

Work quickly but calmly. The sooner an attempt to relocate, or reduce the angle of dislocation, is made, the easier it will be for you and the patient. Everyone will feel better, and the joint will receive an adequate blood supply, if the relocation is successful. You need to get the patient to relax as much as possible. Suggest the patient take deep breaths, and let all the tension go from the painful area. Lightly touch the dislocation, reminding the patient where to concentrate attempts to relax.

Be assured, if you work steadily and gently, the patient's condition will be made better, not worse. Fractures, blood vessel damage, and nerve impairment often associated with dislocations will be improved by a non-forceful relocation. And the evacuation will be easier and safer for everyone involved.

Place yourself comfortably in a position allowing you to pull gentle traction-in-line. Take a firm grip on the arm or leg distal to the injury, pulling in line with the way the patient is holding the extremity. Pull steadily, increasing pull slowly, and not jerking.

Do not use force. Stop if pain continues to increase.

If the dislocation does not relocate after you've pulled traction-in-line for a minute, gently move the extremity toward normal alignment. Maintain traction during the movement. What you're trying to do is manually relax the muscular spasms, and encourage the bones into normal alignment. You can move the bones toward a more normal alignment as long as the patient does not complain of increasing pain, and you're not forcing movement. The muscles, tendons, and ligaments "want" to be back where they belong. You're encouraging them to move back. Most patients will feel the relocation take place and tell you when relocation has occurred.

Patients with a history of chronic dislocations may have a preferred reduction technique, a technique they want you to use. These patients are usually ready, willing, and able to tell you what to do. It would be wise to follow their advice.

Occasionally a dislocation will be complicated enough to prevent relocation. You will have to splint the extremity in the position the patient is holding it. Make the splint as comfortable as possible. Evacuate the patient as soon as you can.

Signs and Symptoms Dislocation:
1. Pain
2. Loss of normal range of motion
3. Deformity (loss of normal symmetry)
4. Characteristic joint position maintained by patient

Upper Body Dislocations

The Mandible (Jaw)

Mandibles can be dislocated by direct force, e.g., a blow, or indirect force, e.g., biting aggressively on a very hard apple. After wrapping something soft and protective around your thumbs, reach gently into the patient's mouth, gripping the back molars. Pull down and forward until relocation occurs. The mandible may be secured with a wide wrap that holds the lower jaw to the upper jaw by extending entirely around the head from bottom to top. The wrap should be easily removed by the patient if he or she feels nausea on the verge of becoming vomit. The patient may require a soft diet for several days.

The Shoulder

Outdoor travelers, particularly paddlers and skiers, often exert sudden force on an already extended arm, forcing the head of the humerus forward and downward. These anterior-inferior dislocations of the shoulder joint are the most common, accounting for over 90 percent of shoulder dislocations. The patient will usually be stabilizing the shoulder in the most comfortable position. Remember that the patient cannot bring the involved extremity across his or her chest to a position of rest. The upper arm will be held away from the body in various positions and cannot be brought into a sling type position. This differentiates a dislocation from a fracture of the humerus, in which instance the patient is invariably splinting the upper arm against the chest wall for comfort. The problem is often recurrent, and the patient can identify the dislocation quite readily. Check circulation, motor, and sensory function to the hand, and also sensory function along the outer aspect of the shoulder. Document findings.

Posterior dislocations of the shoulder are rare. In this instance, the upper arm and forearm will be held across the anterior chest wall and attempts at externally rotating the upper arm away from the chest will be restricted and painful. The assessment is often difficult to make.

The simplest and easiest method for reduction of a dislocated shoulder begins with asking the patient to lie down. Pull steady traction with the arm flexed at 90 degrees, pulling straight-away from the body starting with traction in line with the direction the patient presents the arm to you. Then slowly move the arm under traction until the patient's hand is above his or her head. The final position looks like the patient is ready to throw a baseball. If the shoulder does not reduce, move the arm, still under traction, until the elbow is pointed at the sky. One rescuer can safely perform this technique, but a second rescuer will be useful pulling counter-traction, usually best applied by wrapping some material around the patient just below the level of the armpits (see illustration). This technique may take 10 to 15 minutes. Traction should be maintained until reduction is achieved, or until rescuer and patient tire to the point where traction can no longer be maintained. Unreduced shoulders should be splinted across the chest with padding between the arm and the chest.

A second method is placing the patient prone (face down) and letting the arm hang down towards the ground with 15-20 pounds of weight secured to the hand. This method may be slow and relaxation is critically important, but the muscles will generally fatigue in time, and manual assistance by manipulation of the shoulder is helpful.

After the reduction, immobilize with a sling and two swathes. The sling supports the forearm horizontally in front of the body. One swathe secures the arm to the chest wall with a wrap around the body, and the other secures the elbow to the chest wall.

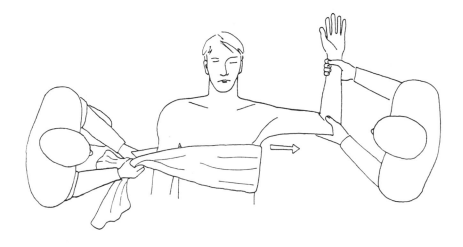

Figure 13-1: Shoulder reduction step 1

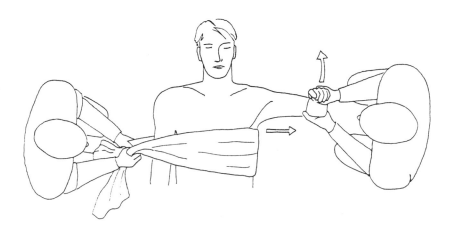

Figure 13-2: Shoulder reduction step 2

The Wilderness First Responder

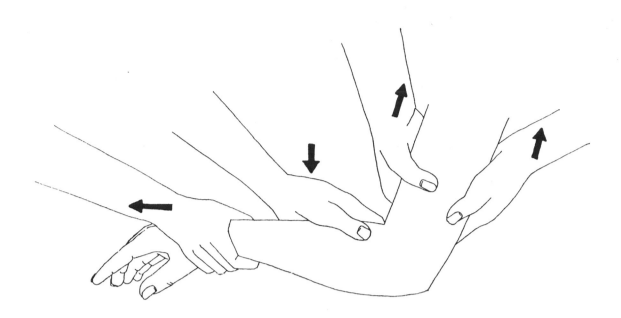

Figure 13-3: Elbow reduction

The Elbow

Look for obvious deformity when compared to the uninvolved side, and restricted flexion and extension of the joint. Most commonly the *olecranon* (bony upper end of the ulna) will dislocate towards the rear, and you will see the resultant bony prominence of the olecranon posteriorly.

Apply traction to the forearm in a partially flexed position with counter-traction applied to the upper arm by an assistant. Apply a slow, steady pull. The patient's ability to flex with elbow to 90 degrees is a sign of reduction. Remember that the joint may also require side pressure for realignment (SEE ILLUSTRATION). Immobilize in a sling and swathe, as described for the shoulder. If reduction is not possible, splint in the position in which the elbow is found.

The Wrist

Wrist dislocations are often difficult to differentiate from a fracture and often difficult to reduce. Therefore, splint immobilization is the treatment of choice. Circulation and neurologic function to the hand is usually not compromised, but, if so, reduction should be attempted with traction-in-line and movement toward normal alignment. Most common neurologic deficit would be median nerve involvement, resulting in numbness over the palmar surfaces of the thumb, index, and middle fingers, and one-half of the ring finger.

The Phalanges (Fingers)

Obvious deformity and limited function are the main assessment factors in dislocated finger joints. Reduction of the common dislocations of middle or distal finger joints is best accomplished by maintaining the digit in partial flexion and actually pushing the dislocated base of the joint back in place while traction is being applied to the partially flexed digit. This is much more successful than attempting to apply traction to a straight digit.

There are two hand dislocations in which reduction is difficult, if not impossible, by closed means. The main one is dislocation of the *metacarpophalangeal* joint (where the finger joins the hand) of the index finger, and the second one the metacarpophalangeal joint of the thumb. The thumb is sometimes reducible closed, but the index metacarpal rarely, if ever. Make one attempt and then quit, immobilizing the joint in a functional position rather than persisting with multiple attempts.

Finger dislocations may be associated with skin disruption. A controversy exists as to management. Recommended is cleansing the open wound as thoroughly as possible and accomplishing the reduction. The patient would benefit from being placed on oral antibiotics, if available and allowable by medical control. Individual circumstances, as always, will dictate the proper choice.

Do not splint a reduced finger to a rigid splint. Tape the injured finger to a non-injured neighboring finger and encourage the patient to flex the damaged finger regularly to promote healing.

Lower Body Dislocations

The Hip

The majority of hip dislocations are posterior. The hip will be moderately flexed, internally rotated, and adducted (brought across the midline toward the opposite leg). Any attempt to extend the hip for splinting or easier transport will be resisted by the patient, and is mechanically nearly impossible to accomplish. The mechanism of injury is a fall in which the hip is flexed and the impact is transmitted longitudinally through the knee, driving the femoral head posteriorly from the acetabulum (hip socket). The mechanism would be similar to that sustained in a dashboard injury in a motor vehicle accident. A climber may dislocate a hip in a fall as he or she makes contact with a rock wall upon reaching maximum rope length and swinging back into the rock face. Remember the typical posture of the posteriorly dislocated hip, which should make it easy to differentiate from a fracture of the proximal femur or shaft which leaves the leg externally rotated. Anterior dislocation of the hip results in a posture of extension, external rotation, and abduction (the thigh is held away from the midline of the body). Again, attempting to extend the hip to a neutral position would be most difficult, if not impossible, and resisted by the patient.

This reduction requires two people, ideally, with one applying counter-traction to the pelvis with the patient lying in a supine position on the ground. The involved hip and knee are flexed to 90 degrees with the rescuer straddling the victim and applying traction in an upward direction. If only one person is available to attempt the reduction, the patient can be placed prone over a log, rock, or bench, and the traction applied downward with the hip and knee flexed 90 degrees. Once reduced, the injured hip must be splinted and immobilized to the uninvolved extremity, and the patient transported in a supine position.

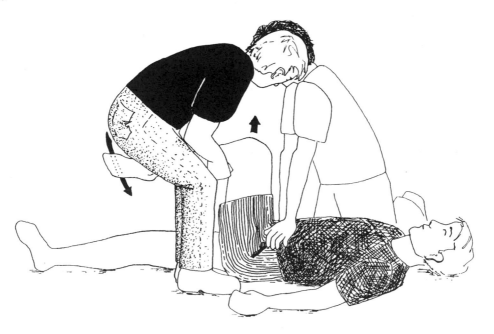

Figure 13-4: Hip reduction

The Patella (Kneecap)

The patella is most often laterally displaced with the knee held in flexion for comfort. Dislocations of the patella are often recurrent and due to pivoting type of injury with partially flexed knee. The patella is not movable and obviously out of place.

Apply gentle traction to extend the leg. Massaging the large thigh muscles often helps in extending the leg. You can place a small pad under the patient's heel to hold the leg in a slightly overextended position. As the knee is extended, the patella will usually reduce itself, although you may have to wait for relaxation and reduction. Keep massaging the thigh. Occasionally a slight nudge of the patella toward normal alignment can be used to shorten the wait. Immobilize the extremity in a splint that reaches well above and well below the knee. With the knee extended and immobilized in a splint, the patient will most often be able to walk well enough for evacuation.

To ease walking, create a crutch, e.g., stick, ice axe, ski pole.

The Knee

A frank dislocation of the knee results from radical tearing of the joint out of its normal alignment, and presents a disaster at best. Major ligamentous disruption is the rule. The knee may not be dislocated at the time of exam, but gross instability is the major clue, vascular impairment a major complement. Check pulses and motor function in ankle and foot.

Observe the joint closely and apply gentle traction to realign the joint as well as possible to benefit damaged neurovascular structures. As with all dislocations, the sooner realignment is established, the better. Splint as securely as possible, making sure not to compromise circulation to the foot. This patient must be carried.

The Ankle

Dislocated ankles are most commonly associated with frac-

tures, obvious deformity, and often grating (crepitus). Vascular impairment to the foot must be assessed by checking circulation, sensation, and motion.

It is important to reduce the degree of deformity as much as possible. Ordinarily this is not difficult due to the gross instability resultant from associated fractures. Often, simply holding the forefoot and allowing the remainder of the extremity to act as the counter-traction will result in improved alignment of the ankle dislocation without much additional effort. Counter-traction by an assistant is helpful. Gentle traction of the heel and foot also helps. Immobilize the ankle with a splint. This patient must be carried.

Toes

Reduction is achieved with the same technique that works for fingers. Splinting is seldom required. Rigid soled boots serve as splints.

Long-term Dislocation Care

Regular monitoring is required to ensure your patient maintains adequate circulation to the injured area. Check often for a pulse beyond the injured joint, and normal skin color and sensations beyond the joint. Give the patient the responsibility of notifying you of changes in her or his condition. Once reduction has been accomplished, encourage the patient to regularly move the damaged joint through a normal range of motion to promote healing.

Most relocated dislocations benefit from 1) RICE—Rest, Ice, Compression, Elevation (see

CHAPTER 14: ATHLETIC INJURIES), 2) immobilization via splinting (SEE CHAPTER 12: FRACTURES), and 3) anti-pain, anti-inflammatory drugs such as ibuprofen until a physician can examine the injury.

Evacuation Guidelines

Patients with dislocations that resist attempts at reduction should be evacuated as soon as possible. Most dislocations should be evacuated for careful medical examination even if they relocate easily. There is always the chance of underlying damage that doesn't show up right away, especially with first time dislocations. Exceptions would include fingers and toes, and chronic dislocations (repeat offenders) that the patient is able to use with reasonable comfort after the relocation.

Conclusion

It's a matter of moments before you have Deborah sitting on a foamlite pad, off the cold snow. Sitting in the snow beside her, you assess her arm on the damaged side, noting there is no numbness or tingling, no loss of normal circulation distal to the injured shoulder. You ask her to lie back, and you assist her into a supine position. Keeping her arm on the injured side flexed, you begin to pull gently in line with the way she held her arm before you took control. As the pressure on the pull is slowly increased, you encourage Deborah to take deep breaths and relax her mus-

cles. She now notices some relief from the intense pain she felt before you started traction in line.

With the patient as relaxed as possible, you begin to slowly move the arm, under traction, up into a position approximately 90 degrees from the body with the elbow still bent and her hand above her head. The final arm position looks something like it would if Deborah was preparing to throw a baseball. You hold that position for several minutes.

With a soft and satisfying thump, the end of her upper arm bone rolls back into its socket.

Deborah's expression changes immediately to one of relief, and she releases a long sigh.

Removing her parka, you construct a sling from the triangular bandage in your first aid kit, a sling supporting the arm on the damaged side. Replacing the parka, you zip it up. The parka becomes a temporary swathe.

With the group sharing out her load, Deborah is able to snowshoe carefully to the van, about two miles distant. A short visit to the hospital reveals nothing extraordinary in her shoulder. She goes home with soreness but no serious damage.

Chapter 14:   *Athletic Injuries*

You should be able to:

1. *Describe the signs and symptoms of the most common wilderness-related athletic injuries including strains and sprains.*

2. *Demonstrate treatment of the most common wilderness-related athletic injuries including strains and sprains.*

3. *Define and describe the treatment for tendonitis.*

4. *Describe ways to prevent athletic injuries.*

It could happen to you

You're two days from the road on your third winter trip following the trackless banks of the Escalante River toward Lake Powell, Utah, but this is your first hike here since the area was proclaimed Grand Staircase-Escalante National Monument, thank you very much President Clinton. It looks the same—startlingly beautiful, chaotic in masterful way—but it feels different now. A designated national treasure. How did you get talked into guiding a half-dozen 14 to 16 year olds?

Evening at the second camp, and Tom, an impetuous teenager full of energy, climbs a rise of sand near the river, runs down headlong, leaps, and crashes. Tweak goes his right ankle. Tom, reluctant to admit a painful mistake, sits quietly holding the ankle when you arrive, called by another member of the group.

After removing Tom's boot and sock for a look at the ankle, it seems almost as you watch the injury puffs up on the outside, darkens like a rain cloud building toward an afternoon shower. Somehow, you think to yourself, you knew this would happen.

Introduction

Muscles, and the tendons that connect muscles to bones, and the ligaments that connect bones to bones, work in concert to provide locomotion, movement of the human body. Under the physical stress of wilderness endeavors, muscles, tendons, and ligaments often suffer traumatic or overuse injuries ranging from mildly annoying to severely debilitating. For the purpose of this discussion, these types of injuries will be called "athletic injuries," well documented among the problems most likely to require treatment in the wild outdoors. Proper intervention by the Wilderness First Responder may well 1) promote healing, and 2) prevent these injuries from getting worse while 3) allowing the patient to continue the wilderness adventure. If the patient must be evacuated, a properly treated athletic injury often allows the patient to leave the wilderness under his or her own power.

General Assessment

As long as the scene is safe, do not move the patient or ask the patient to move until your assessment has been completed. "Walking off the pain," a common patient response to an athletic injury, is a myth that may lead to permanent damage. A patient's eagerness to prove he or she can stay with the group and/or not become a burden to the group may lead to lifelong disability. While keeping the patient in a restful position, LAF at the injury site (SEE CHAPTER 12: FRACTURES):

Look. Is there swelling? Discoloration? The degree of swelling and discoloration is indicative of the degree of damage. You must get down to the skin to assess an athletic injury.

Ask. How much does it hurt? Pain is a primary indicator of the severity of an athletic injury. What happened? How much force was involved? In which direction were the forces applied? Stronger forces against weaker body parts create a greater chance for damage. Did the patient hear a "popping" or "snapping" sound at the moment of stress? Sounds are an indication of damage. Has the patient had similar pain and discomfort before and, if so, what was the cause? The patient often knows what's wrong.

Feel. Is there pain when you press on specific points? Point tenderness is indicative of tears in connective tissues—tendons and ligaments—as well as fractures in bones.

At this point, if you have decided the injury could be "athletic," have the patient move the injury site through it's normal range of motion. Loss of range of motion is a second primary indicator of an athletic injury. Compare the range of motion on the injured side to the range of motion on the uninjured side to help you determine how much has been lost. When muscles, ligaments, or tendons are stressed, does it cause pain? How much pain?

If the patient has tolerated moving the injury without a high level of pain or a substantial loss in range of motion, you, the rescuer, may now move the injury site for the patient. Add stress at the maximum stretch points within the range of motion of the injury site. Once again, assess the level of pain and the range of motion.

If the patient has tolerated your movement of the injury site, allow the patient to attempt to use the injury site—to bear weight on injured ankles and knees, to use shoulders, elbows, and wrists as necessary in order to walk out and/or complete the wilderness journey. If the patient is able to use the injury, the patient, in most wilderness cases, should be allowed to use the injury, if he or she chooses to do so.

The single most important factor related to a wilderness athletic injury is the patient's ability to use the injury.

If at any time in your assessment you suspect the injury is a fracture, the injury should be splinted, and the patient evacuated. In other words, if the patient cannot or will not use the injury, splint the injury and evacuate the patient.

General Treatment

Athletic injuries should be managed initially and as soon as possible with RICE. RICE is an acronym for Rest, Ice, Compression, and Elevation, and these four techniques in combination limit swelling. Swelling delays the patient's return to normal activity more than any other factor. Every minute RICE is withheld could add as much as an hour to the time it will take for healing to occur. RICE also helps prevent further damage.

REST THE INJURY: stop using it. Rest reduces circulation to the injury, thus less swelling. Rest prevents complications that may occur when the injured area is moved.

ICE THE INJURY: cool it with an ice pack, snow pack, soaking in a cold mountain stream, wrapping it in a wet T-shirt and allowing evaporation, etc. Ice constricts blood vessels to limit swelling.

COMPRESS THE INJURY: —with an elastic wrap from distal to proximal (from the end of the extremity toward the heart). Never wrap so tight that adequate circulation is impaired. Compression creates higher pressure on torn tissues, making it more difficult for swelling to occur.

ELEVATE THE INJURY: prop it up comfortably higher than the patient's heart. Elevation reduces swelling by decreasing circulation to the area.

Maintain RICE for 20-30 minutes, then allow the injury to rewarm naturally—12 to 15 minutes—before allowing the patient to test his or her ability to use the injury. The patient's check on the usefulness of injury should be a short "test drive" and *not* sustained use.

If adequate time is allowed for return of normal circulation between treatments, it is difficult to overdue RICE. Although no clinical tests have proven it, empirical evidence suggests that you may use RICE for 20 minutes on, 20 minutes off, 20 minutes on, 20 minutes off, repeated several times immediately following the injury with advantageous results. If the wilderness situation allows, it is recommended to apply RICE to athletic injuries at least several times a day during the first couple of days following the injury, and, better still, until pain and swelling have subsided.

Note: Heat usually exacerbates swelling. Ice—or cold—is the treatment of choice, even if the injury is 48 hours old when you first see it. Heat may be applied once all pain and swelling have subsided in order to loosen up the damaged area for retraining.

Doctors typically recommend taking an anti-inflammatory/ pain-killing drug, such as ibuprofen, for athletic injuries. Indeed, you can think of treatment as RIICE with the second "I" standing for Ibuprofen. The patient may follow the regimen suggested on the drug's label, but many sports medicine specialists recommend upping the dose of ibuprofen to as much as 800 mg every six to eight hours. Maintenance of adequate hydration is essential (SEE CHAPTER 17: HEAT-INDUCED EMERGENCIES).

Athletic Injuries: Types And Treatment

Strains

Strains are injuries to muscle fibers or tendons, resulting when the fibers are stretched too far. Only a few torn fibers, and the injury is usually called a "pull." Many torn fibers produces a "tear." There is usually little or no swelling, no matter the degree of injury, but there may be considerable discoloration, a bruised look. Pain usually subsides when the affected body part is rested, but active use can cause much pain.

Muscle pulls are probably the most common athletic injury. An injured muscle typically spasms, a protective mechanism that shortens the overstretched muscle fibers. Spasms cause pain. RICE, the treatment for strains, will relax the muscle, reducing pain and encouraging healing (see General Treatment). It is critical to remind the patient to start gently stretching the injured muscle as soon as he or she can tolerate the stretching. Gradual, non-violent stretching of the muscle fibers reduces the chance they will heal shortened, a condition that almost always leads soon to a re-injury of the muscle. Full healing is usually indicated by the patient's ability to stretch the muscle without pain and use the muscle through an active range of motion without pain.

Sprains

Sprains are injuries to ligaments. A *first degree* injury, the one most often experienced, stretches but does not actually tear ligaments. There will be pain when the affected joint is moved, stressing the damaged ligaments, and perhaps a little discoloration, but there is little swelling, little instability. With proper care, the patient will be back to normal in one to two weeks. In a *second degree* injury, partially torn ligaments swell and discolor, usually in a very short time. Pain may discourage the patient from stressing the damaged ligaments. Healing time can take as long as six weeks. *Third degree* injuries entail serious ligament tears, typically complete tears. Discoloration may be extreme. Within 30 minutes of injury, most patients will be unable to move the damaged joint due to pain and swelling. The patient could be at day one of six months or more of healing, and many third degree injuries will require surgical intervention. RICE is the treatment of choice (SEE GENERAL TREATMENT).

Note: Both strains and sprains may be associated with fractures and/or dislocations.

Tendonitis

Tendonitis (also acceptably spelled *tendinitis*) is the inflammation of a tendon, a problem unlike strains and sprains in that the injury comes with overuse and not from trauma. Tendonitis can, however, be just as or more debilitating as some strains and sprains.

Almost all voluntary movement in the human body involves tendons transmitting muscular force from muscles to bone and joints. Tendons, as mentioned earlier, are attached to muscles on one end and to bones at an insertion point on the other. On the way from muscle to bone, the tendon passes through a tendon sheath which is attached to the underlying bone. When the muscle flexes it contracts, shortens, drawing the inflexible tendon back toward the muscle. The sheath stabilizes the tendon and acts like a pulley. Without the tendon sheath the tendon would straighten as a rope does when it is tied to a weight and pulled on by someone who wants the weight to move. The tendon sheath keeps the tendon near the bone, increasing the efficiency of the system.

The sheath secretes *synovial* fluid, the same viscous, slimy fluid that keeps joints lubricated. With repetitive motion, such as paddling or hiking, a tendon may get overworked. The sheath tries to keep things running smoothly and secretes more fluid, but the sheath can't expand to hold the increase in fluid, so the tendon gets compressed. The tendon and the sheath swell and inflammation begins. Now the tendon calls for more lubrication and the sheath responds with more fluid and the problem multiplies each time that particular tendon is used. Overuse may also cause a tendon sheath to begin to microscopically tear loose from the bone. In both cases, inflammation—in this case tendonitis—produces insistent pain when the affected tendon is in use.

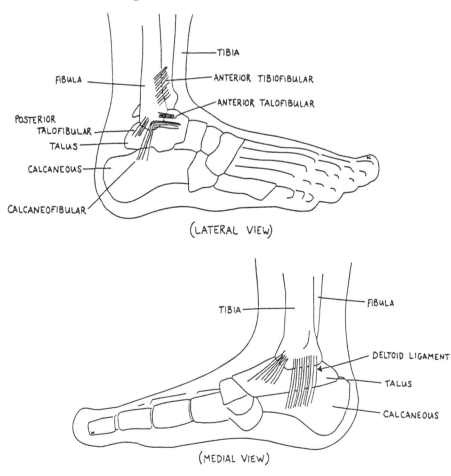

Figure 14-1: Anatomy of the ankle

A more severe type of tendonitis can be had if you ignore the developing problem until calcium salts grow in an inflamed area. The sharp pieces of calcium irritate the bursa sac, the tough bag that surrounds all joints to the keep the lubricating synovial fluid from running away. The irritated bursa starts to overproduce fluid. Eventually, the entire sac becomes inflamed and tense, and the whole joint becomes an agonizing burden to bear. At this point the standard treatment of tendinitis may not work.

The standard treatment is simple: Don't use the joint until it gets better. There is little chance

it will hurt if you do not move the inflamed tendon. Without use, the tendon will finally heal. Application of cold packs three to four times a day for about 20 minutes helps speed the healing by reducing the swelling, and a regimen of an over-the-counter, anti-inflammatory drug will also reduce pain and improve the rate of mending (SEE GENERAL TREATMENT). Some inflamed tendons, especially those of the elbow, respond well to deep massage with your thumb at the point of pain, if the patient can deal with the pain of the massage. Deep tendon massage should move the

tendon one way for better healing, not back and forth.

The wilderness often prevents the best treatment for tendonitis. If your assessment is tendonitis, make every effort to prevent the patient from using that joint for the next few days. When the joint is used, attempt to limit the motion of the joint to within the limits of pain. As an example, a paddler may shorten his or her stroke to reduce pain. Pain-free use stimulates healthy, healing circulation while keeping the joint from stiffening. Persistent pain, especially beyond two weeks, is a signal to ask for a physician's care.

Specific Athletic Injuries

Ankle Sprain

Lateral (outside) ligament damage dominates due to the structure of the ankle which allows little *eversion*, or turning outward, and much *inversion*, or turning inward. Inversion sprains of the ankle are the most common wilderness sprain and, in fact, account for approximately 85 percent of all ankle sprains.

The lower leg's bigger bones, the large tibia and smaller fibula, meet the ankle at the *talus*, an upwardly rounded bone that allows the tib and fib to "rock" back-and-forth on its top. The talus, in turn, "rocks" side-to-side on top of the front of the *calcaneous* (heel bone) at an articulation point called the subtalar joint. This ability to rock allows for freedom of movement when the human body hikes, climbs, or runs. In front of the calcaneous lie two small bones, the *navicular* on the medial aspect of the foot,

and the *cuboid* on the lateral aspect. In front of these two bones are three even smaller bones called the *cuniforms.* These seven—talus, calcaneous, navicular, cuboid, and three cuniforms—are the true ankle bones. The bumps called "ankle bones" are actually the rounded distal ends of the tibia and fibula, bumps called the lateral *malleolus* (the end of the fibula) and the medial malleolus (the end of the tibia).

It takes a complex arrangement of ligaments to secure all these bone-to-bone connections, but six of these ligaments are primary targets for injury. Two of these, the anterior and posterior *tibio-fibular* ligaments, hold the tib and fib together, preventing those bones from being wedged apart by the talus when you take a step. Number three, the *deltoid* ligament, a fan-shaped bunch of fibers, attaches the tibia to bones

on the inside of the ankle. The *deltoid* is wide and tough, allowing little eversion of the ankle. In fact, over-stressing the deltoid is more likely pull off a fragment of bone (an avulsion fracture) than to sprain the ligament. On the outside of the ankle, the other three primary ligaments attach the fibula to the talus and the calcaneous: the anterior *talo-fibular*, the posterior *talo-fibular*, and the *calcaneo-fibular*. These smaller, weaker lateral ligaments allow much more inversion than the deltoid allows eversion and, consequently, they are the ones most often damaged. The ligament in the middle, the calcaneo-fibular, bears the brunt of inversion stress, but, as you can imagine, sprained ankles often involve more than one ligament.

Mild ankle sprains, first degree injuries, can be taped (see below) and the patient will usually be able to move well in the wilderness. Moderate sprains, second degree injuries, can be taped to allow the patient to limp along, self-powered, probably with most of the weight from her or his pack distributed among other group members. Severe ankle damage, third degree injuries, will require splinting and, most likely, carrying of the patient out to definitive medical care.

Since some fractured ankles may show less apparent damage than some badly sprained ankles, persistent pain should send the patient for an x-ray.

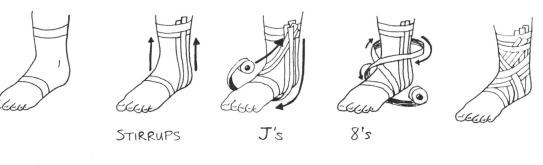

STIRRUPS   J's   8's

(pull up on both
Sides simultaneosly)

Figure 14-2: Ankle taping

Ankle Taping: It's a well-accepted fact that taping reduces the chance of further injury or reinjury to an ankle, but the tape needs to stick well. The support from tape is reduced as the tape loosens. Apply the tape firmly, but not so tight that healthy circulation is reduced. Apply the tape with as few wrinkles as possible. Anchor each strip of tape with a circumferential strip of tape that passes around the lower leg or foot.

Tape works best if applied directly to skin. Tape feels better, especially on removal, if the hair of the ankle and lower leg are trimmed off short first, but hair cutting is not required. You can tape over a thin liner sock if the patient cannot tolerate tape against the skin, but the support will not be as great.

You don't need to tape from toe to calf—mid-foot to four to six inches above the ankle bones is enough. Start by marking the boundaries of the ankle taping area with tape anchors at midfoot and above the ankle bones. Apply stirrups that pull foot up into the ankle. Remember to anchor each stirrup with a strip of tape above the ankle bones. Then apply figure-of-eights to hold the ankle firmly together. Start the "eights" toward the injured side, which is usually the outside of the ankle, to reduce strain on the injured ligaments. Finish by filling in the empty spaces, but leave the heel free (SEE ILLUSTRATION).

Tape provides a flexible splint and, as a splinted extremity, the foot should be assessed before and after taping for adequate circulation, sensation, and motion. The patient may be given the responsibilty of notifyng you if sensations alter in the foot, e.g., tingling, numbness.

As a benefit, taping doesn't seem to be limited to providing support for the ankle. Experts now believe the tape stimulates nerve messages to the brain improving balance and coordination. Athletic tape, made for taping athletic injuries, usually works best, but any tape available, e.g., duct tape, can be used in a wilderness emergency. It is best to remove the tape at night to improve circulation and make RICE more effective.

Achilles Tendonitis

On the other foot, some ankle pain results not from trauma but from overuse and overstretching. Few are the muscles of the foot and ankle, movement of this area being powered by the lower leg via tendons. Too much movement, and more likely in an unfit hiker, may produce tendonitis, Achilles tendonitis by far the most common. The large Achilles tendon runs from the back of the heelbone on its lower end up to the muscles of the lower leg, and is especially at risk for tendonitis during or after a long hike, and even more likely if the hike involved significant elevation gain. The pain of Achilles tendonitis can be startling.

Specific treatment for Achilles tendonitis includes creating a pad, about a quarter inch thick should do, under the heel inside the boot to relieve stress on the

Achilles. Two strips of padding taped in place, one on each side of the Achilles, will further reduce stress.

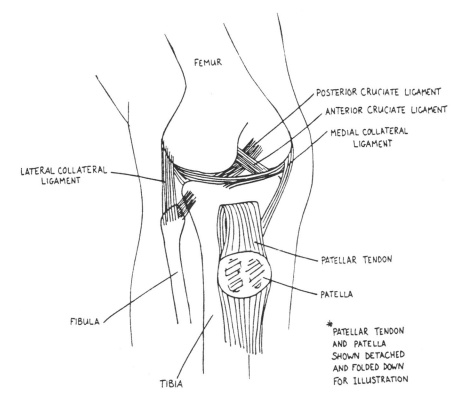

Figure 14-3: Anatomy of the knee

The Knee

Only the ankle has more problems coping with wilderness journeys than the knee. The demands put on the knee are great, and it is highly susceptible to trauma or overuse.

Knees are directly comprised of three bones: the femur, the tibia, and the patella. Another bone, the fibula, attaches behind the tibia, near the knee, but has no specific influence on the joint.

Femurs and tibias articulate, or rub against each other, when legs are in motion. The articulating surfaces of the femur and tibia are semi-flat and, to ensure a secure fit, each knee is padded

with two C-shaped pieces of cartilage, one on the outer half of joint space, the other on the inner half. They, also, absorb some of the shock of movement. They are called the medial *meniscus* and the lateral *meniscus*. Placed strategically in the knee are fluid-filled sacks, called *bursae*, at points of the greatest friction.

The knee is held together by ligaments—four of them. They are attached at the points of highest stress. Connecting the femur to the tibia are the medial and lateral *collateral* ligaments, on the inside and outside of the knee. They provide stability for

side-to-side motion. For back-to-front and front-to-back stability, there are the *cruciate* (crossed) ligaments. They run through the joint space, between the two menisci. Both cruciate ligaments attach on their upper end to the femur, and on their lower end to the tibia, and they are named for where they attach to the tibia. The anterior cruciate ligament (ACL) attaches to the femur at the back of the knee and to the tibia in front, thus preventing the knee from sliding too far forward. The posterior cruciate ligament (PCL) attaches to the femur at the front of the knee and the tibia at the rear, thus preventing the knee from sliding too far backwards.

When in motion, the great muscles of the leg provide additional support to the knee. The *quadriceps* (thigh) muscles are a group of four muscles. They taper down into one tendon that crosses the knee and attaches to the top of the tibia. The patella lives in the middle of this tendon. Three muscles in the back of the leg, the hamstrings, also help support the knee. One attaches to the outside of the knee and the other two to the inside. The *gastrocnemius* (calf muscle) attaches in two places to the back of the femur and, finally, a long thin muscle runs from the groin to the inside of the knee adding a touch more of support.

In addition, a long tough tendon, called the *ilio-tibial band*, runs from the *gluteals*, the muscles of your hindquarters, down the thigh, across the knee, attaching to the outside of the tibia. This band, too, gives a bit of support.

Any force applied to the knee can partially or totally tear a ligament. If the force is applied to the outside of the knee, the medial collateral ligament and anterior cruciate ligament may be involved, as well as the medial cartilage. If the force is applied to the inside of the knee, the lateral collateral could be torn and lateral cartilage may be ruptured. Twisting forces may significantly damage the cruciate ligaments.

During your assessment of the knee, passively test each of the four ligaments holding the tibia to the femur. These tests should be done with the patient sitting down and the leg relaxed. "Relaxed" may be a relative term if the knee is causing a lot of pain. If the patient is unable to tolerate these checks, that knee needs a doctor.

The medial collateral ligament, the one on the inside of the leg, can be checked by holding the ankle, with the knee slightly bent, and pushing from the outside of the knee in. If it's loose or painful, stop pushing.

The lateral collateral ligament, on the outside of the leg, can be checked in the exact opposite way, pushing from the inside of the knee out. Again, looseness or pain is a sign to stop pushing.

The anterior cruciate ligament, one of the two "crossed" ligaments inside the knee joint, can be checked by bending the knee slightly and pulling out on the tibia while pushing back on the femur. Watch for pain and looseness.

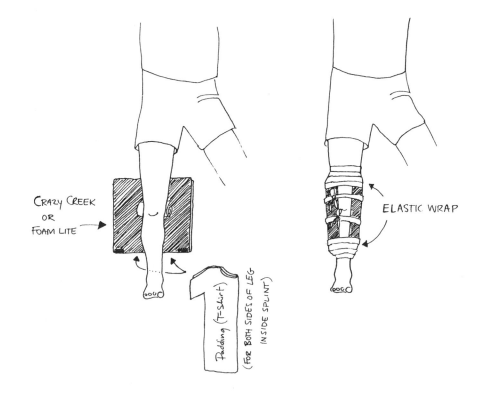

CRAZY CREEK OR FOAM LITE

ELASTIC WRAP

Padding (T-Shirt)
(FOR BOTH SIDES OF LEG INSIDE SPLINT)

Figure 14-4: Walking knee splint

Posterior cruciate damage, which happens in only about one percent of all knee injuries, can be checked simply by lifting the relaxed leg by the ankle and letting the knee sag.

A simple active test for knee function can be performed with a high degree of accuracy, but it should not be performed until passive range of motion is checked. If the patient can stand and walk, do deep knee bends, and jump up and down on each leg individually, the knees are almost always stable enough to remain in the wilderness.

If the knee has been traumatized to the point where it can't be used, the leg should be splinted, with the knee slightly flexed, and the patient should be carried to a doctor. Flexion of the knee can be easily maintained by padding well behind the knee, leaving the knee flexed at about 10 degrees. If the patient feels more comfort with the knee flexed more, add more padding beneath the knee.

If the knee can be used carefully, you can build a splint that stabilizes the knee move while allowing the patient to walk. The patient will probably require some type of crutch. A cylinder splint, one that wraps entirely around the knee, may be used, but patient comfort will usually be increased by creating a splint that leaves the kneecap free. You can make this type of splint by rolling up a sleeping pad from both ends simultaneously, and securing it to the knee with the "jelly rolls," the rolled sides of the pad, against the lateral and medial aspect of the knee. A Crazy Creek Chair® works extremely well as a walking knee splint when placed beneath the knee and folded up around the knee. The stays within the Chair give firm support to both sides of the knee while leaving the kneecap free. Remember: Even a walking knee splint should have sufficient padding behind the knee

The most common source of knee pain is not a sprain but probably overuse of the muscles that support the knee. When they are stressed too much, they tear—a strain—and create a great deal of discomfort. They most often strain near their attachment to the knee. Tendonitis has the same mechanism of injury. Muscle strains and tendonitis are commonly mistaken by the patient, and sometimes the rescuer, as a torn ligament or cartilage. This mistake is very common when the ilio-tibial band (ITB) is involved. Since the band is required for uphill motion, it is often abused when someone is unused to going uphill, or increases their uphill activity, especially if she or he is wearing a pack. Traversing a hillside can also stress the ITB, especially on the downhill leg. The problem, called *ilio-tibial band syndrome*, causes pain primarily where the band attaches to the outside of the knee, simulating a torn lateral collateral ligament.

General knee pain may have other causes including *patellar compression syndrome*, a problem created by too much pressure on the back of the kneecap by too much walking, especially downhill. A dull ache, constant and nagging, is the common complaint. Or, perhaps, the kneecap doesn't run quite correctly in its track. The additional side-to-side motion of the kneecap puts additional stress on its inner surface which eventually causes pain for up to several hours after use. If the pain becomes chronic, never going away, the condition may be *chondromalacia* of the patella. Chondromalacia refers to a disintegration of the cartilage under the kneecap, probably caused by a chemical change stimulated by knee injury or overuse. The cartilage becomes frayed and eroded. Interestingly, the cartilage can't hurt since it has no nerve endings, so the pain must come from inflamed tissue around the cartilage. General knee pain does not to be specifically assessed by the WFR. It can be treated with RICE and a walking splint, and the patient and WFR will need to decide if the wilderness trip must be cut short. A lot of general knee pain doesn't go away in the field, and the patient may eventually require a physician's care. In the meantime, the patient may be encouraged to alter her or his gait and/or use a walking stick to relieve some of the pressure on the knee.

Low Back Strain

It takes surprisingly little stress on the mid to lower back, if the angle is right, to pull muscles. The resulting agony can be surprisingly debilitating. It will probably be several days to weeks before the pain goes entirely away, but almost everyone can make themselves functional in a couple of days by following a recognized routine.

Rest is initially very important. Have the patient rest on his or her side, or on his or her back with thick, relatively stiff padding underneath the knees. Too much rest, however, can soon lead to weakened back muscles. As soon as the patient can tolerate exercise, the patient should be exercising to tolerance. General movement, such as easy walking, is beneficial in the initial phases of the injury. The lower back can be gently exercised by having the patient lie flat on his or her back with the knees raised high and feet flat on the ground followed by lifting the head and shoulders and pressing the lower back into the ground. This "abdominal crunch" stretches the lower back and, over time, strengthens the abdominal muscles, a preventive measure against lower back injury.

Ice the painful region of the back several times a day for several days.

Gently massage the injured muscles several times a day.

Drugs such as ibuprofen often ease pain and promote healing. Patients with a history of lower back pain may wish to consult a physician prior to a wilderness trip with the intention of acquiring a prescription strength muscle relaxant.

If the pain has not appreciably decreased in a week to 10 days, or if pain, tingling, numbness, or paralysis begins to creep down the legs, it's time to forget the wilderness for a while and find a physician.

Shin Splints

Beneath the skin and fat of the lower leg, the muscles lie in seven compartments walled by connective tissue called fascia. Beneath those muscles lies the tibia, which is wrapped in a tough membrane. The shin is the front of the lower leg, everything between the knee and ankle, and any persistent pain in that area is referred to as a "shin splint." Shin splints are a common athletic injury, and it is often impossible to tell what part of the leg is actually damaged.

Compartment syndrome: During exercise, blood flow to muscles increases, and they grow larger. The fascia around the muscles stretches to accommodate the enlargement. With repeated exercise the muscles grow larger and pressure on the fascia increases. In most people this is not a problem, but some people have particularly small muscle compartments. The pressure on the walls of fascia causes them to stiffen, similar to the way callus forms on hands and feet when they are constantly used for rough work. The muscles are compressed against the stiffening walls of fascia causing the pain of a shin splint. Compared to other causes of shin splints, compartment syndrome is relatively easy to diagnose. The pain comes on slowly, gradually filling the compartment. When asked where it hurts, the sufferer will sketch an outline of the muscle on the leg.

Fractures and Tears: Overuse of lower legs can cause small cracks in the bone called stress fractures. Repeated stress on lower legs can damage the tough membrane surrounding the tibia. Twisting or pulling motions can tear muscles, tendons, or ligaments. Just overworking a muscle that is not ready for it can inflame muscle cells and produce pain. Shin splints brought on by stress-fractured bones or torn tissues tend to cause pain most in one specific spot. These prob-

lems also tend to develop with more abruptness.

If your assessment is a shin splint, encourage the patient to take it easy on that part of the body for a while. When pain persists, try periodic icing of the painful area. A nonsteroidal anti-inflammatory drug, ibuprofen usually working the best of those available over-the-counter, may speed healing. If the shin pain keeps getting worse, the patient should consult a doctor.

The Shoulder

Nothing about the construction of that association of three bones at the top of the arm lends itself to long-term anatomical optimism. Shoulders are simply not very stable.

Shoulders may manifest a problem called *impingement*. The pain of impingement typically falls into one of two categories: a result of overuse by repetitive motion, or a result of an impact injury to the shoulder that disrupts normal mechanics.

The humerus, scapula, and clavicle meet at the shoulder, the only joint in the body not held together primarily by ligaments. A few shoulder ligaments prevent the bones from shifting too far in one direction or another but offer little help in keeping the joint snugly in its rightful place. Shoulders are small and shallow ball-and-socket joints. The head of the humerus has little contact with the socket, and the bones stay put because of a group of muscles known collectively as rotator cuff muscles: supraspinatus, infraspinatus, subscapularis, and teres minor. Rotator cuff muscles are not designed to function under the stress applied when the arm rises above a line parallel to the ground. Too much over-the-shoulder exercise, such as sea kayaking, and the muscles can stretch, and the head of the joint can get sloppy within the socket. With the head of the shoulder loose, every time the patient reaches backward over the shoulder, or lifts his or her arm above parallel to the ground, the head slips temporarily out of place.

A simple test tells if the patient is impinged. Ask the patient to lift the arm on the affected side slowly straight out to your side, 90 degrees to the ground. As the patient tries to pass the 90 degree mark, pain hollers "whoa" to the motion.

Rest and anti-inflammatory drugs help the pain of impingement go away… but not the problem. As soon as the patient starts exercising again, back comes the discomfort. The cure involves strengthening exercises for the shoulder.

A shoulder *separation* may result from excessive forces applied to the shoulder. "Separation" is an old term describing an enlargement of the spaces between the bones. Since ligamental disruption is required for separation, the injury is a shoulder sprain, and should be treated as such (SEE GENERAL TREATMENT).

The Elbow

The pain in the elbow comes with overuse of the muscles and tendons used to bend the wrist backward and forward, and may be referred to as "tennis elbow." By palpation, you can usually pinpoint the pain at the proximal end of either the radius or ulna. "Tennis elbow" feels better in some people when they wear a light constricting band about one inch below the elbow to help hold the tendon in place during periods of activity. If the pain remain acute, even with a band distal to the elbow, a splint may be improvised reaching from the palm of the hand to below the elbow to prevent movement.

Prevention

Several factors will help you predict and, perhaps, forestall an athletic injury:

1. Weak or imbalanced muscles. The best way to prevent injury is to get in shape and stay in shape. Individuals with specific weak joints, say a shoulder, should learn and perform exercises specific to the affected joint.

2. Too much body weight. Shed extra pounds to reduce stress on joints, especially lower extremity joints. Carry a lighter pack if you are not in shape for backpacking.

3. Inappropriate or dilapidated footwear. Choose boots that provide adequate ankle support which, in turn, will provide better support for the knee and lower back. Replace worn-out footwear before wearing out an ankle. An inward fold above the heel counter/heel cup can irritate the Achilles enough to cause tendonitis in one day of backpacking. Broken down or poor quality boots can produce pain where other tendons meet the fibula. Boots too stiff, or too tightly

laced, may generate tendonitis at the front of the ankle.

4. Loss of balance. Use a ski pole or walking stick to help maintain balance.

5. Failure to stretch and warm-up muscles before periods of exercise.

6. Previous injury. Follow suggestions one through four even more aggressively.

7. Carelessness.

Evacuation Guidelines

The ability of the patient to use the injury is the key factor in determining the need for an evacuation. All patients with unstable or unusable athletic injuries, injuries that do not permit continuance of the wilderness trip, should be evacuated. Haste is not required or recommended.

Conclusion

On the banks of the Escalante River, you keep Tom at rest while you assess his injury. A pulse is easily palpable in his right ankle, and motion and sensation in the toes of his right foot cause you no concern. The bruising and swelling that first alarmed you doesn't appear quite so bad now that you've calmed down a bit.

Tom describes the accident to you. When his foot rolled in, he felt sudden pain on the outside of his ankle, but he heard no snaps, crackles, or pops. The pain, he says, has started to ease off a little.

As you probe around the injury site, you uncover mild to moderate point tenderness just below the ankle bone, approximately where you think the calcaneo-fibular ligament inserts.

On request, Tom pushes his ankle through its normal range of motion without undue pain. It hurts, sure, but he can "take it." You are relatively aggressive about manipulating his ankle, adding a bit of push to the extremes of the range of motion. Tom winces slightly when you roll his foot in, but you are satisfied the injury is not a major one. When asked to try walking, Tom does so with a slight limp.

In the shade of a cottonwood tree, Tom rests with his ankle propped up on a sleeping bag still in its stuff sack. You compress the ankle with an elastic wrap, applied from the toes toward the knee, and place a plastic bag filled with cold water from the river on the ankle. After 20 minutes, the cold bag comes off.

A 15 minute wait for rewarming, and you ask Tom to try walking again. His limp has lessened, and so, he claims, has the pain.

You will repeat the RICE treatment again before bed, and again in the morning. You will tape Tom's ankle after the morning's treatment. Tom will continue the hike, some of the weight of his pack distributed among the group.

Joe Costello, MS, CSCS, CMT, contributed his expertise to this chapter.

Chapter 15:   Soft Tissue Injuries

You should be able to:

1. *Describe the various types of wounds including contusions, abrasions, lacerations, amputations, avulsions, impaled objects, and punctures.*

2. *Demonstrate the appropriate emergency treatment and long-term care of wounds in the wilderness.*

3. *Describe the appropriate emergency treatment and long-term care of burns in the wilderness.*

4. *Describe soft tissue infections and their management in the wilderness.*

It could happen to you

It was a dark and stormy night near the granite buttress of Fossil Ridge, Colorado, among the scattered and fractured rock surrounding Mill Lake. Your tent mate's vocal complaints about his need to relieve his bladder awaken you.

"I've got to go," he says, scrambling out of his bag.

"Put on your shoes," you suggest over a yawn.

"No," he says, "I'll only be a minute."

A yell of pain, a curse, and your tent mate flops back into your temporary dome-shaped home, tightly gripping his left foot with both his hands. Blood seeps through his fingers, drips onto your bag.

"Stubbed my big toe," he grinds out from between clenched teeth.

Taking a look at the dirty digit, you see a nickel-sized avulsion. Already the blood flow has begun to ease.

Introduction

Soft tissue injuries are among the most common medical problems encountered in the wilderness. In a study at the National Outdoor Leadership School (NOLS), wounds and their complications accounted for one third of all wilderness medical problems severe enough to prevent normal participation in course activities. Burns, including injuries from hot water and open fires, make up another large percentage of wilderness mishaps. Under the rigors of wilderness travel, even apparently trivial wounds may develop an infection. Preventing complications and attaining optimal functional and cosmetic results requires careful evaluation and management of all wilderness soft tissue injuries. Because these injuries frequently occur in remote settings that are hours or days from usual sources of medical care, this task often falls to the prehospital provider. So it is essential that Wilderness First Responders acquire a thorough understanding of the principles of wound and burn assessment and develop the skills necessary to effectively manage wounds and burns in a wilderness environment.

Basic Anatomy Of The Skin

The skin, or integumentary system, is composed of two major layers, the epidermis and the dermis. The thin, overlying *epidermis* protects the dermis from infection and desiccation (drying out). Wounds involving only the epidermis result in little or no bleeding and have a low susceptibility to infection. The *dermis*, the largest organ of the human body, provides most of the tensile strength of skin and contains sweat glands, sebaceous (oil) glands, hair follicles, nerves, and capillaries. Below the dermis, on most of the body, lies subcutaneous fat, sometimes a slim layer, sometimes not. Below the fat lies fascia, the membrane which covers muscle.

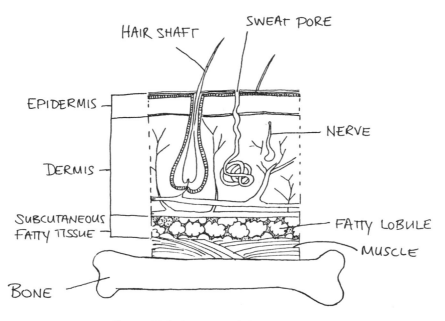

Figure 15-1: Anatomy of the skin

Types Of Soft Tissue Injuries

1. *Contusion*, a bruise.
2. *Abrasion*, a wound in which one or more layers of skin are scraped away.
3. *Laceration*, a cut through the skin. A laceration produced by a sharp object, such as a knife, is sometimes called an incision and generally produces little damage to the surrounding skin. Lacerations from a blunt injury, however, typically result in a tearing or bursting of the skin causing ragged wound edges or star-shaped patterns. Because damage to adjacent skin occurs, these wounds heal more slowly, result in larger scars, and are more prone to infection.
4. *Amputation*, a separation of a body part, e.g., ear, finger, or foot, from the rest of the body. In a partial amputation, sometimes called an avulsion, the distal part is attached by a small piece of skin, muscle, or tendon.
5. *Puncture wound*, the result of an object, e.g., thorn, fang, knife, penetrating the body. These wounds may introduce bacteria into deep tissues and are very difficult to clean adequately. As a result, they are particularly prone to infection. An *impaled object* is a puncture wound with the puncturing object still stuck in it.
6. *Burns*, the result of heat, electricity (e.g., lightning), radiation (e.g., sunburn), or chemicals which damage or destroy skin layers.

General Wilderness Wound Management

A reminder: Perhaps the single most important principle in evaluating an injured patient is to assess the entire patient and not focus exclusively on a specific injury. Every patient should be assessed for serious or life-threatening injuries that may not be immediately obvious. Airway control, maintenance of breathing, circulatory support—including control of life-threatening blood loss—and spine immobilization, all when needed, always take precedence over general wound management. General open wound care, when time to provide care arrives, needs to accomplish three goals: 1) control significant blood loss, 2) prevent infection, and 3) promote healing.

Control of Bleeding

Minor wounds may be allowed, even encouraged, to bleed to a stop, which may provide a cleaner wound. Significant wounds require control of bleeding. Attaining adequate *hemostasis* (control of bleeding) not only facilitates wound assessment and management but, in severe wounds, may be necessary to prevent blood volume depletion. *Hemostasis can almost always be accomplished by applying direct pressure and elevation to the site of bleeding* (SEE CHAPTER SIX: BLEEDING).

Patient Assessment

After significant bleeding is controlled, a detailed history and examination should be performed. It is important to determine when the injury occurred since bacteria begin to proliferate even in relatively clean wounds after approximately six hours. Where the injury occurred provides clues to possible contaminants, e.g., feces, saliva, soil, which increase the risk of infection. Determining the mechanism of injury aids in assessing the extent of the wound and may indicate the need to assess for additional, less obvious injuries. If the patient has known allergies and/or is currently using medications, you should know it before you continue wound treatment.

The tetanus immunization status of the patient should be determined. The bacteria that cause tetanus are ubiquitous. Every patient treated for an open wound should receive immunization against tetanus if 1) the patient has never been immunized, 2) the patient has not received a tetanus booster within the last 10 years, or 3) the patient has a large and/or highly contaminated wound and has not received a booster within the last five years. Tetanus immunization must be received within approximately 72 hours of a wound to be effective. If you serve as an outdoor leader, you would do well to be sure all group members are immunized against tetanus prior to the start of a wilderness trip.

All wounds should be visually assessed for the level of contamination and the presence of foreign bodies. Involvement of important underlying structures such as nerves, major blood vessels, tendons, and joints should be determined, if possible. Motor and sensory function and pulses distal to the injury should be checked before and after wound management.

General Wound Management

A rescuer should be wearing protective gloves and protective eyewear before cleaning an open wound.

All wounds acquired in a wilderness environment should be regarded as contaminated and, therefore, require cleansing to prevent infection and promote healing. When wounds are in hairy areas, closely clipping the hair adjacent to the wound with a pair of scissors facilitates wound management and is preferable to shaving. *Eyebrow hair should never be removed.* An intact eyebrow is necessary for proper alignment of wound edges, and eyebrow hair regrows slowly creating cosmetic problems if removed.

Disinfectants such as isopropyl alcohol and hydrogen peroxide, and soaps and detergents, should not be poured into deep wounds where they damage viable tissue and may actually increase the incidence of wound infection. These substances may be used to wash around a wound prior to wound cleaning, with soap and water working as well or better than anything else.

The most effective and practical method of removing bacteria and debris from a wound utilizes a high pressure irrigation syringe. Irrigation syringes that supply adequate pressure are available commercially in high quality first aid kits. Without an irrigation syringe, you can put water in a plastic bag, punch a pinhole in the bag, and squeeze the water out forcefully, or you can melt a pinhole in the center of the lid of a water bottle with a hot needle, and squeeze the water out forcefully. These and other improvised methods are not nearly as effective, but they may be the best you can do. Simply rinsing or soaking a wound is inadequate to remove bacteria. The cleanest water available, usually water disinfected for drinking with iodine or chlorine, may be used for irrigating, and probably works as well as anything. You can irrigate with water that has been boiled and cooled. Zephiran chloride may be used, or povidone-iodine (10 percent) diluted with ten parts disinfected water to one part povidone iodine. If Zephiran chloride or povidone-iodine are used for irrigation, they must be rinsed from the wound after irrigation, not left in the wound. The tip of the irrigating device should be held just above the wound surface, and the plunger of the syringe forcefully depressed. Be sure to tip the wound in order to irrigate contaminants out and away from the wound. The volume of irrigation fluid required varies with the size of the wound and the degree of contamination. Most wounds require at least a fourth of a liter of water. *Wound irrigation is the single most important factor in preventing infection.*

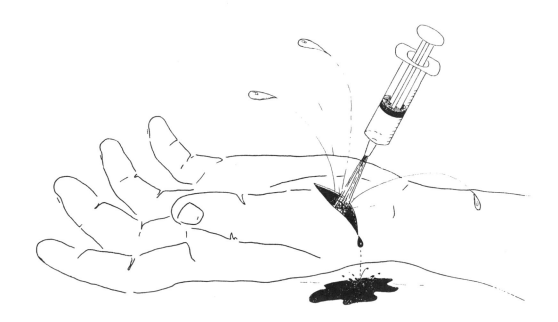

Figure 15-2: Irrigating a wound

Deeply imbedded, visible debris not removed by irrigation may be removed carefully with forceps (tweezers) sterilized by either boiling or open flame, e.g., match or lighter. Carbon, the black stuff, left on forceps after holding them in an open flame is sterile.

For heavily contaminated wounds, applying a one percent povidone-iodine solution to the wound with a sterile gauze pad, after irrigation, may reduce the incidence of infection. Standard stock solutions are 10 percent povidone-iodine and should be diluted as described above before application to an open wound.

Povidone-iodine scrub contains a detergent and should not be used in deep wounds.

After closing and/or dressing (SEE BELOW) a deep wound on an extremity, immobilization by splinting reduces lymphatic flow and the spread of microorganisms. Elevation of the extremity decreases swelling. Both measures reduce the likelihood of wound complications and should be employed whenever possible.

Prophylactic antibiotics are not indicated for most wounds. Many authorities would recommend antibiotics for wounds involving tendons, particularly of the hand, bones, or joint spaces,

and wounds heavily contaminated with saliva, feces, or soil containing large amounts of organic material. If antibiotics are used, they should be started as soon as possible after the injury and a broad-spectrum agent should be chosen such as cephalexin, dicloxacillin, or, if allergy precludes these two, erythromycin. Antibiotics require a prescription, and a physician should be consulted well before you start a wilderness trip. Follow the physician's instructions precisely when using antibiotics. *Antibiotics should never be considered a substitute for a vigorous wound cleaning.*

Wound Healing

If a wound creates a tear through the protective layers of the epidermis, the superficial dermal cells will dry out and die. These dead cells, together with *serum*, the watery portion of blood that seeps from the wound, form the familiar scab or *eschar*. Although wounds heal beneath

scabs, occlusive wound dressings prevent the formation of an eschar by keeping the dermis moist, speeding the growth of new skin and wound healing.

The size and depth of the wound, and several other factors, influence the rate of wound healing. In general, wounds in highly

vascular areas such as the face or scalp heal quickly with a lower risk of infection compared to wounds in less vascular regions such as the distal extremities. The presence of a foreign body or wound infection significantly retards wound healing.

Specific Wound Management

A rescuer should be wearing protective gloves and protective eyewear before cleaning an open wound.

Once irrigation has been accomplished, the eyewear is typically not necessary. In the absence of protective gloves, the rescuer may improvise with clean plastic bags over her or his hands. With relatively minor wounds, in order to prevent sharing germs, the patient may be directed in the management of his or her own wound.

Contusions

Bruises seldom require emergency care, but large bruises benefit from cold, compression, and/or elevation. Substantial bruises should cause you to assess the patient for damage to underlying structures such as bones and organs. Large bruises should be protected from freezing in extremes of cold since a bruised area will freeze sooner than normal skin.

Abrasions

Although scrubbing an abrasion is usually required for adequate wound cleaning, scrubbing wounds damages tissue and should be avoided unless debris cannot be removed with irrigation. A sterile gauze pad is adequate for scrubbing. Scrubbing may be enhanced by using any soap, but all soap should be carefully irrigated from the wound after scrubbing. Green Soap Sponges® are packaged with a soap already in the sponge, making them useful additions to first aid kits. It is important to remove all imbedded debris not only to reduce the risk of infection but also to prevent subsequent "tattooing" (scarring) of the skin. Self-scrubbing is seldom successful due to the high level of pain associated with the nerves exposed by a deep abrasion.

After cleansing, abrasions should be kept moist to avoid desiccation and speed healing. This can be done with microthin film dressings which can be left in place until healing occurs. Without microthin film dressings, topical agents such as antibiotic ointments followed by a dressing of a sterile gauze or a roll of sterile gauze to keep the ointment in place. Tape, an elastic wrap, etc., may be used to hold a sterile gauze pad in place. Ideally, the dressing should be changed twice a day, or at least once a day, and/or any time the gauze gets wet.

Lacerations

Clean, minor lacerations which do not gape open, or gape open no more than half an inch, can be closed with "butterfly" adhesive strips or, even better, with skin closure strips. A thin coat of tincture of benzoin compound applied to the skin around the wound prior to the strips aids in adhesion of the strips. Benzoin is an irritant so take care to keep it out of the wound. Let the benzoin dry for at least 30 seconds before applying the strips. In the absence of benzoin, ethyl-2-cyanoacrylate glue (Super Glue®) may be used. Use of Super Glue® to actually glue a wound closed is not recommended. The closure strips may be applied perpendicular to the wound. Apply one to one side of the wound and another to the opposite side. By using the opposing strips as handles, you can pull the wound edges together, pulling the skin as close as possible to where it should lie naturally,

but without pulling the wound tightly shut. In the absence of butterflys or closure strips, wound closure may be accomplished with whatever tape happens to be available. Adhesive wound closing strips may be left in place until healing occurs. Small wounds cleaned and closed properly with adhesive strips have a very low incidence of infection.

Because optimal conditions for wound care rarely exist in remote settings, suturing or stapling lacerations in the wilderness is controversial. Individuals with advanced medical skills may elect to suture or staple lacerations in low risk, cosmetically important locations like the face after thorough cleansing. However, subcutaneous or deep sutures should be avoided. Heavily contaminated wounds should be treated without suturing.

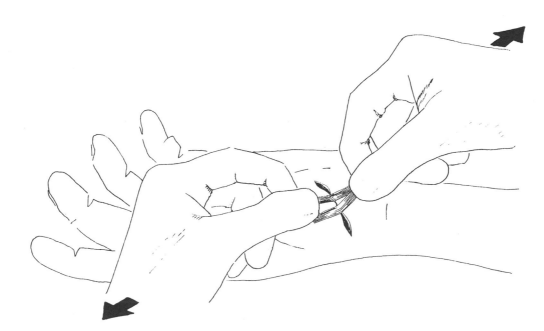

Figure 15-3: Closing a wound

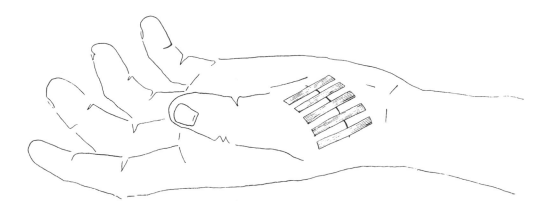

Figure 15-4: Closed wound

After closing, lacerations may be dressed with antibiotic ointment and sterile gauze (see above Abrasions). Alternatively, occlusive microthin film dressings may be used. These dressings prevent eschar formation and provide a humid environment for new cell growth. Because microthin film dressings are see-through, they can be left in place for days, until healing occurs in fact, while allowing monitoring of the wound for signs of infection. These dressings also create a barrier to bacteria and debris which may be particularly important in wilderness settings. If a microthin film dresssing is used, do not apply an ointment under the dressing, a procedure that is 1) unnecessary, and 2) usually causes the microthin dressing to slip off.

Heavily contaminated lacerations left open acquire increased resistance to infection over a three to four day period. After thorough cleansing, the wound should be loosely packed with moistened, sterile gauze and covered with a dry, absorbent dressing. The best solution to moisten the gauze is probably sterile saline, and you could use contact lens solution if you have any available. Sterile water would be next best. Water safe to drink would be third best. The inner moist gauze eventually dries and, when removed, takes some wound debris with it which helps keep the wound clean and open. Unless a wound infection is suspected, the dressing can be left in place until definitive care is available, but, if materials allow, changing the dressings approximately every 12 hours provides

better care. The wound can be sutured—delayed primary closure—in four to five days without impairment in wound healing, which often allows time for return to a hospital.

Amputations/Avulsions

In the case of an amputation, hemostasis is the first priority. The wound should then be irrigated and bandaged as previously described. Do not attempt to reattach the body part. If a detached body part can be easily recovered and the patient can be brought to a hospital within six hours, even longer for fingers and toes, reattachment may be possible. The body part should be quickly irrigated to remove contaminants. The part should then quickly be wrapped in sterile gauze and placed in a plastic bag, if available. Keep the part cold with an ice or cold pack, if available, or by placing the plastic bag containing the body part in a water bottle filled with the coldest water possible. Do not apply ice directly to the body part or frostbite may ensue.

In the case of an avulsion, treat the wound as you would a laceration without completing the separation. Adequate cleaning often requires that you hold the avulsion open during irrigation.

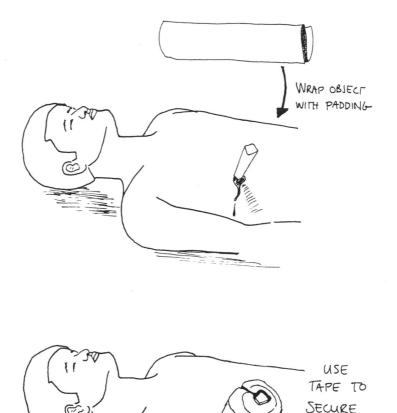

WRAP OBJECT WITH PADDING

USE TAPE TO SECURE PADDING

Figure 15-5: Stabilization of impaled object

Puncture Wounds and Impaled Objects

Puncture wounds carry a particularly high risk of infection. For relatively uncontaminated puncture wounds, irrigation and dressing the wound is the only treatment available, followed by close monitoring for infection (SEE BELOW). For contaminated puncture wounds, treatment should be augmented by evacuation of the patient since infection is almost certain.

Large objects found impaled in a wound should be left in place if you can get to a medical facility with relative ease. Yanking on an object can stimulate serious bleeding and damage underlying structures, especially if the object is impaled in a body cavity, i.e., chest, abdomen, head. The object should be stabilized with padding to prevent movement. The padding should be as high as the object to protect it from being bumped during transport, and the patient should be carried out.

In many cases there is nothing easy about getting to help, and impaled objects sometimes make evacuation very difficult. Removal of impaled objects in the wilderness is an oft-debated subject. They can be impossible to stabilize over rough terrain. Metal objects, such as an ice axe, can suck a significant amount of heat out of a cold patient.

If the object is through a cheek, or in any other way endangering the patient's airway, there is ample agreement on removing it carefully. If the object is loosely imbedded, removal is simple and beneficial to the patient and you, since evacuation is simplified. If the object is in an extremity, removal is often safe. Note the objects shape and angle of entry, and remove accordingly. *Objects impaled in the eye should never be removed.* A patient with an impaled object in the eye should have the object well protected against movement, both eyes should be covered, and the patient should be carried out, preferably propped up at approximately 45 degrees to prevent an increase in pressure in the damaged eye.

Wounds from Bites

Saliva from human and animal mouths contains large amounts of bacteria. All bite wounds should be considered heavily contaminated. The wounds should be copiously irrigated. Following irrigation, one percent povidone-iodine solution, when available, should be added directly to the open wound. Although many bite wounds, particularly dog bites, can be sutured after thorough irrigation and debridement in an emergency department, in the wilderness it is safest to leave bite wounds open. The wound should be loosely packed with moistened gauze and covered with an absorbent dressing, as described above under lacerations. If possible, the bite site should be splinted and elevated. Delayed primary closure can be attempted after return to a hospital.

Bites on the hand, foot, wrist, or over a joint are at high risk for serious infection and should be managed with extreme care. Human bites to the hand, particularly those that occur when a clenched fist strikes a human mouth, are also at high risk for infection. These wounds should be cleaned with the hand as close as possible to the position it was in when it received the wound because the shifting of underlying muscles in hands may trap contamination. Many physicians recommend prophylactic antibiotics for these wounds. If available, the antibiotics should be started as soon as possible after the bite. Penicillin, dicloxacillin, or amoxicillin-clavulanic acid provide good coverage. For penicillin allergic patients, cephalexin or tetracycline can be substituted. Consult a physician concerning antibiotics prior to a wilderness trip, and follow his or her instructions precisely.

Rabies virus infection is more common in wild than domestic animals. Washing a bite wound immediately with soap and water prior to irrigation deactivates the rabies virus on the surface of the wound. All victims of animal bites should be referred as soon as possible to a physician to determine the need for antirabies serum and rabies vaccination (SEE CHAPTER 21: NORTH AMERICAN BITES AND STINGS).

Guidelines For Evacuation

While not a matter of urgency, patients with wounds that hinder the ability to participate in and/or enjoy the wilderness experience should be evacuated. Patients with wounds that require careful closure for cosmetic reasons, e.g., facial wounds, should be evacuated, but delayed primary closure for face wounds can be accomplished in three to five days if the wound has been kept clean and packed open. Patients with wounds that produce shock from blood loss should be evacuated rapidly if the patient does not respond promptly to treatment for shock. *Rapid evacuation* is advised, due to the high risk of infection, for 1) deep and/or highly contaminated wounds, including large imbedded objects and deep puncture wounds, 2) open fracture wounds, 3) wounds that open joint spaces, especially on the hand or foot, and 4) severe wounds from bites and/or from animals that might be rabid.

General Wilderness Burn Management

Burns are among the most painful and emotionally distressing of injuries. Even relatively minor burns may disrupt the wilderness experience of an individual or an expedition. Although burns may result from electricity, radiation, and chemicals, wilderness burns most often result from high heat sources: 1) scalding hot water, 2) open flames, e.g., campfires, camp stoves, or 3) hot objects, e.g., pots. Typically minor, burns may also occur from lightning strikes (SEE CHAPTER 20: LIGHTNING). The most common wilderness burn is a radiation burn from solar rays (sunburn), seldom a serious injury (SEE CHAPTER 31: COMMON SIMPLE WILDERNESS MEDICAL PROBLEMS).

Initial Burn Management

1. *Stop the Burning Process.* The faster the better, within 30 seconds, if possible. Burns can continue to injure tissue for a surprisingly long time. No first aid will be effective until the burning process has stopped. Smother flames, if appropriate, then *cool the burn with water.* Remove clothing and jewelry from the burn area. Do not try to remove tar or melted plastic that has stuck to the wound. If a large percentage of the patient's body has been burned, monitor for hypothermia after cooling.
2. *Manage the ABC's.*
3. *Assess for Associated Injuries,* e.g., fractures, lacerations.
4. *Evaluate the Burn* (depth, extent, pain).

Patient Assessment

Every aspect of burn treatment depends on your assessment of the depth and extent of the injury. Even though this assessment may be an estimate, it will be your basis for deciding how the patient will be managed, whether evacuation is required, and how urgently.

Burn Assessment

Depth	Superficial	Partial Thickness	Full Thickness
Skin Layer	Epidermis	Epidermis/Dermis	All Layers
Color	Bright Red	Red to pale	Pale (for scalds), Charred (for open flame)
Blisters	None	Large, fluid-filled	Dry
Pain	Mild to moderate	Severe	Dull to severe
Healing	Spontaneous 3-5 days	Spontaneous 1-3 weeks	Very slow
Scarring	None	Moderate	Severe

Extent

Use the Rule of Nine's: Each arm represents approximately nine percent of a person's total body surface area (TBSA), each leg 18 percent (the front of the leg nine percent, and the back of the leg nine percent), the front of the body's trunk represents 18 percent TBSA, and the back of the trunk 18 percent, the head represents 9 percent, and the groin one percent. For infants and small children, the head represents a larger percentage and the legs a smaller percentage.

For smaller areas, use the Rule of Palmer Surface: the patient's palmer surface equals about one percent TBSA

Pain

In addition to depth and extent, do not underestimate the value of pain as a burn assessment tool. If the patient is in a lot of pain, that is an indication of the need for a physician's care.

General Management Of The Patient

1. Keep the patient warm. When skin is lost, so is the patient's ability to thermoregulate. Hypothermia will increase the chance of shock.

2. Elevate injured parts.
3. Get the patient to drink as much fluid as he or she will tolerate, unless the patient complains of nausea. Vomiting should be avoided, if possible.
4. Remember: An unconscious patient is unconscious from something other than the burn.

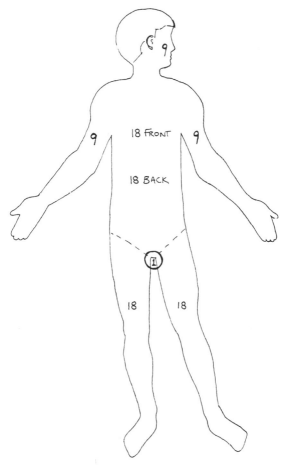

Figure 15-6: Rule of nines

General Management Of The Burn

Caring for the wound itself is often the least important aspect of burn care. All burn wounds are sterile for the first 24 to 48 hours. Burn management is aimed primarily at keeping the wound clean and reducing the pain.
1. Gently wash the burn with slightly warm water and mild soap. It is highly preferable to use an antibacterial soap. Pat dry.

Remove the skin from blisters that have popped open, but do not open blisters. Gently wipe away serum and obvious dirt.
2. Dress burns with a thin layer of antibiotic ointment. Silvadene® cream, a prescription medication, seems to work especially well.
3. Cover the burn with 2nd Skin®, a commercially available product, instead of ointment if the

burn is small enough, or cover with a thin layer of gauze, or apply clean dry clothing. Burns on the face, neck, and hands may be left open to the air. Covering wounds reduces pain and evaporative losses, but do not use an occlusive dressing.
4. When evacuation is imminent, do not re-dress or re-examine the injury. But if evacuation is dis-

tant, re-dress twice a day by removing old dressings, re-cleaning (and removing the old ointment), and putting on fresh ointment and a clean dry covering. You may have to soak off old dressings with clean tepid water.

5. Do not pack wounds or patients in ice. Do not leave wet coverings on burns for very long.

6. Elevate burned extremities to minimize swelling. Swelling retards healing and encourages infection. Get the patient, as much as possible, to gently and regularly move burned areas. Continue regular range-of-motion movement until healing is complete.

7. Ibuprofen is probably the best over-the-counter painkiller for burn pain, including sunburn.

8. If you have no ointment, no dressings, and/or no skill, leave the burn alone. The burn's surface will dry into a scab-like covering which provides a significant amount of protection.

Guidelines For Evacuation

While not a matter of urgency, patients with burns that hinder the ability to participate in and/or enjoy the wilderness experience should be evacuated. Superficial burns, even extensive ones, rarely require evacuation. Partial thickness burns covering less than 15 percent TBSA should receive definitive care, but seldom warrant rapid evacuation.

Full thickness burns need definitive medical care to heal best, but do not usually require rapid evacuation unless they are extensive. Partial and full thickness burns covering more than 15 percent TBSA are a threat to life, requiring rapid evacuation. Any serious burn to the face—indicated by obvious burns, scorched facial hair, black tongue, a dry cough—

may have burned the patient's airway, and should be considered for rapid evacuation, as well as deep burns to genitals, hands, and/or feet. Circumferential burns, burns extending completely around a part of the body, typically swell to the point where circulation is impaired distal to the burn. Circumferential burns warrant immediate evacuation.

General Infection Management

Infection, the multiplication of harmful microorganisms in tissues of the body, is a major cause of death worldwide. In the United States, death from wound infection has been virtually eliminated by the administration of antibiotics. In a wilderness environment, however, organisms invading open wounds added to less than ideal wound cleaning techniques may create a serious and potentially life-threatening infection.

Inflammation

As a wound heals, an unseen barrier develops on the inside of the body, sealing off the wounded area. White blood cells attack entrenched germs that have worked their way inside. Much of the contamination that migrates to the surface and drains out as

white or faintly yellow pus is composed of white blood cells that died in the line of duty.

Some of the contamination is dumped internally into the lymphatic system and carried to lymph nodes where it is picked up by the patient's circulatory system and eventually cleaned out of the blood and excreted from our body. The wound wonderfully maintains itself. This complex body process is called *inflammation*. The wound looks a little red and swollen, feels a little warm and tender. The wound may itch.

Infection

If the bacteria trapped in a wound are too abundant for the inflammation process to handle, infection will occur. The redness

becomes redder, the warmth becomes heat, the swelling continues, and tissue begins to harden past the borders of the wound. Pus will increase in amount and darken in color, typically appearing white, then yellow, then green, then brown. Pain may become great, and mobility of an extremity may be limited. These signs and symptoms usually show up in 24 to 48 hours, but they can develop days after the accident. On the other hand, gas gangrene, the result of an anaerobic bacterium that produces rapidly spreading tissue destruction, can cause death in as little as 30 hours. Gangrenous wounds stir up an abundance of dark, foul-smelling pus.

As infection spreads, lymph nodes can grow large and painful as they attempt to catch and kill the contamination, a condition known as *lymphadentitis*. The principal nodes are located in the elbows and knees, neck, groin, and along the mid-to-lower backbone. Less common in infected wounds, *lymphangitis* produces the red streaks that sometimes appear just under the skin. The streaks move from the wound toward the nearest lymph node as lymphatic vessels become inflamed. Should the infection reach the bloodstream, the result will likely be *septicemia*, some-times called "blood poisoning," and the possibility of life-threatening shock.

Some wounds are more susceptible to infection than others. Wounds on the hand commonly become infected, largely due to less than ideal circulation normally flowing to hands. Flesh torn open by the teeth of animals has a high rate of infection, the bites of cats and humans being especially prone. Infection is likely to result from crushing injuries, burns that open the skin, and severe frostbite. Heavy for-eign body contamination is responsible for many infections, as with an unnoticed splinter of wood buried in a foot or hand.

Any infection, whatever the source, produces similar signs and symptoms once it spreads throughout a human body. The patient develops a fever with accompanying chills and malaise, a fever that typically maintains a temperature of 102 degrees F or higher. Serious infections often cause headache, nausea, vomiting, and/or back pain.

Treatment

1. Open the wound and clean it thoroughly. Soaking the wound in hot water, water as hot as the injured person can tolerate, may be very helpful in the cleaning process. Hot compresses may also stimulate the wound to drain. If scabs have formed, they will have to be removed.

2. Pack the wound open with sterile gauze or clean cloth boiled to make it as sterile as possible. The inner dressings should be wet, the outer ones dry.

3. Provide rest, warmth, a soft or liquid diet, and a high fluid intake for the patient.

4. Give non-steroidal anti-inflammatory drugs, such as ibuprofen, or aspirin, or acetaminophen for fever and pain.

5. Stronger pain killers, if available, are usually indicated.

6. Antibiotics may be indicated if they are available and if the evacuation will be prolonged. A physician should be consulted prior to a wilderness trip for advice on antibiotics.

Guidelines For Evacuation

Rapid evacuation is advised for any patient who does not respond promptly to treatment for infection.

Conclusion

Assuring yourself your tent mate's blood loss is inconsequential, you gather supplies. After putting on protective gloves, you gently but aggressively wash the foot, especially the big toe, clean with soap and water. With an irrigation syringe and plenty of drinkable water, you irrigate the wound clean, lifting the avulsed flap of skin in order to flush as much contamination from the wound as possible. You pat the toe dry with sterile gauze. Smearing tincture of benzoin compound along both edges of the avulsion, you use wound closure strips to secure the avulsed flap as close to its normal anatomical position as possible. After cover-ing the wound with antibiotic ointment, you apply sterile gauze to the site, taping it in place.

Following a brief condemnation of your tent mate for not listening to your sage advise about slipping on his boots before slipping outside, you settle down and try to get back to sleep.

Chapter 16:   Cold-induced Emergencies

You should be able to:

1. *Describe thermoregulation and its relationship to cold-induced emergencies.*

2. *Define and describe the signs and symptoms of hypothermia, frostbite, and immersion foot.*

3. *Demonstrate the treatment for hypothermia, frostbite, and immersion foot.*

4. *Describe the prevention of hypothermia, frostbite, and immersion foot.*

It could happen to you

Heading toward an unnamed lake high in North Cascades National Park of Washington, a June drizzle begins to fall. You've let yourself grow a little out of shape, and you fall behind on the trail, behind Mark who forges ahead. The rain's chill begins to penetrate your clothing, but you can't stop to put on rain gear—you'll fall even further behind. Besides, it's not that cold.

You stumble, almost losing enough balance to hit the ground. For a moment, the rush of adrenaline warms you, but that passes quickly as you move on. You'd like to take a break, and dig out a candy bar. Mark will be worrying about you. You press on. Your water bottle lies forgotten in an outside pocket of your pack.

At last, the surface of the lake spreads out before you, dimpled by rainfall. Mark is already setting up the tent. You drop pack and try to help, but your hands don't seem to work right.

"Never mind," Mark says. "Put on your rain parka."

You fumble your rain gear out of your pack and struggle into it, but you can't get the parka zipped up. Shivers have begun to shake you. Mark zips up your parka, and returns to tent set up, a look of concern wrinkling his forehead.

By the time the tent is set, you have begun to tremble violently, uncontrollably. You hear Mark suggest you crawl into your sleeping bag, but his words have lost importance. You sit and stare through your shivers at the yellow dome-shaped domicile.

Introduction

As a warm-blooded species, humans have the ability to function well in a great variety of environmental conditions, maintaining a core temperature of approximately 98.6 DEGREES F (37 DEGREES C). *Thermoregulation*—heat regulation—is the key to this successful environmental adaptability. Human thermoregulatory centers are located at the base of the brain in the hypothalamus, centers that regulate heat production and heat loss, especially heat loss. The hypothalamus is strongly influenced by nerve impulses from receptors in the skin, and by the temperature of the blood flowing through the receptors. Thus skin is intimately involved in the maintenance of core temperature. Under the direction of the brain, skin has the ability to lose excess heat if the core temperature begins to rise, or to conserve heat if the core temperature begins to fall.

The thermoregulatory centers do their best to balance heat production against heat loss. Heat conservation mechanisms, however, are not as well developed as heat shedding mechanisms. Humans work well in warm climates but survive in cold climates only by using their brains to plan and perform ways to conserve body heat. This means wilderness adventurers are more predisposed to cold-induced emergencies than heat-induced emergencies (SEE CHAPTER 17: HEAT-INDUCED EMERGENCIES). When the thermoregulatory system can no longer maintain an adequate core temperature, life-threatening situations may arise.

Heat Production

There are two major internal sources of heat. Even as you sit quietly reading this book, you are making heat via basal metabolism, the energy necessary to sustain your life at complete rest. The *basal metabolic rate* (BMR) is the constant rate at which a human body consumes energy to drive chemical reactions and produce heat to maintain an adequate core temperature. BMR keeps the core at around 98.6 F (37 C). Food and water are the fuels that are burned, in the presence of oxygen, to maintain the BMR.

When you start doing anything powered by your voluntary muscles, a second heat source kicks in, *exercise metabolism*. Strenuous exercise metabolism may produce 15 to 18 times the amount of heat of basal metabolism, depending on your level of fitness.

In addition to internal heat production, the human body can absorb heat from external sources, from things such as the sun, a fire, another warm body, and, a little bit, the ingestion of hot drinks.

You end up with far more heat than you need on an average day and, if you couldn't shed the excess, you would literally cook in your own juices.

Heat Loss

Four mechanisms allow heat to be lost from the skin. *Conduction* describes heat lost from a warmer object when it comes in contact with a colder object. The most extreme form of conductive heat loss occurs when your warm body falls into icy cold water. On a very hot day, you may not be able to shed heat via conduction, and you might even gain heat from the environment. *Convection* describes heat lost directly into the air. An extreme form of convective heat loss on a cold day is defined by the wind-chill factor which says, essentially, the faster the wind blows, the faster you lose heat into the air. In this case your warm body has heated the air surrounding it, but that warm air is replaced by cold air blowing across it. On a hot day with no wind, you will not shed heat via convection, and, even with a breeze and 92 degrees F ambient temperature, you may not lose heat. *Radiation* describes heat given off constantly by a warm object. You persistently lose some heat into the environment, but you lose it fastest into a black body, e.g., a cloudless night sky. On a cold night you can shed a massive amount of heat via radiation; on a hot, sunny day you can effectively stop losing heat via radiation. *Evaporation* describes the process of a liquid changing into a vapor. As water evaporates it requires energy to convert from a liquid to a gas. In this case the energy is heat, and the evaporation takes place on your skin. This is your most important cooling mechanism.

Hypothermia

When a body loses heat to the environment faster than it can produce heat, the body's core temperature starts to drop—a condition called *hypothermia*. Hypothermia is encouraged by inadequate hydration, insufficient nutritional intake, and fatigue, all common ingredients in a wilderness trip.

Acute Hypothermia

Immersion or submersion in cold water may cause the sudden onset of *acute hypothermia*, an emergency arising in several minutes to perhaps an hour, depending on the temperature of the water (SEE CHAPTER 19: IMMERSION AND SUBMERSION INCIDENTS).

Chronic Hypothermia

The slow onset of *chronic hypothermia*, a condition that takes days to months to show obvious signs and symptoms, is typical of the elderly and often poor and/or homeless who are exposed to less than adequate environmental temperatures. Almost never a wilderness medical problem, the loss of core temperature is so slow some individuals will reach the stage of severe hypothermia without demonstrative shivering (SEE BELOW).

Sub-Acute Hypothermia

Called "exposure" in the "old days," *sub-acute hypothermia*—generalized hypothermia, mountain hypothermia, exposure hypothermia—usually requires an exposure time of at least several hours, perhaps a day or more. Although you might think cold is the dominant environmental factor in sub-acute hypothermia, it is the combination of cold and wet that poses the greatest threat. Well documented are serious cases of hypothermia in Florida and Baja, usually when rain falls under a high wind. Undoubtedly one of the leading causes of wilderness emergencies, sub-acute hypothermia impairs the level of judgment and blunts natural protective instincts.

Mild hypothermia has been termed by some experts as "a case of the umbles": the patient fumbles, grumbles, stumbles and, later, mumbles. Fine motor skills, such as zipping up a parka, decrease. The patient begins to draw inward, becoming less and less sociable. As gross motor skills are affected, a stumbling gait begins. Designed to function optimally at approximately 98.6 degrees F (37 degrees C), the brain will begin to malfunction when its temperature drops below the ideal. In the case of hypothermia, normal thought processes become impaired. Mild hypothermia could be termed "mild stupidity." Patients begin to make poor decisions such as not putting on rain gear when rain begins to fall. Patients typically show increasing confusion and apathy. Mild hypothermia is insidious, affecting the ability of the patient to think, to be aware of its onset, to take care of self.

When the brain first senses heat loss is gaining on heat production, it stimulates the primary defense mechanism against further heat loss—vasoconstriction of the peripheral circulation

(shrinking of the blood vessels in the skin). This vasoconstriction dramatically slows blood flowing to the surface of the skin where it will lose heat into the surrounding environment. The lack of blood causes the skin to become pale and cool.

**Signs and Symptoms
Mild Hypothermia:**
1. Loss of fine motor skills
2. "Mild stupidity"
3. Lack of sound judgment
4. Confusion
5. Apathy
6. Pale and cool skin

If the core temperature continues to fall, the brain will stimulate the muscles to contract and relax—to shiver—a form of involuntary exercise designed to consume energy and produce heat without requiring voluntary work. An average core temperature at the start of shivering is 95 degrees F (35 degrees C). When shivering starts, the patient enters the realm of *moderate hypothermia*. In an effort to rewarm, if the core temperature drops further, the brain will increase the intensity of shivering until it becomes violent. A patient will find it increasingly difficult to speak, to walk, to think. Lack of circulation to the surface of the body may cause the skin to turn a dusky color.

**Signs and Symptoms
Moderate Hypothermia:**
1. Uncontrollable shivering
2. Slurred speech
3. Increased confusion
4. Increased stumbling
5. Cold and pale (perhaps dusky) skin.

Shivering requires an immense amount of energy. If the moderately hypothermic patient is not properly treated, heat rushes from the patient into the environment. Radiative heat will soar into the sky from an uncovered head. Heat will conductively flood into the ground from a uninsulated patient. A breeze will rip heat away via convection. Drop in core temperature will be rapid for an unprotected shivering patient.

When energy stores are depleted, the patient can no longer sustain shivering, a point reached when a core temperature measurement would typically reveal approximately 90 degrees F (32 degrees C). When shivering stops, the patient enters *severe hypothermia*, a condition characterized by increasing muscular rigidity, stupor progressing to unconsciousness, and cold, cyanotic skin. The patient's respiratory rate will slow down and grow so shallow that it may not be detectable. Although the heart rate speeds up, sometimes dramatically, during the phase of rapid temperature loss, it will slow and weaken to the point where it may no longer be palpable in a patient with severe hypothermia. *A severely hypothermic patient may appear dead and yet be alive.*

If you cannot detect breathing, you should begin rescue breathing for a cold patient. If you cannot detect a pulse, you should not immediately begin chest compressions (SEE CHAPTER 5: CARDIOPULMONARY RESUSCITATION).

Note: Core temperatures are approximate and must be taken rectally to be considered of value. Taking rectal temperatures to measure degrees of hypothermia in the wilderness requires a hypothermia thermometer, one that registers lower than a usual thermometer, and is impractical at best. At worst, the process may dangerously expose an already cold patient. It is recommended to use obvious signs and symptoms in determining the treatment for hypothermia instead of rectal measurements. In other words, if someone appears cold, warm him or her up.

> **Signs and Symptoms Severe Hypothermia:**
> 1. Cessation of shivering
> 2. Low level of consciousness
> 3. Muscle rigidity
> 4. Slow and/or non-palpable respirations and pulse
> 5. Cold and cyanotic skin

Treatment Of Hypothermia

Mild/Moderate Hypothermia

For the mild and moderate hypothermia patient, the most important treatment is to change the environment from cold and wet to warm and dry:

1) Immediately replace damp clothing with dry clothing. Remember: The moisture in a hypothermia patient's clothing may not be moisture you can feel. It is safest to assume the patient's clothing is damp. 2) Add extra insulation under and around the patient. 3) Add a windproof/waterproof layer and/or place the patient within shelter from wind and water. Once the patient is thickly bundled in dry insulation, he or she will rewarm. The addition of heat, such as an open fire (when environmentally acceptable and possible), may increase patient comfort psychologically, but it does not increase the rate at which the bundled patient rewarms. A patient violently shivering will rewarm to a normal core temperature without additional heat when he or she is adequately protected against losing the heat being manufactured by shivering. The addition of almost any heat, especially to skin, suppresses shivering, and you do not want to suppress shivering. Shivering inside dry insulation is the fastest trail to rewarming.

The addition of heat via snuggling with a warm rescuer did not increase the rate of rewarming in laboratory tests. In the wilderness, cold patients may *seem* to rewarm quicker when they snuggle inside a couple of sleeping bags with one or two warm bodies. Whether or not the snuggled patient and rescuer or rescuers should be naked versus lightly clothed remains somewhat controversial. Skin to skin transfers heat quicker, but rescuers and patients alike often report feeling more comfortable in light clothing such as long underwear. Light clothing limits moisture transfer, probably the reason for greater comfort.

The addition of heat via heat packs or hot water bottles does increase the rate at which hypothermia patients rewarm. This heat may be applied to neck, armpits, and/or groin, but it works best when applied to palms of hands and soles of feet. This heat should not be applied directly to skin since heat damage may occur on cold skin. Some type of dry material, such as a bandanna, should separate the heat pack from direct contact with skin.

In the absence of adequate dry insulation, you may be limited in your treatment to the addition of external heat sources such as huddling with warm rescuers, building a fire, etc.

A mildly hypothermic patient may be encouraged to exercise once he or she has donned dry clothing. A moderately hypothermic patient typically have too little coordination to be exercised safely, although he or she may be able to perform simple exercises such as sit-ups within a sleeping bag.

To stoke the inner fire of mild and moderate patients, give water and food. Water is probably more important to the patient in the initial stage of treatment. Caffeine and alcohol should be avoided. Food intake should be encouraged, especially simple carbohydrates—sugars—which the body will assimilate most quickly. Warm, sweet liquids, such as a cup of warm Jello®, serve with excellence, adding fluid and simple carbohydrates to the patient.

As long as the patient returns to normal, an evacuation is not required. The patient, however, is often exhausted, requiring a rest day to rehydrate and refuel.

Do not risk a return to a hypothermic condition by pushing a recovered patient to expend too much energy too soon.

Severe Hypothermia

Supplemental oxygen would be of great benefit to the unconscious patient with severe hypothermia. Slow respirations and slow heart rate lead to an insufficiency of oxygen, the eventual cause of brain death. If supplemental O_2 is unavailable, mouth-to-mouth (or mouth-to-rescue mask) breathing, started when breathing is undetectable or barely detectable, may help keep a severely hypothermic patient alive. Cold and stiff and blue? The patient needs O_2. Supplemental oxygen, or at least artificial respirations, should be started as soon as possible, before you aggressively move the patient, even before removing the clothing. Oxygen will give a cold heart a better chance of survival during movement.

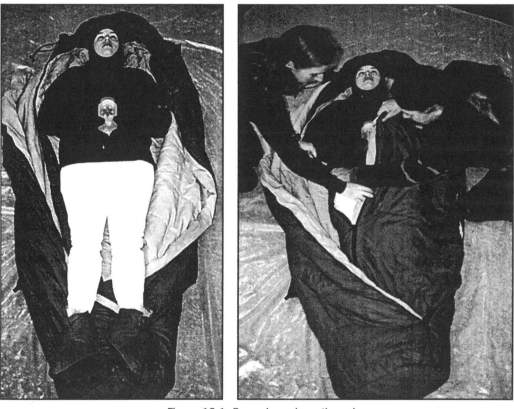

Figure 16-1: Preparing a hypothermia wrap.

Otherwise the severely hypothermic patient gets the same initial treatment as for mild and moderate hypothermia—change the environment—but with the additional requirement of extra gentle handling. Rough handling may actually cause the patient's heart, fragile from the cold, to stop. Gently remove clothing and surround the patient in dry insulation. The thicker the insulation, the better for the patient. If snow or rain is involved, take great care to keep the insulation as dry as possible. Insulation such as sleeping pads must adequately protect the patient from the ground. For maximum results, an occlusive layer—windproof and waterproof—should surround the entire bundle of patient and insulation. The occlusive layer may be a rainfly, a tarp, a sheet of plastic, even large garbage bags. The resulting cocoon, leaving only the patient's face exposed, has been termed a *hypothermia wrap*. Even though it is extremely unusual for a severely hypothermic patient to return to a normal core temperature in the wilderness, he or she has the possibility of surviving a relatively long time, perhaps a couple of days, within an adequate hypothermia wrap. Once again, heat packs may be added, especially to palms of the hands and soles of the feet. Beware of exposing the severely hypothermic patient to extremes of external heat, e.g., open fires, prior to enclosing the patient within a hypothermia wrap. Too much external heat

may drive cold peripheral blood full of metabolic waste products to the cold heart and precipitate cardiac arrest. If evacuation of a severely hypothermic patient is delayed, it is recommended that two rescuers snuggle with the patient inside the hypothermia wrap during the wait. Place the patient in a stable side position, and place a rescuer on each side of the patient.

Note: All hypothermia patients may continue to drop a little in core temperature after you've started treatment, a phenomenon called *afterdrop*. You can't prevent it, but you can be as efficient as possible in your treatment to reduce the effects of afterdrop to a minimum.

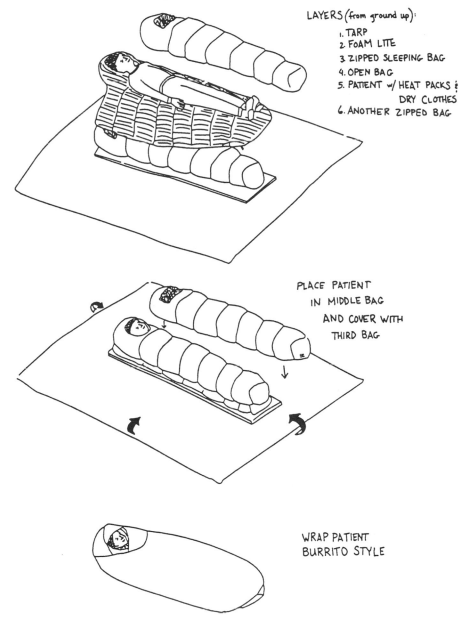

LAYERS (from ground up):
1. TARP
2. FOAM LITE
3. ZIPPED SLEEPING BAG
4. OPEN BAG
5. PATIENT w/ HEAT PACKS & DRY CLOTHES
6. ANOTHER ZIPPED BAG

PLACE PATIENT IN MIDDLE BAG AND COVER WITH THIRD BAG

WRAP PATIENT BURRITO STYLE

Figure 16-2: Hypothermia wrap

Prevention Of Hypothermia

1. Know the environment in which you intend to travel, and travel prepared to prevent hypothermia with adequate clothing, gear, food, and water.
2. Stay well hydrated and well fed.
3. Wear layers of clothing, taking off layers prior to sweating, adding layers back on prior to losing heat.
4. Pace yourself and your group to avoid overexertion with resulting sweat, fatigue, and loss of stored energy.
5. Make sure all members of your party understand hypothermia, and watch each other for early signs and symptoms.

Frostbite

Frostbite is localized tissue damage caused by freezing, a problem most likely to occur at the extremities of the body: ears, nose, fingers, toes. It creates a spectrum of injuries depending on how cold the tissue becomes. Ranging from little or no damage to extensive damage resulting in substantial tissue loss, this spectrum of injuries can be classified in three basic categories: superficial, partial thickness, and full thickness.

Predisposing factors related to frostbite include moisture, low ambient temperatures (which must be below freezing for frostbite to occur), high winds (which speed heat loss), dehydration, and poor nutrition.

True frostbite occurs in two phases, the freezing phase and the rewarming phase. During the freezing phase, blood flow decreases, and ice crystals form in the fluid between cells which draws fluid out of cells, dehydrating them. More damage can occur mechanically as the ice crystals rub against each other. As blood clots form in blood vessels, circulation diminishes causing more destruction. During the rewarming phase, substances are released by the damaged cells that promote clot formation and vasoconstriction, further damaging tissue.

Superficial Frostbite

The initial stage of injury can be termed *frostnip*, considered by some experts to fall short of a true frostbite injury. Skin is white, perhaps waxy, numb, cold to the touch, but still soft and pliable. On rewarming, no damage may be apparent. The outer layer of skin may have been frozen, and may turn red and later peel as sunburn peels. Superficial frostbite is, in fact, similar in physiology to a superficial burn (SEE CHAPTER 15: SOFT TISSUE INJURIES).

Frostnip is rewarmed optimally by submerging the affected body part in warm water, water heated to 104 to 108 degrees F (40 to 42 degrees C). If the water circulates around the affected part, even better. In the wilderness, however, warm water is often impractical, at best, but skin-to-skin rewarming is safe and effective. The cold skin should be in contact with warm skin. For example, a cold finger can be cradled in a warm armpit, or cold feet placed against a warm belly. Do not massage cold tissue, or place it near a strong radiant heat source, both of which may increase damage.

Every attempt should be made to prevent refreezing the area. Ibuprofen will ease pain and speed healing. Aloe, applied topically, may aid in healing.

Partial Thickness Frostbite

The first true frostbite is partial thickness frostbite, an injury affecting a partial thickness of the skin, similar to a partial thickness burn. Some signs and symptoms of a partial thickness injury mimic a superficial injury: Skin white, waxy, numb, cold to the touch. The affected skin, however, will feel harder than frostnipped skin, and it will dent when you push on it. The dent may linger.

As with superficial frostbite, rewarming should be accomplished by submerging the affected part in warm water (104 to 108 degrees F/40 to 42 degrees C) to maximize healing. Skin-to-skin thawing is acceptable in the wilderness. Once again, no massage, no strong radiant heat, give ibuprofen, and use aloe when it is available.

When partial thickness frostbite is rewarmed, a fluid-filled blister, sometimes called a bleb, forms. Blebs can form in minutes to hours, perhaps as long as 48 hours, after rewarming. Bleb formation is often the deciding factor in whether you are treating superficial or partial thickness frostbite. If the fluid is relatively clear, the damage to tissue did not go very deep, and hope for the patient's tissue is generally high. Only a little skin, perhaps, will be lost. If the fluid filling the bleb is reddish, the damage penetrated deep, into the vasculature, and the loss of tissue will probably be higher. If the fluid is deep red or reddish-blue, the damage is significant, and substantial loss of tissue is likely. Blebs should be protected with dry dressings. Care should be taken to prevent rupture of the blebs which turns closed wounds into open wounds. Ruptured blebs should be covered with antimicrobial ointment and sterile dressings. All care should be taken to prevent refreezing of blebs. Since circulation is impaired, tissue that has been thawed suffers more extensive damage when it refreezes. If you can keep the affected part elevated above the level of the patient's heart, you may improve the outcome for the patient.

Full Thickness Frostbite

If frostbite is not treated in the partial thickness state, it can progress to full thickness frostbite, sometimes called *deep frostbite*. Deep frostbite can be recognized because the affected area is colorless and frozen solid. It may be described as "wooden" by the patient. Full thickness damage feels icy cold to the rescuer, and completely numb to the patient.

It is impossible in the wilderness to detect how far freezing has extended into the tissue. In other words, a toe might be only frozen solid on the surface, or it might be frozen through the bone. Proper treatment might save part of an extremity.

This type of severe frostbite is extremely painful when rewarmed, too painful to use. Severely frostbitten feet, once rewarmed, typically prevent the patient from walking, a consideration when the patient must then be carried from a remote and frigid environment. Instead of rewarming, it is usually best to insulate the frozen tissue well to prevent any further freezing or rewarming, and then evacuate the patient as rapidly as possible to definitive care.

Note: Controversy and complications surround the wilderness management of full thickness frostbite. It is not known how long tissue can be kept frozen without increasing the damage, but it is strongly suspected that destruction of tissue is related to length of time frozen. Furthermore, keeping deep frostbite frozen is far from easy. Since frostbite often occurs in association with hypothermia, the treatment for hypothermia often causes the frostbite to thaw. Treatment for hypothermia must take precedence since it creates a potential threat to life. With an otherwise healthy patient, even the heat generated by activity during an evacuation may be enough to slowly thaw deep frostbite. Perhaps the best that

can be said is this: You should try to keep deep frostbite frozen until you've reached the best situation possible for rewarming.

In extreme situations, full thickness frostbite may be rewarmed in the field. Rewarming should be rapid without being damaging. The best method, as with less serious frostbite, involves soaking the frozen tissue suspended in circulating water pre-heated to 104 to 108 degrees F (40 to 42 degrees C). Too much heat should be carefully avoided. Too much time in the warm water is not a problem. You cannot "overthaw" but you can "underthaw." You'll need to monitor the temperature of the water. It cools off quickly, necessitating the addition of more warm water fairly often. Watch for indications of adequate rewarming: The flush of pink to the affected area, and the flush of severe pain on the patient's face. The skin will later turn deep red, perhaps cyanotic, or mottled. The black, dried, dead look of mummification may develop rapidly. Once rewarming is accomplished, the affected parts should be air dried, covered with an antimicrobial ointment, and kept elevated. Pain-killing drugs would benefit the patient. Ibuprofen may speed healing, and should be given to the patient prior to thawing. Refreezing must be avoided. Trauma, even mild trauma such as walking on thawed feet, must be avoided. Evacuation of the patient should be given priority consideration.

Prevention Of Frostbite

1. Wear adequate cold weather clothing, including boots, and keep it all as dry as possible.

2. Avoid constricting clothing, especially tight boots.

3. Wear mittens instead of gloves.

4. Avoid skin contact with cold metal and cold gasoline, both of which could cause frostbite on contact.

5. Stay well hydrated.

6. Maintain a high calorie diet.

7. Watch other party members for the early signs of frostbite including white patches on the face.

8. Pay attention to your fingers and toes, and stop and treat frostbite early, while it still causes tingling and pain, and before it goes numb.

Immersion Foot

Immersion foot, or trench-foot, is a common cold weather, non-freezing injury resulting from prolonged contact with cold and moisture that causes inadequate circulation with resulting tissue damage.

Trenchfoot is divided into three phases. Phase one, the pre-hyperemic phase, or just-before-increased-blood-flow phase, is the period of time when blood vessels are contricted by the cold and wetness inside the shoe or boot, and too little oxygen is carried to the cells of the foot. When you check the foot, it is cold to the touch, there may be a bit of swelling, and discoloration is evident (usually white or bluish). The patient may complain of numbness or tenderness. When the foot is rewarmed, the damaged tissue usually looks red, and feels sensitive, and the discomfort may last from hours to days. This phase can occur in less than 12 hours of exposure.

Phase two, the hyperemic phase or increased-blood-flow phase, is the period when the cells of the foot have become damaged by the lack of adequate circulation, the blood vessels open back up, and the tissue swells with excess fluid. Patients complain of tingling pain that never lets up. A foot check will reveal swelling. On rewarming, blisters form, and, later, ulcers where the blisters have fallen off revealing dead tissue underneath. In severe cases, gangrene will result. Suffering may last from two to six weeks, and medications for pain are often prescribed. This phase typically takes at least 12 hours of exposure to occur.

Phase three, the posthyperemic or recovery phase, may last weeks to months. The swelling subsides, and the foot takes on a normal appearance once again. During this phase, the patient may complain of increased perspiration in the foot, increased sensitivity to cold, and varying degrees of pain, itching, and paresthesia (a creeping, tingling, prickly feeling). The damaged foot may be more susceptible to cold injury in the future.

Here's what should be done if you think you, or a companion, are developing trenchfoot. Stop and carefully dry the cold foot or feet. If the foot looks dirty, carefully wash it before drying it. Keep it elevated above the level of the foot-owner's heart while you gently rewarm the foot with passive skin-to-skin contact. No rubbing or placing the foot near a strong heat source such as a fire or stove, both of which can damage the tissue of the cold foot. Start the patient on a regimen of over-the-counter anti-inflammatory drugs (aspirin or, even better, ibuprofen), following the directions on the label. Remember it will probably take 24 to 48 hours before the severity of the damage is fully apparent. If you end up with a painful, obviously swollen foot that develops blisters, that patient needs the attention of a physician. Whether or not that patient can walk out to a physician will be determined by the patient.

Trenchfoot is encouraged by poor nutrition, dehydration, wet socks, inadequate clothing, and the constriction of healthy blood flow in the feet by too-tight shoes and socks. Make sure your boots fit with plenty of room for the socks you choose to wear. Keep a dry pair of socks on hand at all times, preferably packed in a plastic bag to make sure they stay dry. Don't add more socks if your feet get cold—get bigger boots, or boots with more insulation, or add insulation to the outside of your boots with gaitors. People who sweat heavily are more susceptible, and an antiperspirant spray can reduce sweating and thus reduce the risk of trenchfoot. Periodically, preferably twice a day, dry your feet and gently massage them before stuffing them back into boots. Do not sleep in wet socks.

Evacuation Guidelines

Any patient treated for mild or moderate hypothermia who recovers may safely stay in the wilderness. Any patient treated for severe hypothermia requires rapid yet gentle evacuation. A patient with frostbite who develops blebs and/or dusky or blue-gray skin should be evacuated. A patient who is assessed with full thickness frostbite should be evacuated. Most patients with immersion foot, unless the problem is mild, should be evacuated.

Conclusion

In North Cascades National Park, Mark helps you into the tent. Unrolling a sleeping pad, he fluffs out your sleeping bag while you fumble ineffectively with your clothing. Mark has to help you undress and wiggle into dry pile pants and pile sweater. Once you've crawled into your sleeping bag, your friend spreads his bag over you for additional insulation. He leaves the tent, returning soon with your wool stocking cap, the one you left lying unused in your pack.

Firing up the stove, Mark brings water to a boil, pours a cup, drops in a bag of peppermint tea and two teaspoons of sugar. By the time the tea is ready, your shivers have diminished to an occasional tremor. You sit up and gratefully sip the tea, feeling assured you'll see tomorrow's dawn.

Murray Hamlet, DVM, contributed his expertise to this chapter.

Chapter 17:   Heat-induced Emergencies

You should be able to:

1. *Describe the signs, symptoms, treatment, and prevention of dehydration.*

2. *Describe the signs and symptoms of heat cramps, heat exhaustion, and heat stroke.*

3. *Demonstrate the treatment for heat cramps, heat exhaustion, and heat stroke.*

4. *Describe the prevention of heat cramps, heat exhaustion, and heat stroke.*

It could happen to you

The group you're guiding on this August trip down the Wild and Scenic Chattooga River looks a little older than your average clients, but their enthusiasm is undiminished by age. You raft past the point in the Ellicott Rock Wilderness where Georgia, North Carolina, and South Carolina meet. Although the movement of the raft you're oaring, one of two rafts traveling together, creates a breeze that makes you feel relatively cool, you know the high temperature, somewhere in the 90s, and high humidity, not far behind the temperature, are sending your body's need for water skyrocketing. You lean on an oar, unclip your water bottle from where it rides near at hand, and take a big swig. You told the clients to drink up throughout the day during your pre-put-in talk, and you hope your example is noticed.

Towards mid afternoon, however, jovial David, an overweight man in his late 50s, quick to laugh, doesn't seem as jovial any-more. He begins to act strange—slightly disoriented and very argumentative. He states rather firmly that he is hot, tired, and very thirsty. By the take-out, David becomes more disoriented and combative, insinuating, in a nasty way, that you've ruined his day. His skin looks unusually red. On shore he begins to halluci-nate, swinging at invisible large black birds. He is convinced the birds are "going for my eyes."

Introduction

Of the two environmental temperature extremes, heat and cold, the human body is better adapted at dealing with heat. With virtually hairless skin filled with abundant sweat glands, powered by a cardiovascular system of marvelous endurance, humans function well when the mercury rises. You are not, however, a foolproof design. Over-heating can ruin your day—and your life.

To understand heat illness requires an appreciation of the fundamentals of human ther-moregulation, body heat produc-tion vs. body heat loss (SEE CHAPTER 16: COLD-INDUCED EMER-GENCIES). As the body core tem-perature begins to rise, the excess heat is absorbed by the blood. As the thermoregulatory centers in the brain detect the increase in blood temperature, the brain causes the peripheral circulation, the vasculature of the skin, to dilate, or open up. This dilation of peripheral vascula-ture increases blood flow to the skin where the blood can be cooled. At the same time, to fur-ther increase the rate of heat loss from the skin, the brain stimu-lates the sweat glands to produce sweat. The evaporation of sweat from the skin increases the rate of cooling many times. As long as you can sweat and the sweat can evaporate, you can continue to cool efficiently. If for some reason, either the sweating mechanism begins to fail or the sweat cannot evaporate, then the cooling mechanism will fail. On hot, very humid days, for instance, cooling becomes extremely inefficient because sweat cannot evaporate, and it is relatively easy to overheat.

Sweat consists primarily of water with some electrolytes, specifically sodium and chloride ions which are necessary for normal body function. It is this combined water depletion—*dehydration*—and electrolyte depletion that forms the basis of a spectrum of problems with one general name: Heat illness.

Dehydration

Without water, there could be no life—at least no life as you know it. As a developing embryo, you nestled in a watery bed and your body weight averaged around 80 percent water, an average that dropped to approximately 74 percent by birth. As an adult, you gurgle along at somewhere around 62 percent water overall, and healthy blood, the red tide of life, surges at between 85 and 90 percent water.

Water puddles inside every one of your cells, and flows through the microscopic spaces between cells. In water, oxygen and nutrients float to all parts of your body, and waste products are carried away. When your kidneys remove wastes from your body, those wastes have to be dissolved in water. Digestion and metabolism are water-based processes, and water is the primary lubricating element in your joints. You even need water to breathe, your lungs requiring moisture to expedite the transfer of oxygen into blood and carbon dioxide out of blood. Sweat, as mentioned, is mostly water. The water in your blood carries heat from warmer body parts to cooler areas of your anatomy when you are exposed to cold. In short, if you aren't well hydrated, you won't be able to stay healthy, maximize your performance, or even maintain joy at being outdoors.

The water in your body, the fluid that keeps you alive and active, leaves you at an alarming rate. Estimates vary widely, but an average person at rest on a normal day loses between two and three liters of water. One to one-and-a-half liters rushes out as urine, and another one-tenth liter in defecation. Moisture is lost from the act of breathing, more than half a liter per day, and that rate increases in dry winter air.

Then there's sweat. The fluid lost in perspiration can climb to one to two liters per hour during periods of strenuous exercise. Compared to watching TV all day, one hour of exercise may demand approximately a 50 percent increase in the amount of water your body uses.

How can you tell you're running low on water? At first the signs are subtle. You'll get a mild headache, and then start feeling tired. Down merely one-and-one-half liters, your endurance may be reduced 22 percent and your maximum oxygen uptake (a measure of heart and lung efficiency) can be lowered 10 percent. And your thirst mechanism, that feeling of "Gosh, I need a drink of water", doesn't kick in until you're about one to one-and-one-half liters low. Down three to four liters can leave your endurance decreased to 50 percent and your oxygen uptake reduced close to 25 percent. By now, if you're observant, you'll have noticed your urine has turned a dark yellow. You may suddenly find yourself seriously dehydrated: Disoriented, irritable, rapid pulse, completely pooped.

Dehydration can be classified into three levels.

MILD: dry mucous membranes (lips and mouth), normal pulse, darkened urine, mild thirst.

MODERATE: very dry mucous membranes, rapid and weak pulse, darker urine, thirst.

SEVERE: very, very dry mucous membranes, an altered level of consciousness (drowsy, lethargic, disoriented, irritable), no urine, no tears, and shock (indicated by rapid and weak pulse, rapid breathing, and pale skin).

Heat Cramps

On the minor end of the spectrum of heat-induced emergencies are heat cramps, a painful spasm of major muscles that are being exercised. Heat cramps are often associated with heat exhaustion (SEE BELOW). Those most often cramped are people unacclimatized to heat who are sweating profusely. Heat cramps are poorly understood, but probably result not only from the water lost in sweat, but also the salt lost in sweat. Rest, and gentle massage and stretching of the affected muscles usually provides relief. Drinking water, preferably with a pinch of salt per liter added, is advisable. Heat cramps do not often occur in someone who is adequately hydrated. Once the pain is gone, exercise may be continued. If the cramps return and/or worsen, a day of rest with adequate water and food is the recommended treatment.

Heat Exhaustion

Heat exhaustion is characterized by headache, dizziness, nausea, rapid pulse, rapid breathing, and, of course, exhaustion. Dehydration is the primary threat, and the patient is experiencing the early stage of shock, compensatory shock (SEE CHAPTER 7: SHOCK). Thirst is a common complaint. Sufferers are so sweaty they often feel cool, grow goose bumps, and complain of chills. Core temperature may or may not be elevated.

Treatment should include 1) changing the patient's environment from hot to cool, e.g., moving the exhausted person to a shady spot, pouring water on his or her head, fanning, and 2) orally rehydrating the patient with water, preferably with a pinch of salt and, perhaps, a couple of pinches of sugar. Some experts prefer using an electrolyte-balanced drink such as Gatorade®, but the drink should be watered-down three or four times for more rapid absorption in a resting person. It will take about an hour to get a liter of fluid back into circulation. Heat exhaustion is not physiologically damaging, but it should be treated aggressively before it progresses to a more serious condition.

Signs and Symptoms Heat Exhaustion:
1. Headache
2. Dizziness
3. Nausea
4. Increased heart rate
5. Increased respiratory rate
6. Fatigue
7. Thirst
8. Pale, cool skin

Heat Stroke

On the serious end of the spectrum lies heat stroke, a problem that kills approximately 4000 people in the United States every year, a true life threatening emergency. Death has been known to occur within 30 minutes of assessment.

There are two varieties of heatstroke. In *classic heat stroke*, the patient is usually elderly or sick, or both. Temperature and humidity have been high for several days, and the patient has dehydrated to the point where his or her heat loss mechanisms are overwhelmed. You might say the patient simply ran out of sweat. Skin gets hot, red, and dry. He or she lapses into a coma and, if untreated, dies.

In the wilderness, you are far more likely to encounter the second variety, *exertional heat stroke*. The patient is usually young, fit, and unaccustomed to heat, sweating but producing heat faster than it can be shed. Signs include, primarily, a sudden and very noticeable alteration in normal mental function: Disorientation, irritability, com-bativeness, hallucinations or bizarre delusions, incoherent speech. Skin is hot and red, but wet with sweat. Rapid breathing and rapid heart rates are almost universal. Loss of coordination and, later, seizures are common. Clinically speaking, the patient's core temperature has risen to at least 105 degrees F (40.5 degrees C), and this rise in core temperature is the primary threat. Cardiovascular and neurologic collapse, if they haven't happened already, are imminent.

**Signs and Symptoms
Heat Stroke:**

1. Altered level of consciousness
2. Increased heart rate
3. Increased respiratory rate
4. Loss of coordination
5. Seizures
6. Hot, red, wet skin.

Rapid cooling is required to save the patient's life, and the best method includes removal of clothing, covering with wet cotton clothing, and vigorously fanning, all of which increases evaporative heat loss. Massaging of arms and legs, and ice packs at the neck, groin, and armpits increase heat loss. Easing the patient into cold water is less effective and often dangerous since she or he is difficult to manage, and may drown. In the absence of an abundance of water, concentrate on cooling the head and neck of the patient. The process of cooling is often lengthy.

Since heat stroke patients are dehydrated, rehydration is critical. Unfortunately, getting the patient to drink is typically impossible due to the decreased level of consciousness. With impaired mental condition, it is inappropriate to force fluids. Continue cooling externally in hopes the patient will recover enough to begin oral rehydration.

Heat stroke patients should be seen by a physician as soon as possible, which means a rapid evacuation, when possible, is appropriate. During the evacuation, the cooling process may have to be maintained. With a patient who seems to have recovered, too much internal heat can cause breakdowns in some body systems that show up later, a cause for evacuation even if your treatment appears successful. Since relapses into heat stroke are not uncommon for recovered patients, all patients should be closely monitored until he or she is turned over to a physician.

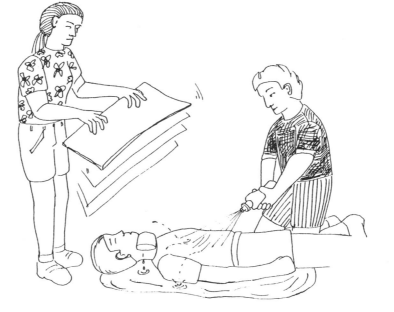

Figure 17-1: Patient being cooled

Prevention

Since internal water is used faster than the need for replenishment is felt, water should be consumed at a disciplined rate. There's considerable benefit from starting each day with an ingestion of a large volume of water, about half a liter. Following that, the International Sportsmedicine Institute recommends one-half to two-thirds ounce of water per pound of body weight per day, ingested periodically throughout the day. Figured in liters, that's about three to four liters per day for the average-sized person. Drink water with meals and snacks, to encourage digestion, and suck down a few swallows before bedtime to replace what you'll lose in sleep.

You should be pounding down water on an even more disciplined schedule when you travel outdoors. Since the human body can only absorb so much water at one time, the rate of ingestion should be matched, as closely as possible, to the rate of absorption. Most people fall into a rate-of-absorption range of one-quarter liter per one-quarter hour. That means, for maximum efficiency and well-being, drink about one-quarter liter of water every 15 minutes during periods of exercise. In some conditions you will lose water faster than you can replace it. In those conditions, rest breaks, during which fluid is consumed, become important.

Fluid has to get out of your stomach and into your small intestine to be absorbed. Some research indicates cold water, water at a temperature in the low 40s F, is emptied from the stomach at a higher rate than water at other temperatures. Ten years ago it was widely accepted that, if a drink contained more than two or three percent sugar, the rate of emptying from the stomach was considerably slowed and, thus, absorption was slowed. Current research has shown that, even though stomach emptying is slowed somewhat by sugar, the absorption rate from the small intestine is increased by slightly sweetened drinks. Tests indicate that a drink of six to eight percent sugar (specifically glucose, maltodextrin, or sucrose) gets absorbed as fast as plain water during periods of hard exercise with the added benefit of supply-ing energy for improved physical performance. Fructose ingestion does not seem to improve absorption or performance.

A balanced diet meets even the most active person's requirements for electrolytes, but there are small advantages to having a tiny bit of salt in a drink when you're active. For one, salt helps you retain water during exercise and, for another, salt stimulates the need to drink. Too much salt, of course, would be counter-productive, causing you to need more water than normal. "Sports drinks," with measured amounts of sugar and salt, are commercially available almost everywhere.

Note: Salt tablets are too concentrated, and should be avoided. They draw water into the stomach to dilute the salt, while the sufferer needs the water out in the circulatory system where it is used to help maintain a normal core temperature.

There are some beverages that, even though they contain water, just don't work well, and may be counter-productive, for hydration. Caffeinated drinks, such as coffee, stimulate fluid loss through urination. Three cups of coffee supply only about two cups of water to your body. Alcohol is a toxin that draws water out of your cells to "water down" increasing blood toxicity. You must drink eight ounces of plain water just to balance one ounce of alcohol. Fruit juices contain too much sugar to meet your body's demands for fluid during exercise.

You cannot train yourself to need less water. In fact, the harder you work, the more water you need. To prevent dehydration, follow these recommendations:

1. Drink a half-liter of water first thing each morning.

2. Drink one-fourth liter of water or a sports drink every 15 to 20 minutes during periods of hard exercise.

3. Drink water with meals and snacks to ensure adequate digestion.

4. Keep track of your fluid consumption and drink at least three to four liters of water every day.

5. Drink even more in winter, when your need is great and your thirst mechanism at its most sluggish.

6. If you drink alcohol, chase it with plain water, approximately eight ounces of water per ounce of alcohol to maintain hydration.

7. Monitor your urine: Clear and copious describes normal, healthy urine output.

As a group leader, maintain a pace that allows everyone to adapt to the heat. If anyone feels the symptoms of heat exhaustion coming on, the group is going too fast. It is especially important to maintain a gradual pace early in the hot, humid season. The thermoregulatory system will become more efficient as it gets used to hot weather. It takes approximately 10 days to two weeks for a human body to adapt to heat and humidity. Remember: The elderly, the very young, the very muscular, and the very overweight take longer to acclimatize to heat.

Take a break during the hottest part of the day, the middle afternoon hours. Wear cotton clothing that lets air pass through and sweat evaporate. Wear a brimmed hat or cap that provides shade for face and head.

Avoid drugs known to contribute to heat induced emergencies: alcohol, antidepressants, antihistamines, some anesthetics, cocaine, and amphetamines.

Guidelines For Evacuation

Evacuate all patients treated for heat stroke, even if the patient appears to have recovered. Patients successfully treated for heat cramps and/or heat exhaustion need not be evacuated.

Conclusion

With the help of other clients on the Chattooga River, you take control of David, lowering him to the ground in the shade of a tree near the bank. He is wearing shorts, a T-shirt, and a PFD. Removing the PFD, you soak David with water from the river. Using the PFD as a fan, you aggressively fan the patient.

Under your direction, two other clients remove their PFDs and join the fan club. You direct a third client to keep pouring water over the patient, and a fourth client to massage David's arms and legs.

When the second raft arrives, you ask the second guide to call for help immediately on the radio waiting in the company van parked at the take-out. David's signs and symptoms show no improvement, and you know you'll be aggressively cooling him until medical assistance arrives.

Chapter 18:   Altitude Illnesses

You should be able to:

1. *Define and describe acclimatization.*

2. *Describe the signs and symptoms of acute mountain sickness, high altitude pulmonary edema, and high altitude cerebral edema.*

3. *Describe the treatment for acute mountain sickness, high altitude pulmonary edema, and high altitude cerebral edema.*

4. *Describe ways to prevent altitude illnesses.*

It could happen to you

You're at the airport in Gunnison, CO. The plane brings clients from Florida, California, New York, and Texas—six excited teenagers. After a brief welcoming speech, you load the van and drive the group to the camp you work for near Crested Butte, CO, at an elevation of over 9,000 feet above sea level.

On the morning of the second day of the week-long experience, after lessons in hiking and camping, after lessons in outdoor cooking, after lessons in expedition behavior, you lead your group out of camp toward the really high country. The hike is washed in sunshine, and the group stays together well. No

stragglers. You set tents and establish a cooking area on bare ground near the edge of an alpine meadow at 11,200 feet.

On the third morning Ashley asks for a private conversation. She slept poorly. Her nausea erupted into vomit just before dawn. Her head "throbs."

"I can't go on," she says.

Introduction

The medical problems collectively referred to as "altitude illnesses" are the result of hypoxia, insufficient oxygen in the blood for normal tissue function, a result of the decreased barometric pressure at higher altitudes. When you go up, the barometric pressure goes down, the concentration of oxygen in the air decreases, and the chance of altitude illness climbs.

Since there is a measurable increase in ventilation and

decrease in aerobic exercise performance above 4,000 feet elevation, "high altitude" can be said to start at that point. Complications seldom occur, however, below 8,000 feet. In defining terms, consider 8,000 to 12,000 feet as high altitude, 12,000 to 18,000 as very high altitude, and 18,000 plus as extreme high altitude. At 18,000 feet the barometer reads one half that of sea level, making the inspired pressure of oxygen also one half. You effec-

tively get 50 percent less oxygen with each breath.

The human body will adjust to dramatic changes in barometric pressure, given enough time. Altitude illnesses—which range from mildly disturbing to completely fatal—are determined, primarily, by three factors: 1) how high the patient goes, 2) how fast the patient attains a specific altitude, and 3) predisposing factors such as genetics and previous upper respiratory illnesses.

Acclimatization

The rate of *acclimatization*—the process of physiologically adjusting to altitude—differs with individual physiology and the specific altitude attained, but most people will adjust enough to prevent illness if they spend two to three days in the 8,000 foot to 12,000 foot range, and not gain more than 1,000 feet of sleeping altitude each successive day. For instance, if you slept at 14,000 feet last night, you can climb beyond 15,000 feet the next day, but you should drop back down to no more than 15,000 feet to sleep. Critical to acclimatization is adequate hydration and nutrition. Climbers in camp who mix rest with periods of light exercise seem to acclimatize faster than climbers who rest only.

Acclimatization is a complex physiological process, but, in general:

The first stage of acclimatization, and the most important means of adjustment, is increasing ventilation. Heavy breathing increases the oxygen content of the blood, thus getting more oxygen to body tissues. Remember: It is okay to pant. This stage starts immediately with full acclimatization for a specific altitude taking six to eight days.

In the second stage, the heart rate speeds up and systemic blood pressure increases. After approximately seven to 10 days at a specific altitude, heart rate and blood pressure decrease, but never return to sea level values.

The third stage is a stimulation of bone marrow to produce more red blood cells, which increases the capacity of blood to carry more oxygen, and the final stage occurs on a cellular level with capillary density increasing, muscle cells shrinking, and mitochondria—the intracellular "furnaces" where food is burned in the presence of oxygen to create energy—increasing. These cellular changes get more oxygen into action quicker and easier.

It takes about six weeks to reach 90 percent of maximum of red blood cell production at a specific altitude. On the average, however, 80 percent of overall acclimatization is complete at ten days, but 95 percent is not reached until six weeks.

Acclimatization is lost at approximately the same rate as it is gained—significant loss at two weeks, most of it lost by six weeks—but the main point is this: If you take time, you will almost always adjust to higher altitudes.

Acute Mountain Sickness

All altitude illnesses are degrees of the same inability to adjust to lower concentrations of oxygen in the air. The most common form of altitude illness—sometimes called *acute mountain sickness* or AMS—produces symptoms that can appear in as little as six hours and usually within 48 after a rapid ascent to an altitude of 8,000 feet or more, and ranges in severity from mild to moderate in the grand scheme of debilitation. Headache is the first complaint. Other symptoms include *anorexia* (loss of appetite), nausea, *insomnia* (inability to sleep), *lassitude* (in this case, psychological weariness), and unusual fatigue. Vomiting may occur. Patients are typically short of breath on exertion, a shortness of breath that quickly goes away with rest. Skin may become cyanotic (bluish to purplish).

Peripheral edema, swelling of the face, hands, or feet, may or may not accompany AMS. A patient may show signs of peripheral edema without showing any significant other signs or symptoms of AMS.

AMS does not cause physiological damage, but the signs and symptoms do indicate that the patient is not acclimatized to a specific altitude.

Signs and Symptoms AMS:
1. Headache
2. Anorexia
3. Nausea
4. Perhaps vomiting
5. Insomnia
6. Lassitude
7. Unusual fatigue
8. Shortness of breath on exertion

Note: The signs and symptoms of AMS could also indicate dehydration, hypothermia, infection, carbon monoxide poisoning, a hangover, a drug overdose, and other problems. A patient at high altitude, however, should always have AMS considered as a possible problem.

Ataxia

Ataxia is a loss of muscular control leading to difficulty in maintaining balance. A simple check for ataxia calls for the patient to stand straight up with his or her boots pressed together, with hands pressed into the sides of the thighs, with eyes closed. If the patient wobbles or starts to fall, and has to open his or her eyes to regain balance, the patient is ataxic. You may also ask the patient to walk a straight line touching the heel of the front boot to the toe of the back boot with each step. If the patient can't walk the line, the patient is ataxic. *Ataxia is the single most useful sign indicating the patient is progressing from a mild/moderate altitude illness to a severe altitude illness.*

High Altitude Pulmonary Edema

The most common severe form of altitude illness, the form most often causing death, is *high altitude pulmonary edema* (HAPE), an illness that typically shows up within three days of reaching a specific altitude. Fluid, for reasons not totally understood, seeps out of the pulmonary (lung) capillaries and begins to fill the alveolar spaces. The patient begins to drown.

A patient with HAPE develops shortness of breath unrelieved by rest. Breathing is often accompanied by gurgling sounds audible to the naked ear, especially in later stages of the illness, caused by the fluid in the lungs. In earlier stages of the illness, you may hear the sound as "crackles" through a stethoscope. The sound appears most often in the right side of the chest, but commonly on both sides, and without a stethoscope can sometimes be heard with an ear pressed against the chest wall of the patient. As fluid continues to collect in the lungs, the patient develops a cough, dry at first but increasingly productive, eventually producing a frothy, pink-with-blood sputum. The heart rate will increase, and skin is typically cyanotic. Chest pain may be expected as a complaint. Fluid may build up to the point where the patient suffocates to death.

Signs and Symptoms HAPE:
1. Shortness of breath (even at rest)
2. Crackling and/or gurgling breath sounds
3. Increasingly productive cough
4. Increased heart rate
5. Chest pain

High Altitude Cerebral Edema

In a case of high altitude cerebral edema (HACE), fluid collects around the patient's brain (cerebrum). HACE and HAPE may occur in a patient at the same time. While HAPE typically develops over a longer period of time, HACE can appear suddenly—seemingly within minutes—and kill quickly.

Ataxia may be dramatic with HACE patients. Even sitting up may be impossible. A severe headache should be expected with HACE, a constant throbbing unrelieved by rest and/or medication. Lethargy, weakness, and vomiting are common. As pressure on the brain continues to increase from fluid build-up, watch for severe personality changes including hallucinations and combativeness. Seizures, unconsciousness, coma, and death may follow.

Signs and Symptoms HACE:
1. Ataxia
2. Headache
3. Lethargy
4. Weakness
5. Vomiting
6. Personality changes
7. Coma

Treatment For Altitude Illnesses

Since you can't predict who will deteriorate from mild to severe altitude illness, a patient must stop ascending until the symptoms resolve. It is at this point the majority of life-threatening mistakes are made. The Important Rule is: *Don't ascend until the symptoms descend*. The dead are almost universally among those who broke the Important Rule.

Light exercise increases respiratory drive, and may relieve mild symptoms of AMS. In 24 to 48 hours, a healthy person will usually adjust enough to a given altitude to relieve the symptoms of acute mountain sickness.

Acetazolamide, e.g., Diamox®, is a drug that almost always speeds the resolution of mild to moderate acute mountain sickness. The drug, available in the United States by prescription only, is also taken to prevent mild altitude illness, which it does effectively for most people without masking the symptoms of severe altitude illness—in other words, acetazolamide has not been proven to prevent HAPE or HACE. It increases the rate of breathing and, thus, increases arterial oxygen. If you plan to carry and use acetazolamide, do so under the supervision of a physician, and ask about side effects, e.g., numbness or tingling

in the lips and fingertips. A patient treated successfully with acetazolamide may continue to ascend, but the patient's symptoms should improve before continuing to ascend. It is recommended that the patient keep taking the drug for the duration of the climb.

For any patient with ataxia, immediate descent is recommended. For any patient with a headache that grows worse despite rest and ibuprofen or another painkilling drug, immediate descent is recommended. For any patient with increasing shortness of breath at rest, immediate descent is recommended. Descend 1,000 to 3,000 feet, or until the patient notices relief of symptoms.

If your assessment is HAPE, immediate descent is the treatment of choice. In addition to descent, the patient will best be served by supplemental oxygen. Nifedipine, e.g., Procardia®—a drug that reduces blood pressure in the pulmonary system—may be given according to prearranged instructions from a physician.

If descent is delayed, the patient will probably benefit greatly from being placed in a portable hyperbaric chamber such as the Gamov Bag. Igor Gamow (pronounced Gam-off), in the mid 1980s, developed a portable hyperbaric chamber for use at high altitude. The device is an elongated bag made of sturdy nylon. The increased internal pressures achieved with a simple foot pump simulate descent of several thousand feet, relative to the real altitude. The device is lightweight and easy to transport when folded into a small carrying bag. Though oxygen is not used to inflate the bag, a patient can receive supplemental oxygen while undergoing "descent" within the bag. There are even windows so that a stricken mountaineer will not suffer as much from claustrophobia during treatment. Hyperbaric treatment should be used to prolong life until descent is possible, and *not* to allow unhealthy climbers to keep ascending.

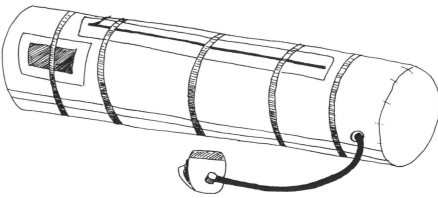

Figure 18-1: Gamov Bag

If your assessment is HACE, immediate descent is critical. Dexamethasone, e.g., Decadron®—a steroid that may reduce

pressure on the brain—may be given according to prearranged instructions from a physician. A portable hyperbaric chamber

may also be of great benefit to a patient with HACE.

Prevention

As mentioned earlier, most people will adjust to altitude given enough time. Staged ascent is the key to acclimatization and, therefore, the key to preventing altitude illnesses. Above 10,000 feet, most people should gain no more than 1,000 feet of sleeping altitude per 24 hours (SEE ABOVE ACCLIMATIZATION). As a group leader, pace your group to the speed of the slowest acclimatizers.

Adequate hydration is critical to the prevention of altitude ill-nesses. You should drink enough water to keep your urine output clear and copious.

A high calorie diet is essential for the energy needed to ascend and acclimatize. A diet of 70 percent or greater carbohydrates, since they require less oxygen to metabolize, may aid in the prevention of altitude illness, but probably will not serve much in terms of prevention under 16,000 to 17,000 feet.

Avoid respiratory depressants, such as sleeping pills and alcohol, especially during the first two or three days at high altitude.

Training that is going to prepare you for altitude must be done at altitude, but physical fitness prior to ascent is a bonus in the game of safety and enjoyment. Fitness does not, however, protect against acute mountain sickness. Fitter persons may actually be more susceptible, almost undoubtedly because they tend to go up too fast.

Evacuation Guidelines

Immediate descent should be initiated for any patient suffering altitude illness associated with ataxia, HAPE, and/or HACE. If the patient recovers from the illness upon descent, further evacuation to definitive medical care is not required.

Conclusion

Near the alpine meadow above Crested Butte, CO, you ask Ashley to stand straight and tall, to press her palms into the sides of her thighs, to press her feet together, and to close her eyes. She easily accomplishes the task without the slightest loss of balance. Ashley has no difficulty breathing, and her breath sounds, to your naked ear, are normal.

Instead of gaining more altitude today, you decide to spend a second night at this camp, and use the day to teach skills scheduled for higher up. You encourage Ashley to hydrate, strongly suggesting she drink at least four liters of water during the day. You remind her how important it will be for her to eat well, even though she may not feel hungry. You tell her she will feel better, and acclimatize quicker, if she is active around camp today. You plan to monitor Ashley throughout the day, ready to descend if her condition deteriorates, but your confidence is high that this trip will continue.

Colin Grissom, MD, contributed his expertise to this chapter.

Chapter 19:   *Immersion & Submersion Incidents*

You should be able to:

1. Describe the safest approaches to an immersed or submerged person.

2. Describe the treatment for immersion hypothermia.

3. Demonstrate the treatment for a drowned person.

4. Define a near-drowned person, and describe the treatment for a near-drowned person.

It could happen to you

Another oppressively hot, sultry, summer day, and you're enjoying the shade cast by a old oak along the shore of a quiet pond in southeastern Arkansas. Your cane pole extends out over the clear water, the bobber at the end of the line unmoving, the worm on the hook undoubtedly having gasped his last breath long ago.

Three boys, maybe high school age, maybe younger, have given up on the fish, and now dive delightedly into the cool water. When you look up at a cry from across the water, you see two of the boys on shore, gesturing wildly.

About six body lengths from shore, turbulence in the still water catches your attention. A dash around the small pond, and you walk into the water, carrying a long stick you picked up from the edge of the forest. You'll reach with the stick, offering it to the boy if you find him capable of grasping it.

You find him sure enough, just below the surface, his foot caught in a tangle of submerged roots. You detect no movement. Releasing the stick and diving in, you are able to free the boy and swim with him to shore, dragging him the last few yards of shallows. Face up on the shore, the boy remains unresponsive.

Introduction

A patient whose nose remains above the surface of the water—a patient, in other words, who can breathe—is someone experiencing immersion. A patient whose nose has been below the surface of the water for a substantial amount of time—a patient who cannot breathe—is someone experiencing submersion. In recent years drownings, deaths following submersion incidents, have ended approximately 9,000 lives every 12 months in the United States, keeping it second or third as a cause of accidental death. Almost all the deaths had one thing in common: The victims never intended to be in the water. They planned to stay in the boat or on shore.

Several other factors related to deaths-by-drowning shed a bit of light on why some of them died. 1) Many of the dead were non-swimmers. 2) Most of the drowned victims were not wearing personal flotation devices (PFDS). 3) Some of them were whitewater paddlers not wearing helmets who hit their heads on the way down. Some of them were wearing helmets and hit their heads on the way down.

4) At least one study estimates that more than half of the dead had alcohol or some other mind-altering substance "on board." 5) Immersion hypothermia, the loss of core body temperature and the resulting loss of coordination from being immersed in cold water, was a factor in a large number of drownings (SEE BELOW). 6) Males drown far more often than females with males outnumbering females 12-to-1 in boating related drownings.

Near-drownings, submersion incidents in which the patient survives the underwater experience for at least 24 hours, have increased to the point where an estimated 80,000 will occur this year.

Perhaps the most sobering estimate accompanying immersion and submersion incidents is this: Many of the dead or permanently debilitated, some experts guessing as many as six out of seven, could have been saved by immediate and proper actions by rescuers.

Few, if any, rescue scenes carry more risk for the rescuers than an immersion or submersion incident. The water threatening the life of your intended patient may suddenly threaten your life. The scene is not safe until all persons are safely out of the aquatic environment. An appropriate order of events determining how you attempt to rescue the patient from the water should be Reach, Throw, Row, Tow, Go. *Reach* first to a struggling immersed person from a secure position. If you can't reach him or her with your arm or leg, extend your reach with a stick, paddle, piece of clothing, etc. If your reach is not long enough, *Throw* the person something that floats. He or she may be capable of swimming to shore with the aid of flotation. If throwing does not work, you may be able to *Row* or paddle to the person in a stable water craft, or you may be able to toss a line to the person, and *Tow* him or her to safety. To *Go*, swimming to a drowning person, is to risk your life. Panic lends the struggling person great physical power and determination. Go only if you are well trained and capable.

Immersion

Sudden immersion in very cold water may precipitate an acute type of hypothermia, *immersion hypothermia*, that comes on quickly, usually in minutes to less than an hour, depending on the temperature of the water, the size of the patient, what the patient is wearing, and other factors. In general, the patient should receive proper treatment for hypothermia (SEE CHAPTER 16: COLD-INDUCED EMERGENCIES). In addition to standard hypothermia treatment, the cold water immersion patient should be handled gently, even though he or she may be conscious and capable of walking, and should be dried and well insulated before being exposed to high external heat sources. Well documented are cases where extremely cold patients have been pulled from icy water only to die when they were placed immediately in very warm environments. A possible explanation is that rapid external rewarming drove potassium rich, cold blood to the hearts of the patients, causing the hearts to stop.

On rare occasions someone will suddenly die after being thrown into frigid water, a problem sometimes called *immersion syndrome*. The cause of death, not exactly understood, may be a reaction of the heart to rapid cooling, or the inhalation of icy water, or a combination. The amount of time someone can remain under cold water and still recover is often surprising, especially if the patient is very young and the water is very cold. In July of 1988, near Salt Lake City, Utah, a two-and-a-half year old girl was submerged for approximately 66 minutes in a frigid mountain creek. When she was found, CPR was started and continued in route to the hospital. With surgical intervention, she had a complete recovery.

Drowning

Those who die during a submersion incident typically go through a series of events that vary little from individual to individual. The person panics and struggles fiercely while holding his or her breath. The heart rate speeds up and the blood pressure rises. Involuntarily swallowing water is common. Swallowed water may or may not cause vomiting. The drive to breathe becomes overpowering, and the person inhales water. Most people have an involuntary constriction of the muscles of the upper airway, a *laryngospasm*, which keeps the water out of the lungs.

Asphyxia, an inadequate intake of oxygen, causes a loss of consciousness. Respiratory arrest and then cardiac arrest soon follow. At some point the laryngospasm relaxes, water enters the lungs and begins crossing cell walls, entering the blood stream. Persons whose lungs are full of water are referred to as "wet" drownings, and they comprise the majority of the drowned. Ten to 15 percent of drowned persons will have a secondary laryngospasm accounting for a "dry" drowning.

When the patient is pulled from the water, treatment must begin immediately. Artificial ventilation should start as soon as it is determined there is no breathing. Artificial breathing can even be done while the patient and rescuer are still in the water if the rescuer is stable. e.g., standing in shallows. At this writing, the Heimlich maneuver is not recommended as a means of clearing the airway prior to artificial breathing for drowned

patients. Just start breathing for the patient. Fresh water submersions have a statistically better chance of survival because the fluid moves more rapidly from the lung to the bloodstream. Salt water may even draw fluid from the blood into the lungs.

Once on a stable surface, e.g., land, a boat deck, determine if the patient's heart is beating. If it isn't, start chest compressions.

Cervical spine injury should be considered in some drowned patients, such as patients who have dived into shallow water, drowned while surfing, drowned by flipping a kayak or canoe in whitewater. Use the jaw thrust to open the airway, and treat for

spine damage if your CPR works (SEE CHAPTER 8: SPINE INJURIES).

Expect the patient to vomit. When vomit erupts, roll the patient immediately on his or her side, sweep out the vomitus, roll the patient back over, and continue CPR.

If you resuscitate the patient, treat for hypothermia. Hypothermia should be assumed in all immersion and submersion incidents, and the patient should be treated accordingly.

Note: Since a drowned patient is not rigid from the cold as in severe terrestrial hypothermia, chest compressions should never be withheld from the drowned patient without a pulse.

Near-drowning

A near-drowning is a submersion incident in which the patient survives the underwater experience for at least 24 hours, but does not necessarily go on to live a long, healthy life. Many near-drowning patients either swallowed and/or inhaled water. It takes very little water in the lungs to have profound effects on

the patient. Vital body fluids are washed out, and unhealthy material in the water is absorbed into the body. Pneumonia, tears in weakened lung tissue, chemical imbalances in the blood, and other related problems may result in death days, weeks, or months later. Some near-drowning patients suffered respiratory

and/or cardiac arrest and were resuscitated. Near-drowners will probably be hypothermic, and should be treated accordingly. Everyone who has almost drowned should be hurried to a medical facility as soon as possible to be evaluated by a physician.

Prevention

Many drownings are preventable accidents. All you add to the water is a few drops of sound judgment. What you save the potential patient from, according to those who describe "near misses," is something mighty unpleasant.

1. Learn to swim.

2. Avoid swimming, and diving, in unsafe areas.

3. Never swim alone.

4. Wear a PFD while in a water craft and, as a water-based trip leader, insist all party members also wear a PFD.

5. Do not ingest mind-altering substances prior to swimming or boating.

6. Cross wilderness rivers at safe fords with open run-outs, and

   a) post someone downstream to aid anyone washed into the flow,

   b) loosen pack straps and hip belt before crossing to make getting out of the pack easier for anyone who is washed into the flow,

   c) wear boots for better balance,

   d) use a long stick or pole as a "third leg" for balance, and/or

   e) cross in linked groups.

Evacuation Guidelines

Almost all patients should be evaluated by a physician following an accidental submersion incident, especially if the patient was removed unconscious from the water, required resuscitation, exhibits difficulty breathing, complains of shortness of breath, and/or reveals a history of lung disease. A patient remaining unconscious after a submersion incident should be evacuated as soon as possible.

Conclusion

On the shore of the small pond in Arkansas, you look, listen, and feel for breathing in the young man. Finding none, you give two full breaths, mouth-to-mouth. A pulse check at the carotid artery reveals a strong heart beat. You return to artificial respirations, blowing in one breath after the patient's chest deflates following the preceding rescue breath. Within moments, it seems, the patient sucks in a gasping rush of air on his own, and gags. You roll the young man onto his side just as vomit flies across the muddy shore.

Since he continues to breath on his own, you maintain him in a stable side position. One of the other boys retrieves your day pack from near where your fishing pole still rests on the opposite bank. Your jacket, brought just in case, now covers the nearly-drowned young man.

It's not far to your car, probably less than 200 yards. With the help of the other boys, you carry your patient to your car, and drive him to the nearest hospital.

Chapter 20: Lightning Injuries

You should be able to:

1. *Describe the mechanisms of lightning injuries including direct strike, splash, contact, ground current, and blast effect.*

2. *Describe the most common lightning injuries.*

3. *Describe treatment for the most common lightning injuries.*

4. *Describe how to reduce the chance of lightning injury to a minimum.*

It could happen to you

A July storm, rolling in around 1:30 AM, brings heavy rain and booming claps of thunder to your campsite near Carter Notch in the White Mountains of New Hampshire. After a particularly close lightning strike, one that splits a tall tree in half, you make a quick tent-by-tent check on your young clients. As you move toward the last tent, a scream shifts you into high gear.

"Help. She's dead! She's dead!"

You crawl into the tent, to the side of a 13-year-old girl. The flash of the next strike paints an eerie mosaic of shadow and light on her immobile features. Her head and left shoulder still lie off her sleeping pad where they had been when the ground current swept under the tent.

Introduction

Lightning occurs most often on hot days when warm, moist air rises rapidly to great heights forming dark clouds filled with static electricity. As a charge accumulates on the bottom of the cloud, an opposite charge develops on the top of the cloud and on the ground below the cloud. When the difference between charges reaches a potential greater than the ability of the air to insulate, lightning reaches out to equalize the difference.

The bolt of electricity is a direct current that may reach 200 million volts and 300,000 amps, with a temperature of 14,432 degrees F (8,000 degrees C). The bolt may reach out miles in front of a storm, perhaps more than seven miles (11.3 km), and move through a channel eight centimeters wide.

Lightning flashes out approximately eight million times per day worldwide, or 100 times per second. It can run inside the cloud, cloud-to-cloud, and ground-to-cloud, but the one most likely to cause injury to humans runs cloud-to-ground. Lightning kills more people in the United States every year than almost all other natural disasters combined, placing second only to flash floods. Injuries usually occur between May and September, and those who die are usually working or playing outdoors.

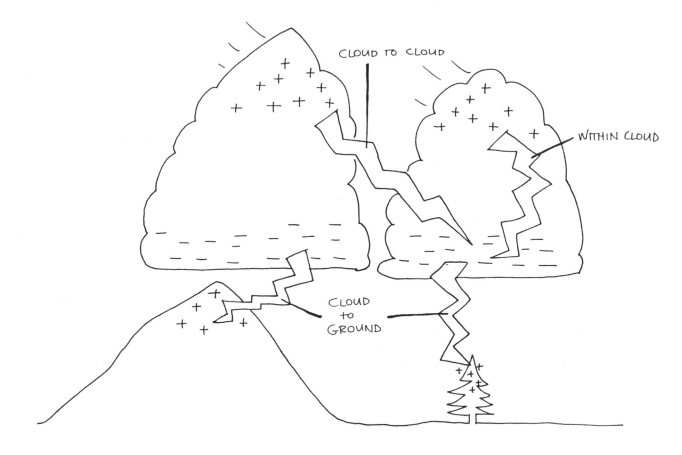

Figure 20-1: Lightning strikes

Mechanisms Of Injury

Injuries directly caused by a lightning strike may be classified in one of five mechanisms of injury:

Direct Strike: As the name implies, the bolt of lightning hits someone directly. Most often struck is a person out in the open—hikers crossing an alpine meadow, anglers on the shore of an exposed lake. Unable to find shelter, the person may become the tallest "object" around. The person is often standing near or in contact with a conductor, particularly a metal object such as an exterior-frame backpack, an ice axe, or a bicycle. If the metal object is carried at shoulder height or higher, the chance of attracting a direct strike is even greater. Direct strikes carry a large potential for death.

Splash or Side Flash: : The lightning strikes something more immediately appealing than the human, e.g., trees, shelters, but "splashes" through the air to hit someone whose body offers less resistance to the electrical charge than the object receiving the direct hit. Side flashes may occur from person to person.

Contact: Lightning, either by direct strike or splash, hits something with which someone is in direct contact.

Ground Current: : The electrical charge radiates out from the strike point either along the surface of the ground, similar to the way waves spread in circles from a rock thrown in a lake, or along conducting routes such as root systems or drainages wet from the rain that is probably falling. A person on the ground in line with the current may attract enough electricity to cause injury. Someone standing or walking with feet spread creates a "stride potential," encouraging the charge to enter one leg and exit the other.

Blast Effect: Although not an injury resulting directly from contact with electricity, the blast of the shock wave of air that explodes out from a near lightning strike can throw someone with enough force to cause traumatic injury.

Types Of Injuries

Virtually unpredictable in the ultimate effect lightning will have on a human body, lightning injuries vary from minor to major, including death.

Cardiac Arrest: The current of lightning upsets and sometimes stops the natural rhythm of the heart. If the heart is healthy, it often restarts on its own, but it may fail to start up again because it is too damaged, or it may restart and stop again if the heart suffers prolonged oxygen deprivation, i.e., the patient fails to start breathing again.

Respiratory Arrest: The area of the brain that controls respiratory drive and the muscles used for breathing have been shut down by the charge of electricity. This arrest of breathing may be prolonged, leading to a second cardiac arrest when cardiac activity spontaneously returned after an initial cardiac arrest.

Neurologic Injury: The patient is most often knocked unconscious by the charge, and some patients will suffer temporary paralysis, especially in the lower extremities. Seizures and/or the inability to remember what happened may result.

Burns: It is rare to have serious skin and muscle burns after a lightning strike, but superficial burns—linear, feathery, fernlike—are common. If the burn is deep and penetrating, the patient usually has much more to worry about than the burn. The treatment for lightning burns is the same as any burn treatment (SEE CHAPTER 15: SOFT TISSUE INJURIES).

Blast Injuries: The impact of the blast effect can cause just about any trauma you can imagine: Fractures, head injury, spinal injury, dislocations, chest and abdominal injuries.

Other Trauma: : Post-lightning strike patients complain most often of ringing in the ears, or loss of hearing, that usually resolves in hours to days without permanent damage. Rupture of an eardrum, however, is common, and deafness is not impossible. Ears may bleed. Temporary loss of sight is not unusual, but blindness is rare. Patients are often bothered by insignificant nausea and vomiting for a brief time.

Management

Two factors make the management of patients struck by lightning unique. One is the *triage* of multiple patients—the sorting of patients when a group has been injured—and the other is the efficacy of CPR. First, in standard triage, rescuers are taught to give priority to those still alive, and let the dead stay dead. It is the simple guideline of "the greatest good for the greatest number." After a lightning strike, however, the still, silent, dead patients are very often recoverable, and need to receive immediate attention. The moaning wounded can wait. If a patient does not suffer cardiopulmonary arrest, he or she will survive. Second, CPR done appropriately can bring many pulseless, breathless, post-lightning strike patients, perhaps as many as 80 percent, back to life since the patients are often simply "shorted out" and otherwise physiologically sound. Even if the patient has a pulse, rescue breathing is often required, sometimes for a prolonged period, to save the patient.

Beyond these two unique aspects, the basic management principles apply. When the scene is safe, perform an initial assessment followed by a focused assessment. Treat injuries as necessary.

Prevention

1. Know weather predictions and weather patterns for your intended region of wilderness travel. If storms are predicted and/or if storms typically strike, for instance, in mid afternoon, avoid lightning-prone areas when storms are most likely to occur.

2. Learn to read weather. A developing storm tends to move very fast. Clouds in the distance can be hanging over you, spitting lightning, with astounding suddenness. When you see the flash of lightning, start counting, "one one-thousand, two one-thousand," and so on until you hear

the thunder. Sound travels at approximately one mile per five seconds. If you get to "five one-thousand" and hear the boom, you are one mile from the storm. Lightning has been known to fatally strike a human six to seven miles (ten or more kilometers) ahead of a storm. Take preventive steps early.

3. Avoid likely target areas: a) a high exposed area, such as a ridge, b) an open area, such as an alpine meadow, c) on or near a large body of water, d) an isolated tall object, such as a tree, and e) metal objects, unless you can get inside the object, such as a truck or van.

Note: Paddlers, including sea kayakers, rafters, and other small craft operators should move to shore or well away from shorelines, at least 200 feet away, whenever possible. You may, however, find yourself in a narrow canyon without the possibility of moving well away from shore. If safe moorage is possible, it is still recommended to seek a shoreline since thunderstorms are typically accompanied by high and potentially dangerous winds. If safe moorage is not possible, the fact that the bottom of canyons are seldom struck by lightning is in your favor.

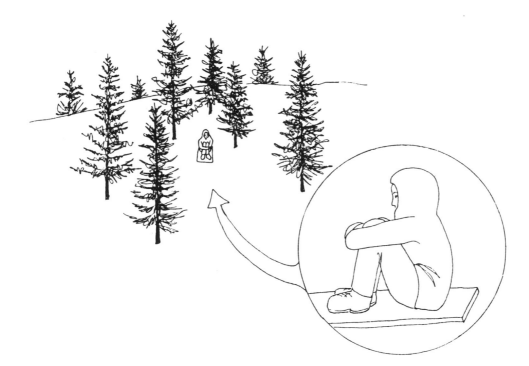

Figure 20-2: Lightning protection position

Note: Rubber tires on a car or truck do nothing to protect you. Since electricity stays on the outside of metal, taking the path of least resistance, being inside a car or truck does protect you.

4. Currents of electricity run like currents of water, from high to low, so stay out of ravines and other low spots that collect water. Deep dry caves are safe, but stay away from the entrance where lightning may jump the opening where water drips. Shallow wet caves and overhangs are generally considered unsafe.

5. Dense forest cover and thick stands of small trees of relatively uniform height should be considered your best bet for safety.

6. In a tent, stay completely on your sleeping pad and out of contact with the sides of the tent.

7. Lightning, ground current especially, can injure entire "huddled" groups. Spread groups out, at least several meters between individuals, to minimize the number who may be harmed by a strike and to maxi-

mize the number who may be able to respond to the injured.

8. Sit on your sleeping pad, or some other non-conductive object, and make yourself as small as possible. Huddled in a ball, keeping your feet close together, gives the least potential differences in the separate points of your body.

Lightning Demythed

1. Lightning *will* strike in the same place twice, and many more times than twice.

2. Lightning is *not* stored by a human body.

3. Lightning strikes *before*, during, and *after* a storm.

4. Lightning *can* cause serious internal injury while leaving no external signs.

5. Lightning *can* cause serious injury that doesn't show up until long after the strike.

Evacuation Guidelines

Evacuate survivors of lightning strikes even if no loss of consciousness occurred. Problems, especially problems involving the neurological system, e.g., mental and motor functions, can show up days later.

Conclusion

Near New Hampshire's Carter Notch, you kneel beside the 13-year-old girl, assessing for breathing, and finding none. You give her two full breaths. A five second check for a carotid pulse reveals pulselessness. You initiate chest compressions.

You have no sense of time, but it seems after only minutes of ventilations and compressions, she regains a pulse but not spontaneous respirations. You continue rescue breathing for several minutes before she gasps out a ragged breath on her own. For the next hour, you are by her side, periodically giving artificial respirations to supplement her weak breathing. Around 2:30 AM she starts to shift restlessly, blink her eyes, moan.

The storm beats fiercely at the camp for an hour more. Once you assess the environment as safe, your associate group leader, who knows the area well, hikes out for help with two stronger members of the party. You wait in trepidation, glued to your patient's side. Storm clouds make a helicopter evacuation impossible, but a rescue team hikes in. At approximately 11:00 AM, the girl is packed in a litter and on her way to the nearest road. Although the strength of her breathing and heartbeat diminish during the morning, although she lapses back into a coma, she remains alive, and fully recovers after a three week stay in the local hospital.

Chapter 21: North American Bites And Stings

You should be able to:

1. Describe the signs and symptoms of the most dangerous bites and stings common to North America.

2. Describe the treatment of the most dangerous bites and stings common to North America.

3. Describe the prevention of the most dangerous bites and stings common to North America.

It could happen to you

Cries from her tent bring you in a rush from where you're preparing dinner in the Sipsey Wilderness of northwestern Alabama. You find a member of your party, a young woman named Bethany, in extreme discomfort, curled into a fetal position, complaining of "the worst cramps you can imagine" in her abdomen and lower back. Sweat drenches her, and her skin appears flushed, feels warm. You suspect a fever. You open your mouth to ask what's wrong, but, before you can speak, she opens her mouth to splatter the tent wall with vomit. Her pulse races at 110, and seems weak to you.

Thinking appendicitis, or a rare and fatal gastroenteritis, or the imminent birth of an alien, you quickly organize the group and abandon the campsite in favor of a mercifully short carry to the car and a rapid drive to the hospital.

Introduction

The bites and stings humans receive from other animals vary greatly in severity depending on the type of animal, e.g., big vs. small, venomous vs. non-venomous, the reason for the attack, e.g., cornered and afraid vs. hungry, and the way the human acts during the confrontation, e.g., runs away vs. fights back. Despite the variations, similarities do exist in the damage done by bites and stings, and general principles have been established for the management of the wounds received from wild creatures.

In order of significance, treatment for bites and stings should include 1) making sure the scene is safe, 2) immediately stopping serious blood loss, if appropriate, 3) immediately cleaning the wound against the introduction of microorganisms, and 4) managing the patient and the wound to reduce the effects of envenomation, if the animal was poisonous.

Spiders

Few people are gladdened to learn that almost all spiders, worldwide, carry venom which can be injected through nasty fangs. On the positive side, only a few dozen species have a bite harmful to humans because 1) the spider injects too little venom or 2) the spider's fangs cannot penetrate human skin.

Black Widow

One of the most venomous spiders, the black widow, at least four species of which are common in the United States, bears the tag "cosmopolitan," a spider found around the globe. Only the shiny female, up to one inch in average length (two to 2.5 cm), poses a threat, and she packs more danger in every drop of venom than any other creature in North America. The typically red—but not always red—"hourglass" shape on her abdomen helps identify her. She has been found in every state but Alaska, secreting her tattered web under logs and large pieces of bark, in stone crevices, in trash heaps and outbuildings, or deep in clumps of heavy vegetation. Rarely aggressive, she may be touchy during springtime mating and egg-tending days.

Her drop of poison is tiny, a huge boon to bitten humans. Patients almost never feel the bite, although some have reported immediate sharp pain. There may be little or no redness and swelling at the site initially, but a small, red, slightly hard bump may form later. Within 10 to 60 minutes symptoms usually begin to occur. Pain and anxiety become intense. Severe muscular cramping often centers in the abdomen and back. Burning or numbness characteristically disturb the patient's feet. Watch for headaches, nausea, vomiting, dizziness, heavy sweating—all common reactions.

Even though patients claim it feels like death is imminent, black widows kill very few humans, only two to four during an average year in the United States, and the dead are almost always the very young, the very old, or the very allergic.

You the rescuer need to keep the patient as calm as possible, a course of action that "applies" perhaps your best first aid treatment. If you can find the bite site—which may show up as a faint red mark—wash it, and apply an antiseptic such as povi-done-iodine. Cooling the injury, with ice if possible, with water or wet compresses if necessary, will reduce the pain. Cold also reduces circulation which slows down the spread of the venom. Medications for pain, if available, would be appropriate.

Evacuation to a medical facility is strongly advised, especially if you are unsure what is causing the symptoms, just in case complications arise. Most people will receive painkillers and eight to twelve hours of observation. Youngsters, oldsters, and the very sick may be admitted for longer. Antivenin is available if needed.

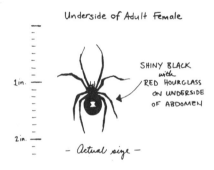

Underside of Adult Female

SHINY BLACK with RED HOURGLASS ON UNDERSIDE OF ABDOMEN

1 in.

2 in.

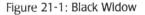

— Actual size —

Figure 21-1: Black Widow

Recluse

The most common serious spider bite in the United States comes not from the venom of the black widow, but, instead, from the solitude-seeking recluse (fiddleback, violin spider). Generally pale brown to reddish, with long slender legs averaging about an inch (two to three cm) in length, they most often have the shape of a violin on the top front portion of their body. The head of this "fiddle" points toward the tail of the spider. Unlike the black widow, both sexes of recluses are dangerous.

The recluse prefers the dark and dry places of the South and southern Midwest, but travels comfortably in the freight of trucks and trains, and probably can be found in all 50 states. They don't mind the company of humans, and set up housekeeping underneath furniture, within hanging curtains, and in the shadowed corners of closets. In the wild lands they hide the daylight hours away beneath rocks, dead logs, and pieces of bark in forests all over America. They attack more readily in the warmer months, usually at night, and only when disturbed. Curious children are their most frequent victims.

Like most spiders, their bite is often painless. Having relatively dull fangs, the serious wounds they inflict are usually on tender areas of the human anatomy. Within one to five hours, a painful red blister appears where the fangs did their damage. Watch for the development of a bluish circle around the blister, and a red, irritated circle beyond that: The characteristic "bull's-eye" lesion of the recluse. The patient may suffer chills, fever, a generalized weakness, and a diffuse rash.

Sometimes the lesion resolves harmlessly over the next week or two. Sometimes it spreads irregularly as an enzyme in the spider's venom destroys the cells of the patient's skin and subcutaneous fat. This ulcerous tissue heals slowly and leaves a lasting scar. In a few children, death has occurred from severe complications in the circulatory system.

As with many spiders, without an eight-legged corpse as evidence, it is difficult to be sure what is causing the patient's problem. Initially, there is little to be done other than calming the patient, applying cold to the site of the bite for reduction of pain, and keeping the wound as clean as possible. Medications for pain, if available, would be appropriate. Any "volcanic" skin ulcers should be seen by a physician as soon as possible. Antibiotic therapy may be necessary if the site becomes infected.

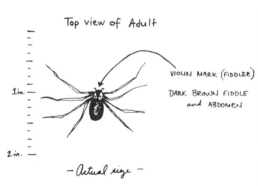
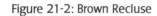

Figure 21-2: Brown Recluse

Hobo Spider

The hobo spider is an import from Europe that has spread, at least, across the Northwest. All hobo spiders are brown with gray markings and eight conspicuously hairy legs. The leg span reaches from one-half inch to 1.5 inches (1.25 to 3.75 cm). A herring-bone stripe pattern in brown, gray, and tan often appears on the abdomen. Hobo spiders have been mistaken for recluses, but hobos lack the violin shape (see above). Laboratory tests have shown that the female's bite is far more toxic than the male's, but it is difficult to tell at which sex you are looking.

The bite of a hobo will probably produce a blister that ulcerates and takes several months to heal. Approximately 50 percent of patients complain of headaches, muscle weakness, visual disturbances, and/or disorientation. Since the signs and symptoms are similar, hobo bites are often blamed on the recluse spider.

Bites from hobo spiders are rare. They tend to avoid large cities and congregate in small towns and rural communities. They like it under houses and deep in woodpiles and clumps of debris. Indoors they may lurk any place that is not regularly cleaned. You will probably never find one out in the far, untrammeled places. They don't bite unless trapped against the skin of an unsuspecting human with no way to escape.

First aid for hobo bites is the same as for recluse bites (SEE ABOVE).

Tarantula

Despite a fierce appearance, North American tarantulas are relatively harmless. Pain, seldom more than moderate, typically follows the bite. Later signs and symptoms are rare. Washing the bite site is encouraged. Cold and/or medications for pain would be appropriate treatment.

Prevention of Spider Bites

1. Do not try to pick up or capture spiders.
2. Check places you intend to put your hands and feet before exposing your body part to a bite.
3. Gather firewood before dark, or do it carefully while using a flashlight.
4. In spider country, keep your tent zipped up.
5. If you must move around in the dark, wear boots or camp shoes, and use a flashlight.
6. Take a look in your boots before stuffing in your feet in the morning.

Reptiles

Although venomous snakes may inflict a large number of bites in the United States every year, deaths are unusual. As many as 14 patients may have died in a single 12 month period, but the average is far lower. Those who die are usually very young or very old.

Ninety-nine out of every 100 poisonous snake bites are received from pit vipers—rattlesnakes, copperheads, and water moccasins. The few remaining bites come from North America's only other venomous family, the coral snakes.

Pit Viper

They don't all have rattles, but all pit vipers do have distinctly triangular heads, cat-like pupils, heat-sensitive pits between eyes and nostrils, and danger squirting from two very special teeth, hinged to swing downward at a 90-degree angle from the upper jaw. The jaw opens alarmingly wide, allowing the venom to be ejected down canals within the fangs and into the tissue of a prey or enemy. The amount of venom and the toxicity of the venom determine the danger to the bitten. For instance, the poison of the Mojave rattlesnake is approximately 44 times more potent than the Southern Copperhead's.

Pit viper venom is generally yellowish, odorless, and slightly sweet to human taste buds. It evolved from the snake's saliva, which makes sense when you remember the purpose is to acquire and utilize food for the snake, not to deal death and destruction to large, inedible mammals who stumble over the low lying reptiles. The venom attacks the nervous and circulatory systems of the snake's prey. In a mouse that can spell death in a few minutes. How dangerous is this venom to a human? Depends on the age, size, health, and emotional stability of the patient, whether or not the patient is allergic to the venom, where the patient was bitten (near vital organs being the most dangerous), how deep the fangs go, how upset the snake is, the species and size of the snake, and the first aid given to the patient. Arizona is the most likely place to die of a snakebite, with Florida, Georgia, Texas, and Alabama filling out the top five.

One rattlesnake bite in four carries no venom. The other three may vary from insignificant to mild to moderate to severe envenomation. Mild envenomations hurt, swell, turn black and blue, and sometimes form a blister at the site. Moderate envenomations add swelling that moves up the arm or leg toward the heart, numbness, and swollen lymph nodes. A severe envenomation might add big jumps in pulse rates and breathing rates, profound swelling, blurred vision, headache, lightheadedness, sweating, and chills. Death is possible.

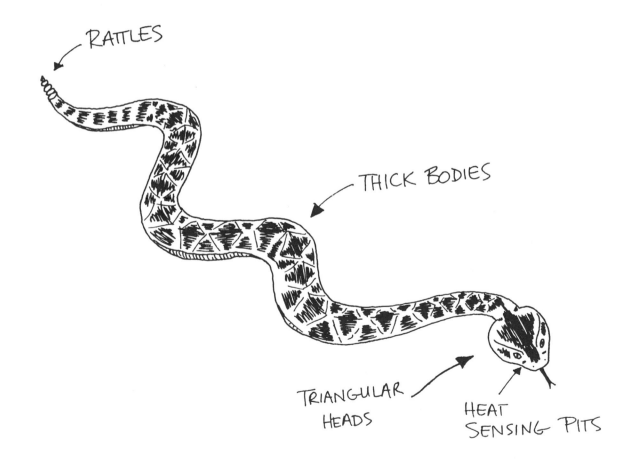

Figure 21-3: Rattlesnake

Coral Snake

Brightly banded in red, yellow, and black, all coral snakes of the United States are described by a particular color sequence: "Red on black, venom lack; red on yellow, kill a fellow." In other words, red bands bordered by yellow bands equals dangerous. Short, fixed fangs in the front of a small mouth make it all but impossible for coral snakes to bite anything on humans other than a finger, a toe, or a fold in skin, and they often have to hang on and chew to do damage. Envenomation ranges from the mild end with localized swelling, nausea, and vomiting, to the severe end with dizziness, weakness, and respiratory difficulty. Since it takes up to 12 hours for signs and symptoms to reach the point where the patient wants help, early evacuation of known bitten persons is strongly advised. Antivenin should be started as soon as possible to be most effective. Little first aid works other than keeping the patient calm and cleaning the wound.

Lizards

Only two lizards, worldwide, are considered venomous enough to end the life of a human. Unfortunately, meetings with both are possible in the Southwest of the United States. The Gila Monster and the Mexican Beaded lizard bite when they are picked up or stepped on. They have powerful jaws to compensate for primitive teeth and no means to inject the poison. They lock on while the venom drools into the wound. You may likely be required to heat the underside of their jaws with matches or a lighter to break their grip. There may be a great deal of local swelling and pain.

Treatment for Reptile Bites

Calm and reassure the patient, putting her or him physically at rest with the bitten extremity immobilized (splinted) and kept lower than the patient's heart. Before splinting, the wound should be gently washed, and rings, watches, or anything else that might reduce the circulation if swelling occurs should be removed.

Evacuate the patient by carrying—or going for help to carry them—or, if the patient is stable, by slow walking. If the patient is many hours from medical care and/or if severe symptoms develop rapidly, e.g., severe pain, severe swelling, the patient should be placed at rest and activity kept to a minimum. The patient should drink as much water as possible in frequent small amounts, unless vomiting is a problem.

If you think of it, attempt to identify the biting creature, but not if it puts you or anyone else at risk. If the species is known, there is a high probability that antivenin is available if needed.

The rest of the recommended treatments for reptile bites concern actions you should NOT take instead of actions you should take. Do NOT cut and suck. Mechanical suction (NOT mouth suction) may be valuable if used in the first three to five minutes after the bite. Suction should be applied for 30 minutes via the Sawyer Extractor®. Do NOT give painkillers unless the patient is very stable, showing no signs of getting worse. Painkillers may mask important symptoms. Do NOT apply ice or immerse the wound in cold water. Some snake venoms may be driven deeper into human tissue by the application of cold, and some envenomated tissue may be easily damaged by cold. Do NOT give alcohol to drink, do NOT apply a tourniquet or even a constricting band, do NOT electrically shock the patient—actions which cause much more harm than good.

Note: Constricting bands, such as an elastic wrap, applied from proximal to distal to the bite site prior to splinting, may be useful in the field treatment of coral snake bites. At this writing, however, use of any constricting band remains controversial.

Prevention of Reptile Bites

1. Do not try to pick up or capture snakes or lizards.
2. Check places you intend to put your hands and feet before exposing your body part to a bite.
3. Gather firewood before dark, or do it carefully while using a flashlight.
4. In snake country, keep your tent zipped up.
5. Wear high, thick boots while traveling in snake country.
6. When passing a snake, stay out of striking range, which is about one-half the snake's length.
7. If you hear the "buzz" of a rattler, freeze, find it with your eyes without moving your head, wait for it to relax the strike position, and back away slowly.

Scorpions

Loving the night, as most spiders also do, and hiding by day, scorpions all sting with the tip of their "tail"—the last few segments of their abdomen. From small species that reach maturity at three-fourths inch (about 2 cm) to humongus nine-inchers (23 cm), scorpions have crab-like pincers used only to hold and tear apart their prey. Insects are their primary source of food.

Most victims report no more pain than that inflicted by a irritated honeybee. An attack of the species *Centruroides* may be different. In North America only the *Centruroides* is a known killer of humans. They are usually old-straw-yellow or yellow with dark longitudinal stripes, and reach from about one to three inches (two to 7.5 cm) in length. Their pincers are long and slender as opposed to bulky and lobster-like. The sting, immediately and exquisitely painful, is increased by a light tap on the site. Deaths have almost exclusively been in small children, the elderly, and the severely allergic. This scorpion is only found in Mexico and the extreme southwestern United States.

First aid for any scorpion sting should involve cooling the wound which allows the body to more easily break down the molecular structure of the venom. Cooling also reduces pain. Use ice or cool running water if available. On a warm night, a wet compress will help. Keep the patient calm and still. Panic and activity speed up the venom's spread. If the scorpion was *Centruroides*, post-sting manifestations may include heavy sweating, difficulty swallowing, blurred vision, loss of bowel control, jerky muscular reflexes, and respiratory distress. These serious signs are cause for quick evacuation to a medical facility. Antivenins are available in many areas where dangerous scorpions live.

In the Southwest, most stings occur May through August. The victims are usually putting on clothing, walking barefoot in the dark, or picking up objects (like firewood) off the ground. By following the simple rules of spider avoidance (see above), you will contact few scorpions.

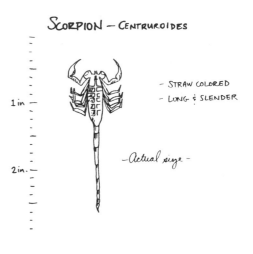

SCORPION — CENTRUROIDES

- STRAW COLORED
- LONG & SLENDER

1 in —

2 in. —

— Actual size —

Figure 21-4: Scorpion

Ticks

Ticks come in two basic sizes—tiny and hard to find, and big and easy to find. A relative of the spider, the tick crawls around on its unsuspecting host on eight tiny legs, looking for the right spot to settle down for a few days. It may search for hours. With specialized pincer-like organs, it digs a small wound in his host. Into the wound goes a feeding apparatus called a hypostome, and its relatively powerful sucking mechanism allows the tick to feed on the blood of the host. Anchored firmly in the wound, it feeds for an average of two to five days, sometimes longer, depending on the species, and drops off weighing hundreds of times more than when it first arrived. In the host it often leaves a reminder of its visit, disease-causing microorganisms. Worldwide, only the mosquito spreads more illness than the tick.

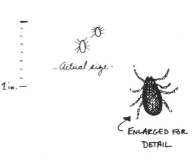

— Actual size —

1 in. —

ENLARGED FOR DETAIL

Figure 21-5: Tick

Lyme Disease

First diagnosed in Lyme, Connecticut, the corkscrew-shaped bacteria, *Borrelia burgdorferi*, a spirochete carried by some ticks, has spread to almost all states, still in heaviest concentrations in the Northeast and upper Midwest, and along the coast of northern California. The tick must be attached for approximately 48 hours in order to spread Lyme disease.

The warning signs of Lyme disease include: 1) Two days to five weeks after the bite, a well-defined rash appears—a ragged bull's-eye, red surrounded by lighter shades—in 60 to 80 percent of patients. The rash appears anywhere it pleases, unrelated to the bite site, in several places at once, disappearing to reappear in different spots. 2) Flu-like symptoms, with a fever, headache, fatigue, and a stiff neck occur before or after the rash. Rash and illness disappear in a few days to weeks. 3) Extreme, chronic fatigue with irregular heart beat and partial numbness or paralysis can occur weeks to months later in a few sufferers. This stage can be very serious. 4) Swelling and pain in joints, especially the knees, may start up to two years later. Any joint can be affected, and the arthritis may move from joint to joint with periods of remission. A blood test will show if you have the disease, but only in later stages.

Lyme disease is not fatal, although it is possible to die from cardiac complications associated with the disease. Without antibiotic treatment, however, it can lead to lifelong arthritic problems.

Rocky Mountain Spotted Fever

Montana's Bitterroot Mountains first recorded Rocky Mountain spotted fever, caused by the parasite *Rickettsia rickettsii*, but it spread from coast to coast. After feeding for approximately three hours, infected ticks may pass the disease. Three to twelve days later, the patient develops a spotty rash, usually beginning on the hands, feet, wrists, and ankles. The spots migrate over the arms, legs, face, and abdomen. Severe headaches are common, with stiff neck and back, and general muscle aches. The characteristic fever rises during the first days, and remains high. If untreated, approximately 20 percent of the victims will die. Almost everyone will recover with antibiotic treatment.

Colorado Tick Fever

All the Rocky Mountain states have recorded patients with Colorado tick fever, as well as western Canada and South Dakota. A virus produces the sudden fever with muscle aches and headache that develops three to six days after the bite of the tick. Diarrhea, vomiting, and stomachaches are common signs and symptoms. The patient often recovers and relapses several times in the course of the illness. It is very rarely fatal, although sufferers report feeling so crummy they wish they could die.

Tularemia

Another bacteria, often borne by ticks of the South and Southwest, causes the high fever and flu-like symptoms of tularemia. A decaying wound at the site of the bite is common. Antibiotics will defeat the bacteria.

Tick Paralysis

At least 43 species of ticks, worldwide, have been known to cause tick paralysis, with more cases showing up in North America than anywhere else. A venom in tick saliva causes the problem, which appears to be a block to nerve messages, and children are affected more often than adults. The patient may first be restless and irritable with complaints of numbness or tingling in hands and feet. Ascending paralysis develops over the next 24 to 48 hours. Once the tick is removed, the patient recovers, almost always without complications. Any patient with an ascending paralysis and without a known cause should be inspected carefully for an imbedded tick.

Tick Removal

Quick tick removal is necessary to reduce the chance of disease transmission. Forget those ineffective and possibly dangerous ways of smearing them with petroleum jelly, nail polish, or gasoline, or burning them out with a match. Using bare fingers to pull them out works, but it's not the best way. You can crush the tick, propelling the tick's juices into the patient. A pair of tweezers should be in your first aid kit. If the tweezers are fine-pointed, all the better. Grasp the tick near the skin and pull out gently. No twisting, yanking, or squeezing. After the tick is out, scrub the area gently with alcohol, an antibiotic ointment, or soap and water. What if your removal technique leaves tick mouth parts in your skin? If your pull is straight and slow, the mouth parts very rarely detach from the tick. Even if they do, the chance of getting Lyme disease from just the mouth parts seems to be nonexistent. Save the tick, preferably without touching it with your hand, if you would like to have it checked for disease. Make note of the time and your location to keep with the removed tick.

Prevention of Tick Bites

1. Tick checks, several times a day if you're active outdoors in tick season, are extremely important. Obviously, considering a tick's inclination to tuck itself into hard to see areas, a partner will add much to an adequate check. Free roaming ticks on your skin can be easily and safely lifted off. Imbedded ticks should be immediately un-imbedded (SEE ABOVE).
2. If you wear light-colored clothing and tuck your pants into your socks, you stand a great chance of recognizing and removing the dark-colored tick before it reaches your skin.
3. Two repellents have proven effective in keeping ticks off: DEET (N,N-diethyl-meta-toluamide), the active ingredient in most repellents, may be applied to skin. A concentration no greater than 35 percent DEET is recommended. Permethrin, a spray repellent, should be applied to clothing. Although tests indicate permethrin does not harm skin, it doesn't work on skin. On clothing, however, it dries and actually *kills* ticks (and mosquitoes) on contact. The long lasting effect of permethrin will allow you to treat your clothes prior to many trips and leave the spray can behind.

Bees, Wasps, Yellowjackets, Hornets, Fire Ants

Bees, wasps, yellowjackets, hornets, and fire ants (*Hymenoptera*) are related largely due to their habit of injecting a venom when they sting. Most humans find the pain extremely annoying, and that's the end of the story. Every year, for an estimated 50-100 people in the United States, the sting causes, usually in less than an hour, the end of life. Some experts guess the fatality rate runs even higher. Death almost always results from anaphylaxis, a severe allergic reaction.

Stings cause immediate pain, followed by redness and swelling, followed by itching. With any of these insects, 10 or more stings could cause vomiting, diarrhea, headache, fever, muscle spasms, breathing difficulty, or convulsions; 100 or more could cause cardiac arrest. Ice packs generally ease the pain and swelling. Mild to moderate allergic reactions characterized by hives, facial swelling, and dizziness, can be treated with an oral antihistamine. If severe difficulty breathing results, only an injectable drug, epinephrine, available by prescription in pre-loaded syringes, reverses the reaction (SEE CHAPTER 28: ALLERGIC REACTIONS AND ANAPHYLAXIS).

Honeybees, non-aggressive by nature, lead the swarm as a source of fatalities in humans. As many as 15 percent of all humans may have some sensitivity, often mild, to bee venom, and the bee, unlike other *Hymenopterans*, has a barbed stinger that rips out of the insect and stays in human skin, continuing to pump venom for up to 20 minutes. The famed "killer" bees, near relatives of honeybees, are edging into the extreme southern U. S. from Latin America where they've attacked several hundred people with fatal results. Killer bee venom is no more potent than honeybee venom, but killers are noted for mass attacks by hundreds of individual bees. Evidence suggests there is no significant difference in the amount of envenomization whether the stinger is scraped out or pinched and pulled out. The amount of envenomization does increase the longer the stinger is left in, and, therefore, bee stingers should be removed as rapidly as possible. Interesting to note, neither honeybees nor killer bees are Native Americans, having been imported from Europe and Africa respectively.

Wasp family members, including hornets and yellow jackets, unlike bees, are predators and scavengers who are attracted to meat and decaying matter. Their dirty stingers have a higher rate of infection, and the site of their stings should be thoroughly cleaned. One of these insects is capable of multiple stings, but deaths in humans rarely occur.

Step on a fire ant bed, which typically contains up to 25,000 ants, and 30 seconds later you're covered in hundreds. As other ants do, fire ants bite, but that's only the first part of the attack.

Holding on with mandibles, fire ants arch their backs, jab in their stingers located in the end of their abdomens, release their venom, pull out their stinger, rotate, jab in their stinger. Unless you intervene, each ant will create a ring of burning stings. The venom causes local tissue destruction which produces, within 24 hours, a fluid filled bump that itches horribly for a week or more. Fire ants, another imported insect, are well established in at least 11 southern states, and fire ant victims seeking medical attention have soared in number to as high as 85,000 in one year. Deaths, due to anaphylaxis, may run as high as 30 per year.

If confronted by a bee or two, or a wasp, stay calm and back away slowly. They don't like rapid movements, especially swatting movements. If attacked by a swarm, run for dense cover, lay face down, and cover your head with your hands. If attacked by a hoard of fire ants, running and swatting are both approved methods of fighting back. Bright colored summer clothing seems to attract winged insects. Tan, light brown, white, and light green appear to have no special appeal. Food left uncovered around camp is a no-no. Insect repellents work.

Centipedes

Some centipedes, but no millipedes, have venom glands and fangs that can penetrate human skin. Burning pain and swelling may result. Redness and discomfort may persist for a couple of weeks, perhaps more. Although most centipede bites heal without specific treatment, oral antihistamines and/or topical hydrocortisone may relieve the symptoms.

Rabies

Only mammals get rabies, and it acts in this way: The virus travels at a constant speed from the bite site to the spinal cord, and up the cord to the medulla where it replicates. Once it replicates in the brain of a human, death is assured. It then travels back out along the nervous system. The animal becomes infectious after the rabies virus collects in the saliva glands. It is transmitted to other mammals through bites that tear the flesh. The incubation period in humans, the time from bite to brain, varies with individuals and with the bite site. Ten days is probably the minimum, but some patients have presented years after the inoculation. An average individual would incubate the virus for about three weeks after a bite on the face, and about seven weeks after a bite on the foot.

Annually in the U.S. about one million people are treated for animal bites, including those inflicted by other humans. Twenty to 25,000 of these people will be treated for rabies. Each year somewhere between zero and three cases of human rabies will actually be diagnosed, and the diagnosis will be made postmortem (after death).

Statistics from the United States, Canada, and Mexico give evidence of the primary reservoirs of rabies. The major hosts are skunks (43 percent), followed by raccoons (28 percent), bats (14 percent), cattle (4.6 percent), cats (3.0 percent), and dogs (1.7 percent). The rest of the carriers were a few wolves, bobcats, coyotes, groundhogs, muskrats, weasels, woodchucks, foxes, horses, and a rare human. The significant statistic for outdoor enthusiasts to note is 96 percent of the rabies virus in the United States is carried by wild animals.

Infected animals can spread the disease without biting. If their saliva contacts a mucous membrane (the inner surface of lips or the eye) or an already open wound, the disease may result. There are several well-documented cases of transmission by corneal transplant from an infected human.

Rabies produces general early signs and symptoms: headache and fever, cough and sore throat, loss of appetite, fatigue, abdominal pain, nausea, vomiting, diarrhea. Patients also report a tingling sensation at the bite site. Once in the central nervous system, the virus makes the patient anxious, irritable, depressed, disoriented, unable to sleep, and prone to hallucinations. The patient may complain of stiff neck, double vision, and visual sensitivity to light. You may notice muscle twitching and, later, seizures. The final stage includes bizarre behavior like aimless unreasonable activity, biting at those who approach, and drooling. Painful muscle spasms in the throat result when the patient tries to eat or drink. The pain leads to avoidance of swallowing, and thus drooling. Some patients will have throat spasms at the sight of water, and so the name *hydrophobia* (fear of water) became attached to rabies. As the nervous system deteriorates, patients become paralyzed, slip into a coma, fail to breathe adequately, and die.

Treatment

Immediate care for the bite of any animal, including rabid animals, needs to concentrate on cleaning the wound. Wash it vigorously with soap and water. Aggressive washing, which can deactivate the rabies virus, does more than other first aid treatment. Rinse the wound thoroughly. The sooner cleaning takes place, the better.

As soon as possible, have the wound checked by a physician. Tetanus shots and/or antibiotics may be recommended to prevent bacterial infections. The doctor might suggest the rabies vaccine. Fortunately, the current Human Diploid Cell Vaccine against rabies works every time in minor exposures. Human Antirabies Immunoglobulin is also required in more significant exposures. A series of five relatively painless shots have replaced the old painful abdominal injections. To be most effective, the shots should be started within 72 hours of the bite.

How do you decide if the biting animal had rabies? There is only one sure way: Have the brain of the animal tested for presence of the virus. This is often impossible. Without the head, five other questions should be asked: 1) Was the animal one of the highly suspect species? 2) Was the attack provoked? Rabid animals tend to attack without provocation. Trying to pick up or feed a wild animal and having it take a nip out of your finger is a very natural and unsuspect action. Having it leap from the shadows at your throat is an unprovoked and suspect attack. 3) If the animal was a pet, what is its vaccination status? 4) What is the geographical incidence of rabies in the area of the attack. 5) How did the animal behave in general? Loss of natural timidity and weird behavior are important non-clinical signs of rabies infection in animals.

When in doubt, get the expensive shots. If you make the wrong choice, you have accepted the death sentence. Once the clinical symptoms of rabies begin, you will almost assuredly die.

Plague

Between 1347 and 1350, the Black Death, caused by the bacteria *Yersinia pestis*, began somewhere in Asia and eventually rubbed out about 25 million Europeans (roughly one-third the population). Nine-tenths of the people of England were permanently laid low. Before those devastating years, even in BC days, reports of the ravages of plague were known and feared. In recent years, plague has been on the rise in the western United States.

Carried by rodents and passed primarily by the bite of rodent fleas, both rodent and flea are killed by the bacteria, an unusual aspect of this disease. Black rats are especially susceptible, and *Rattus rattus* is blamed for the Black Death of 14th Century Europe. In the United States, deer mice and various voles maintain the bacteria. It is amplified in prairie dogs and ground squirrels. Other possible reservoirs include chipmunks, marmots, wood rats, rabbits, and hares.

Hikers and campers are at mild risk if they hang around rodent-infested areas. Coyotes and bobcats are known to have transmitted plague to humans after the animals were dead and the humans were skinning them. Skunks, raccoons, and badgers are suspect. Sick people transmit plague readily to other people. Meat-eating pets that eat infected rodents (or get bitten by infected fleas) can acquire plague. Dogs don't get very sick, but cats do. There is only one known case of plague being passed to a human by a dog, but several cats have passed the disease to humans by biting them, coughing on them, or carrying their fleas to them.

Several forms of plague exist, but the three most common are *bubonic*, septicemic, and pneumonic. Buboes are inflamed, enlarged lymph nodes, and they give bubonic plague its name.

After an incubation period of two to six days, patients usually suffer fever, chills, malaise, muscle aches, and headaches. Blackened, bleeding skin sores gave a name to the "Black Death." The *septicemic* form may appear similar but does not give rise to buboes. Gastrointestinal pain with nausea, vomiting and diarrhea is common. The *pneumonic* form results most often from inhaling droplets that contain the bacteria, but it can develop from bacteria that got into your blood. Coughing often produces blood in the sputum.

If plague is suspected, the patient should be isolated. Use body substance isolation. Do not inhale air the patient has exhaled. Tranport the patient immediately. Fatalities are common. Antibiotics are required. Prevention includes avoidance of rodents, avoiding touching sick or dead animals (if you must touch them, wear rubber gloves), and restraining dogs and cats while traveling in infected areas.

Hantavirus Infection

Strong evidence names the deer mouse as the primary reservoir for hantavirus. It's been found in pinyon mice, brush mice, western chipmunks, and other rodent residents, primarily in the southwestern United States. Rodents don't get sick, but they carry the germs in their saliva, urine, and feces for weeks. Inhaling aerosolized microscopic particles of dried rodent saliva, urine, or feces gets the virus into humans where it causes an extremely dangerous respiratory syndrome. So far, approximately one-half of diagnosed cases have died. Rodent bites could possibly transfer the disease, but human-to-human transference does not occur. There has been no known insect-to-human transference. Most inhalations occur in dwellings where rodent droppings have collected.

Infected humans appear to have the flu—fever, ache-ridden muscles, headache, cough—then, suddenly, lungs fill with fluid and patients suffer respiratory failure.

To avoid hantavirus: 1) Avoid contact with all rodents and their burrows. 2) Do not use enclosed shelters unless they have been cleaned and disinfected. 3) Do not pitch tents or place sleeping bags near rodent burrows. 4) Use tents with floors or sleep on ground tarps that extend two to three feet beyond sleeping bags. 5) Store food away from rodent contact. 6) Promptly and appropriately dispose of all trash and garbage.

Bears

There are three recognized species of bears in the United States and Canada. In the far north lives the great white polar bear (*Ursus maritimus*). The most widespread is the black bear (*Ursus americana*). Black bears may be jet black to creamy yellow, average 300 pounds but may reach 600 pounds, have no hump and a straight profile. The third is the brown bear (*Ursus arctus*), currently divided into two subspecies: Kodiak brown (*U. arctus middendorffi*) and the grizzly (*U. arctus horribilis*). Brown bears may be dark brown to blond, average 500 to 900 pounds but may reach 1400 pounds, and have a prominent shoulder hump and a dish-face profile.

Statistically, your chances of being killed by a bear are slim, but, to reduce the chances to an absolute minimum, here are three basic rules concerning bears:

1) Hike and camp in a manner designed to avoid bears. In known bear country, avoid areas that are used often by bears— trails with bear tracks and bear scat, trails along salmon streams and through berry patches, trails through dense brush and thick forest, especially at night. Avoid areas that smell of decaying meat. Bears like to cover their uneaten food lightly and camp nearby to finish it off later. If possible camp in the open. Cook food at least 100 yards from sleeping sites. If camping near a river, sleep upriver from the cooksite. Night breezes tend to blow down river, pushing the food smells away from the sleeping bags. Camp cleanly. Avoid wiping food-stained hands and utensils on clothing. Avoid spilling food on the ground. Avoid fish and greasy food. Pack food and other odorous stuff, e.g., toothpaste, soap, in a separate bag so the smells don't get into pack and clothing. Hang the food at night, if possible, out

of bear-reach from the ground and from the trunk of the tree. All food residue should be packed with the food, not burned. Dishes should be cleaned even further away from the tents than the cooksite, and kept packed with the food. Although no evidence indicates bears are attracted particularly to menstruating women, menstrual wastes should still be stored away from camp, possibly bagged securely in plastic and hung with other odorous material.

2) Travel in a group large enough to ensure a measure of safety. Bears like a measure of safety, too, and have not attacked a group of four or more in recent history.

3) Strive to never surprise a bear. Bears, particularly grizzlies, do not accommodate people up close and personal. Mother bears need even more room. Push their comfort zone, and they tend to either attack or run away. Once smelling or hearing humans, almost all bears will run away. Traveling with the wind and making noise help make bears aware of human proximity.

A surprised bear who has seen the surpriser cannot be predicted to act in a certain way. Hopefully, he or she will turn and run. If the bear doesn't run, speak in a calm, quiet voice. Back away slowly, but do not run. Running encourages the bear to play chase, a game bears win. If the group of people is four or more, it usually works best to maximize the threat to the bear. The people should stand close together, raise their arms, speak in a reasonably loud and assured voice, identifying themselves as humans, the age-old nemesis to the bear. Statistics say the bear will retreat.

Bears who feel threatened turn to the side, displaying their size. They will often woof aggressively. They may charge toward the threat, and suddenly stop. These are invitations for the human to retreat. It is advisable to do so, but, remember, no running. It is best to back off slowly and keep speaking in a calm voice (which may be difficult by now). Humans without backpacks may benefit from turning to the side while backing off, an act which makes you look smaller and less intimidating.

Climbing a tree is seldom worth the effort. Black bears climb like squirrels, and grizzlies will climb into the lower branches at a very fast rate. Avoid eye contact with the bear, an act of aggression.

If the bear actually attacks, different tactics are called for depending on the species of bear. Black bears seldom attack seriously unless they are hungry. They are not used to having food fight back, and it is statistically best to counter-attack, doing all possible to convince the black bear to dine elsewhere. If the bear is a grizzly, assuming a least-threatening posture—playing dead—is the best tactic. Curl up to guard vital parts, clasping hands protectively behind neck. Fainting is not a bad idea. The brown bear may take a few bites, but then leave you alone. Those playing dead should remain so until the bear is well away. There seems to be no reasonable response to a polar bear's attack.

Patients surviving bear attacks should have serious blood loss stopped. The wound should be adequately cleaned and bandaged (SEE CHAPTER 15: SOFT TISSUE INJURIES).

Dangerous Marine Life

Below the dancing surface of the ocean, which covers about 71 percent of the earth, live four-fifths of the world's living organisms. Some of these creatures are potentially dangerous to humans. Generally, risky aquatic life can be divided into three categories: 1) those with big teeth, 2) those that envenomate, and 3) those that sting with nematocysts.

Those With Big Teeth

Of all fish worldwide, sharks elicit the greatest fear. Their triangular teeth are continually migrating forward to fall out and be replaced by new ones growing in the back of their crescent-shaped mouths. The result is an orifice always full of razor-keen weapons capable of removing large amounts of tissue from a prey's body. They account for the most human deaths annually from aggressive marine life. Even so, the number of shark attacks each year averages only between 50 and 100 in all the seas of the earth. It seems safe to go back in the water considering the ratio of sharks to people who swim off shore.

If you work or play in the oceans of the United States, your chance of being shark food is perhaps one in five million.

There are steps you can take to reduce the risk of attack even more: 1) Swim in groups. 2) Do not swim at dusk or during the night in infested waters. Those are the times sharks feed. 3) Wear bright or gaudy-colored swimsuits or wet suits that reduce the chance of being mistaken for something sharks like to eat. 4) Avoid turbid water where shark eyesight will be impaired. 5) Avoid thrashing and splashing and other erratic movement and noise that attract attention. Sharks hunt with vibration receptors as well as their eyes. 6) Be watchful if you are a successful spear fisher. Sharks also use their sense of smell, and are attracted to blood and other body fluids in the water.

If a shark seems interested in you, face it and swim away slowly. Avoid the crawl stroke, the butterfly, and other quick swimming styles. Stick to a breast stroke or easy side stroke. If the shark charges, curl into a ball. If it seems intent on taking a bite out of you, kick and punch at the eyes, nose, and gills.

In warmer waters, swimmers sometimes run the risk of toothy contact with barracudas or moray eels. Barracudas seldom attack humans, but when they do it is swift and fierce, and usually in murky water where they have become confused. Their big V-shaped mouths, with long pointed teeth, can do much damage. The glitter of shiny paraphernalia and jerky swimming movements may attract the barracuda. Moray eels do not bite unless threatened. Their sharp teeth and powerful jaws tend to hold a victim so strongly that the eel has to be killed to be

removed. Divers are at risk if they stick their hands into coral holes and rock crevices where eels like to lurk in wait for more tastier morsels than humans.

Patients surviving an attack by sea life with big teeth should have 1) blood loss stopped, and 2) wounds thoroughly cleaned. Humans tend to deal poorly with marine bacteria, and wound infections from marine bites carry a high risk of infection. Any wound that breaks the skin should be seen by a physician as soon as possible.

Those That Envenomate

Venomous sea creatures are almost always non-aggressive organisms that bite after being stepped on or handled unknowingly. The most likely of these animals to become the victims of human carelessness are stingrays and sea urchins. Contact usually produces local burning pain, followed by redness, swelling, and aching (and bleeding in the case of the stingray who has large barbs on the end of its tail).

The wound should be cleaned immediately with sea water. Explore the clean wound and remove any loose piece of the creature that may be stuck in the patient. Cleaning will also remove some of the venom, and, if the water is cold, relieve some of the initial pain. Scrubbing the wound with a povidone iodine solution can help reduce the effects of the venom. As soon as possible, soak the wound in hot water. This may further remove venom and pain. Once the early pain has eased, the application of heat should not increase it. Check again for debris in the wound. These injuries carry a

high risk of infection. When the wound has dried, cover it with a sterile dressing and bandage it loosely. With all marine-related cuts, a loose bandage is best, allowing the wound to drain. Monitor the patient for signs of infection (see Chapter 15: Soft Tissue Injuries). Prophylactic antibiotics are typically recommended due to the high incidence of infection.

Hawaii is the only state with venomous sea snakes. Reptiles in every sense of the word, they breathe air but can remain submerged for hours. Commonly ranging from three to four feet in length, individuals have been measured to nine feet. They flatten out toward the rear, and propel themselves forward and backward with undulating motions, like delicate ribbons waving in sea currents. Attacks are rare, unless they are provoked. Their short fangs deliver a relatively mild bite, but the venom is very toxic. Developing in minutes to hours, the patient complains of nausea and non-specific feelings of illness. Anxiety increases. Pain grows, with partial paralysis possible. Difficulty breathing may follow. Heavily envenomed patients develop a growing intensity of signs and symptoms, and may lapse into a coma. One in four victims die without antivenin.

Treatment in the field consists of removing the patient from the water, and calming him or her down. Hysteria and movement increase the activity of the poison. Place a light constricting band, not a tourniquet, close to the bite and between the wound and the patient's heart. Cutting and sucking is dangerous and non-productive. Evacuate the patient as soon as possible to a medical facility.

Those With Nematocysts

Coelenterates, a group that includes all the jellyfish, form an enormous phylum of sea creatures with around 9,000 named species. Some of them are harmful to humans, with common names that sometimes reflect the risk they pose: fire coral, stinging medusa, Portuguese man-of-war, sea wasp, sea nettle, hairy stinger, stinging anemone. They all share a stinging organelle, called a nematocyst, that lives encapsulated in a cnidoblast on the tentacles of the coelenterate. The cnidoblast has a trap door (the operculum) with a trigger (the cnidocil) that opens the door. Filled with venom, the nematocyst has a sharp, coiled, thread-like appendage which springs out when the trigger is touched, lodging in the patient.

The reaction in humans will range from mild to severe. Mild reactions are immediate, and include stinging, burning, itching, and sometimes local numbness to touch. The stung area may acquire a bruised appearance that lingers for days. A moderate reaction progresses to headache, nausea, and vomiting. Severely reactive patients have difficulty breathing that may lead to loss of consciousness, convulsions, and the possibility of death.

Since the leading cause of death is drowning in the ensuing panic, removal of the patient from the aquatic environment is of immediate importance. Once safely out of the water, the irritated area of the patient's skin should be rinsed with sea water. Rinsing with fresh water may stimulate the nematocysts that have not fired to do so. Physically lift off any tentacles that still cling to the patient, but do so without touching the tentacles with a naked hand. The organelles that aren't rinsed off should be "fixed" so they will cease to envenomate. A wash of vinegar seems to work best. Alcohol, ammonia, or urine have been used successfully. Meat tenderizer, mixed with one of the liquids to form a paste, and applied to the skin, is an effective fixer. Keep the fixer on until the pain goes away. It might take as long as a half an hour.

The final step in treatment is to remove the imbedded nematocysts. They can be rubbed off with sand and sea water, shaved off with a knife, or scraped off gently with anything that has an appropriate edge. Persistent itching can be relieved with corticosteroid cream. The patient should be watched over the next 24 hours for signs of a severe allergic reaction.

Evacuation Guidelines

A patient treated for a bite or sting from a known venomous animal should be evacuated to definitive care. A patient treated for anaphylaxis, even though he or she seems to have recovered, should be evacuated. Any suspicion of rabies calls for an evacuation of the patient. Large animal bite wounds and/or animal bite wounds showing signs of infection call for an evacuation of the patient.

Conclusion

When the bite occurred was never known. It caused no immediate pain. What bit her was never established beyond the shadow of a medical doubt. The physician in charge discovered a red, hardened bump on her right lower leg and recorded the high probability of a black widow envenomation. The patient's stay in the hospital included medication for the pain, a watchful eye for more severe reactions such as difficulty breathing, and nothing more as far as treatment went. After a few days, she was released with complete recovery.

Chapter 22:   Diving Emergencies

You should be able to:

1. *Describe the signs and symptoms of the most common* SCUBA *diving emergencies including barotitis, barosinusitis, pulmonary overinflation syndrome, arterial gas embolism, and decompression sickness.*

2. *Describe the appropriate care for the most common* SCUBA *diving emergencies.*

3. *Describe prevention of the most common* SCUBA *diving emergencies.*

It could happen to you

You're learning to SCUBA dive in the warm waters off Kona, Hawaii. With successful completion of the basic course behind you, you're about 40 feet down, about a quarter mile from land, a student in an Open Water Diver course. Near you a second student floats suspended beneath the waves. The instructor is on the boat somewhere above, waiting at a pre-arranged pick-up spot.

You take a compass bearing from the device on your right wrist, and kick off in a southwesterly direction. The second student heads in a different direction. He will follow a different underwater course to arrive at the same pick-up spot.

A moray eel pokes its head from a crevice in a rock wall, jerks back in as you swim past. Colorful fish of a dozen species scurry away at your approach.

Nearing the anchor chain of the instructor's boat, the point where you'll slowly ascend to the surface, you see the second stu-

dent swimming toward the same spot when he suddenly stops, stares at you a moment, takes a quick look at the air pressure gauge on his left wrist, and begins to swim rapidly upward. The first words you hear when your head breaks into sunshine come from the second student and sound distressed. He complains of chest pain and difficulty breathing. The instructor leans over the side, telling you, in an urgent whisper, to hurry on board.

Introduction

SCUBA—a word so well known many people have forgotten it stands for self-contained underwater breathing apparatus. SCUBA diving has swelled in popularity to the point where there are well over three million active recreational divers in the United States, and more than 300,000 new divers are trained each year.

For healthy, well-trained, and well-equipped individuals, SCUBA diving is a very safe activity. It is, however, an activity with some inherent risks. The most common risks are associated with the changes in air pressure, sometimes rapid changes, divers must deal with, sometimes descending, sometimes ascending. Improperly treated, some of the medical emergencies associated with diving can cause permanent disability or death.

Physical Principles Of Diving

When a SCUBA diver descends beneath the surface, the ambient pressure increases because of the weight of the water. Water, much more dense than air, creates pressure changes that are substantial even for small changes in depth. At a depth of only 33 feet, the pressure is two atmospheres, or twice the pressure at sea level.

Body tissues consist primarily of water, which is not compressible, so body tissues are not significantly affected by the changes in pressure that occur at depths down to 100 feet, the maximum depth at which most SCUBA diving is done. Gases, however, are compressible, so the gas-filled spaces of the body are directly affected by changes in pressure.

Gas Laws

Knowledge of three gas laws is fundamental to understanding why pressure-related diving medical emergencies occur. Knowledge of these laws is *not* a critical part of knowing how to handle the emergencies, but the laws are presented here for reference.

Boyles's law states that the volume and pressure of a gas are inversely related to its pressure at a constant temperature. In other words, when the pressure on a gas increases the volume decreases, and the converse is true. This law explains the basic mechanism for all types of barotrauma (SEE BELOW).

Dalton's law states that the pressure exerted by each of the individual gases in a mixture of gases is the same as it would exert if it alone occupied the same volume. Alternatively, this law states that the total pressure of a mixture of gases is equal to the sum of the partial pressures of the component gases. Since the biologic effects of a gas depend on partial pressure, Dalton's law is fundamental to an appreciation of decompression sickness (SEE BELOW).

Henry's law states that the amount of gas dissolved in a fluid is proportional the partial pressure of that gas in contact with the fluid. This law explains why a more inert gas, e.g., nitrogen, dissolves in a diver's body during descent and, conversely, is released from tissue with ascent.

Types Of Barotrauma

Air pressure within the middle ear, sinuses, lungs, and other gas-filled spaces of the body is normally in equilibrium with the environment. If something obstructs the free passage of air into and out of these spaces, then a loss of equilibrium will develop. Tissue injury may occur. Such injuries are collectively referred to as *barotrauma*.

Overall, barotrauma is the most common problem for SCUBA divers. Barotrauma can be categorized according to whether it occurs during descent or ascent.

Barotrauma of Descent

Barotrauma of descent, or "squeeze" as it is known to most divers, results from the compression of gas in enclosed spaces as ambient pressure increases with descent underwater. The ears and nasal sinuses are most often affected. More than one type of barotrauma may be present at the same time.

Barotitis (ear squeeze) affects essentially all divers at one time or another and is the most frequent type of barotrauma. Although the external ear can be affected, this is unusual unless the patient was wearing a hood or ear plugs making the ear canal a closed space. Much more common is middle ear squeeze, or *barotitis media*, which results when the diver fails to equalize pressure in the middle ear because of closure or dysfunction of the eustachian tube (the tube from the middle ear to the throat that allows for compensation in pressure changes). Divers usually notice a sense of fullness in the ear, followed by increasingly severe pain. *Vertigo* (dizziness caused by a disturbance in equilibrium) is a common complaint. Blood may leak from the ear, and the *tympanic membrane* (eardrum) may rupture, resulting in *tinnitus* (ringing in the ear) or hearing loss, depending on the severity of the injury. Nausea may be a complaint.

The field treatment for middle ear squeeze is abstinence from diving or other pressure exposures until the condition has resolved, and the use of oral decongestants, e.g., pseudoephedrine, to shrink swollen mucus membranes and help open up the eustachian tube. A combination of an oral decongestant and a long-lasting nasal spray, at least for the first two or three days, is usually most effective. Analgesics (painkillers) may be given as needed.

Although far less common, inner ear barotrauma is much more serious than middle ear barotrauma because of a possible permanently disabling injury. Inner ear barotrauma typically results from the sudden or rapid development of markedly different pressures between the middle and inner ear. These different pressures may result from an overly forceful Valsalva maneuver, a common and typically safe maneuver to equalize pressure in the middle ear by pinching the nose shut and holding the mouth shut and forcefully expelling air, or from an exceptionally rapid descent during which the middle ear pressure is not equalized.

The classic triad of symptoms indicating inner ear barotrauma is roaring tinnitus, vertigo, and deafness. A feeling of fullness or "blockage" of the affected ear, nausea, vomiting, pallor, sweating, disorientation, or loss of coordination may be present. The onset of these symptoms may occur soon after the injury or may be delayed many hours, depending on the specific type of inner ear injury and the diver's activities during and after the dive. The essential point, however, is that any SCUBA diver with a hearing loss should be considered to have inner ear barotrauma until shown otherwise, and should be seen by a physician as soon as possible.

Just as with the ears, the nasal sinuses may also fail to equalize pressure during descent, thus resulting in *barosinusitis* (sinus squeeze). The frontal and maxillary sinuses are most often affected. Sinus squeeze usually causes pain in the affected sinus, and the diver may notice bleeding from the nose or the mouth. Your examination may be unremarkable or may elicit tenderness when you lightly tap over the affected sinus.

Treatment of sinus squeeze is similar to that for middle ear squeeze and consists of the use of decongestants, analgesics, and abstinence from diving until the condition is resolved. Antibiotics are usually indicated in cases of frontal sinus squeeze because of concerns about complications resulting from frontal sinusitis. Consult a physician.

**Signs and Symptoms
Ear/Sinus Barotrauma:**

1. Pain in the affected area
2. Bloody or unusual fluid leaking from the ear or nose or mouth
3. Vertigo
4. Tinnitus and/or hearing loss
5. Nausea and/or vomiting

Barotrauma of Ascent

Although less common than squeezes, SCUBA divers may also suffer barotrauma of ascent, which is the reverse process of what happens in the squeeze syndromes. The only type of barotrauma of ascent that occurs with any real frequency is the *pulmonary overinflation syndrome.*

A dramatic demonstration of Boyle's law, pulmonary overinflation syndrome results from the expansion of entrapped air in the lungs. Air entrapment usually occurs because of breath-holding during ascent, e.g., the diver ran out of air and/or the diver panicked. The net effect leads to alveolar rupture and air filling extra-alveolar locations. Pulmonary overinflation syndrome usually presents with gradually increasing substernal chest pain, difficulty breathing, and difficulty swallowing. Subcutaneous emphysema—bubbles of air trapped beneath the skin—may be present. You may be able to auscultate decreased breath sounds.

The treatment for pulmonary overinflation syndrome usually consists only of observation and abstinence from further diving for four to six weeks after the condition has resolved. In severe cases, hospitalization may be necessary. Administration of supplemental oxygen may hasten resolution of the condition. An important point, except in exceedingly rare situations, is that recompression is contraindicated because of the fear of causing further pulmonary barotrauma.

Arterial gas embolism (AGE)—air bubbles entering the bloodstream—is the most serious complication of pulmonary barotrauma of ascent and, indeed, the most dramatic and serious medical emergency associated with SCUBA diving. Next to drowning, a gas embolism entering the brain is the leading cause of death in SCUBA divers. An arterial gas embolism typically presents just before or within ten minutes of surfacing from a SCUBA dive.

Manifestations of arterial gas embolism are many, but they tend to be dramatic, the brain being affected most often. Loss of consciousness, seizures, blindness or other visual disturbances, inability to speak, confusion, vertigo, headache, weakness (including hemiplegia), and various sensory disturbances are the most common signs and symptoms. The patient may appear to be having a cerebrovascular accident—a stroke (SEE CHAPTER 25: NEUROLOGICAL EMERGENCIES). Sudden loss of consciousness in any SCUBA diver within 10 minutes of surfacing should always be considered to be attributable to a gas embolism until proven otherwise. If gas bubbles affect the heart, the patient may appear to be having an acute myocardial infarction—a heart attack (SEE CHAPTER 23: CARDIAC EMERGENCIES).

All patients suspected of suffering a gas embolism must be referred for recompression, i.e., hyperbaric (high pressure) oxygen treatment, as rapidly as possible. This is the primary and essential treatment. As soon as possible, all patients should be given high-flow supplemental oxygen.

The majority of patients have definite signs and symptoms of neurologic injury when first evaluated, but a significant number manifest spontaneous recovery, at least initially. Nonetheless they must still be transported for recompression treatment because it is impossible to fully exclude damage, and many of these patients deteriorate over the next few hours, often to a worse condition than at first.

In contrast to previous recommendations, it is now recommended that in the field and during transport, patients should be maintained supine. Placement in the left-side/head-down position is no longer recommended because of the uncertain benefit of such a maneuver, concerns about causing or aggravating cerebral edema (especially if left in the head-down position for longer than 30 to 60 minutes), and increased respiratory difficulty associated with being in such a position.

Other Disorders

Decompression Sickness

Decompression sickness (DCS), or, as it is more often called, "the bends," is a multisystem disorder that results when the nitrogen from breathing compressed air that accumulated on descent— explained by Henry's law—collected in the blood in a greater concentration than can be returned to a gas and breathed out on rapid ascent. Gas bubbles then form in the blood and other tissues. Bubbles cause mechanical effects, such as blockages in blood vessels. The overall effect is to decrease tissue perfusion.

The manifestations of DCS are many, with the musculoskeletal system and central nervous system being most often affected. Joint pain is the single most common symptom of DCS and occurs in about three-fourths of patients. The joints most often affected are the shoulders and elbows, although any joint may be affected. The pain is usually described as dull and is usually located deep in the joint. Movement of the joint worsens the pain.

Neurologic manifestations of DCS are less common. Because of the random manner in which bubbles may affect the central nervous system, essentially any symptom is compatible with neurologic DCS, but the lower thoracic, lumbar, and sacral portions of the spinal cord are most often affected, and consequently paraplegia (paralysis of the lower extremities) or paraparesis (partial paralysis of the lower extremities), lower extremity *paresthesia* (numbness or tingling), and bladder or bowel dysfunction are the most common symptoms of neurologic DCS.

Anyone who manifests symptoms after a SCUBA dive that cannot be adequately explained by other conditions should be presumed to have DCS until proven otherwise. Such a patient should be transported for recompression treatment without delay. All patients suspected of having DCS should be started on high-flow supplemental oxygen as soon as possible, and other life support measures should be given according to the patient's specific condition.

Note: In both AGE and DCS, patients should be transported to the recompression chamber as rapidly as possible. In some cases this means an air evacuation. In such situations the patient should be subjected to the least possible pressure reduction so as not to cause further bubble formation or expansion of existing bubbles. Depending on the specific circumstances, e.g., weather, geography, transport distance, available aircraft, either helicopters or fixed-wing aircraft may be used if they can be safely flown at less than a 1000-foot altitude or if they have a cabin that can be pressurized to less than a 1000-foot altitude.

Nitrogen Narcosis: Rapture of the Deep

Several diving-related problems may develop as a result of breathing gases at a higher than normal atmospheric pressure. Among these is *nitrogen narcosis*, a result of the anesthetic effect of nitrogen at elevated partial pressures. There is considerable variability in susceptibility to nitrogen narcosis, with symptoms usually becoming evident at approximately three atmospheres or 100 feet down. At depths of 200 feet, divers suffering nitrogen narcosis are usually so impaired that they can do little or no useful work. Loss of consciousness begins to occur at depths deeper than 300 feet.

Nitrogen narcosis is a reversible condition that has manifestations similar to alcohol intoxication, including impaired judgment, giddiness, poor concentration, incoordination, and slowed motor response. Nitrogen narcosis completely resolves with ascent to shallower depths, and divers often do not notice or recall the adverse effects.

The real importance of nitrogen narcosis is not in its occurrence per se, but in its ability to impair a diver's judgment and memory, thereby possibly precipitating an accident. This possible confounding factor always must be considered when taking a diving accident history, especially when there is a history of diving deeper than 100 feet.

Note: DAN—Divers Alert Network—maintains a medical emergency hotline, 24 hours a day, in Durham, NC, at (919) 684-8111, and a non-emergency advisory line at (919) 684-4544.

Prevention Of Diving Emergencies

1. Use Valsalva maneuvers to equalize pressure in ears and sinuses.
2. Refrain at all times from breath-holding.
3. Monitor carefully the volume of air in your tanks.
4. Monitor carefully your depth, and do not exceed prescribed times at specific depths.
5. Avoid rapid ascents. Base ascent rates on depth of dive and time at depth.

Evacuation Guidelines

Any patient assessed with arterial gas embolism or decompression sickness should be evacuated as soon as possible. Any patient suffering increasing difficulty breathing and/or sudden unconsciousness should be evacuated as soon as possible.

Conclusion

By the time you've removed your mask, fins, and tank, and stored them on board the boat lying off Kona, the instructor has the second student in a position of comfort, breathing 100 percent oxygen from the emergency cylinder he keeps below deck. The patient's condition appears stable, but he tells you he'd rather not take any chances. Heading back toward shore means drawing closer to a hospital. Better safe than sorry.

Mark Crawford, EMT-P, USAF Pararescue, Retired, contributed to this chapter.

Chapter 23: *Cardiac Emergencies*

You should be able to:

1. *Describe coronary artery disease and the risk factors related to coronary artery disease.*

2. *Define and describe the treatment for angina, myocardial infarction, and congestive heart failure.*

It could happen to you

The snowshoe trips you lead in the snowy Cascades east of Seattle leave after breakfast and return to the lodge in time for dinner. All a client has to do is show up. No prerequisites. No medical forms to fill out. Equipment is supplied by the lodge that pays your salary.

Robert, call me "Bob," seems like a nice fellow and appears, generally, to be in good health. But by mid morning, Bob has fallen behind the group. You drop back to check on him.

It's cold, but not enough to explain the paleness of his face,

not enough to justify the pain in his eyes.

"Feels like someone parked their snowmobile on my chest," he pants out in a ragged whisper. "Must be that rich breakfast they fed us at the lodge."

Introduction

Heart attacks lead to more deaths than any other cause in the United States, and wilderness enthusiasm does not provide immunity. Coronary arteries, the vessels leaving the aorta and supplying blood to the heart muscle itself, are very susceptible to injury to their lining. The general term is *arteriosclerosis*, several conditions in which the arteries thicken, harden, and otherwise lose their elasticity. *Atherosclerosis*, probably the most common form of coronary artery disease,

is a gradual clogging of the arteries from fatty deposits and other debris. As the arteries narrow, less blood passes through to reach the heart. Decreased blood flow may lead to several cardiac emergencies, including myocardial infarction ("heart attack").

Encouragement for clogging comes from dietary saturated fat and cholesterol, cigarette smoking, lack of exercise, obesity, and *hypertension* (high blood pressure). Heredity and aging are factors. Diabetes predisposes a

person to coronary artery disease. Oral contraceptives in women over 40 seem to encourage heart attack. Males have more heart disease than females but not by a large number.

You'll notice some of these factors are uncontrollable: heredity, age, gender. On the positive side of things, however, many of the factors are controllable. With consciousness and dedication to prevention, any individual can reduce his or her chance of coronary artery disease.

Types Of Cardiac Emergencies

Angina Pectoris

Caused by interruptions in adequate blood flow to the *myocardium* (heart muscle), a result of narrowed arteries, *angina pectoris* usually comes on with physical or emotional stress, or heat or cold stress, events that increase the work load on the heart. *Angina* pectoris, however, can occur without unusual stress.

Angina pectoris means "pain in the chest," and is more often referred to simply as angina. But sudden chest pain, ranging from a mild ache to crushing pressure (often described as "squeezing, tightness, constricting," or sometimes "burning") is only one of several typical signs and symptoms. The patient may report the pain radiates to the left side of his or her body: shoulder, arm, neck, jaw. Shortness of breath, nausea, and vomiting are not uncommon. Heavy sweating, pale cool skin, and complaints of dizziness or lightheadedness may be a part of your assessment. Indigestion is routinely suspected by the patient.

Signs and Symptoms Angina:
1. Chest pain
2. Shortness of breath
3. Nausea
4. Vomiting
5. Pale cool sweaty skin
6. Dizziness

Since the heart is starved for oxygen, a high flow of supplemental oxygen would be of great benefit. Do what you can to calm and reassure the patient, keeping him or her comfortable and physically at rest. Comfort includes maintenance of normal body core temperature.

Ask about medications. Angina sufferers may be carrying *nitroglycerin* in tablets or spray. Nitroglycerin works by reducing the demands on the heart and dilating the coronary arteries, allowing more blood to pass through. If it has been prescribed to your patient, and if the expiration date has not been reached, help the patient use the drug. Most local protocols ask you to contact medical control in order to gain permission to help the patient take nitro. In the wilderness, out of touch with any medical control, the patient will benefit greatly from your assistance. Most patients carry tablets and most prescriptions call for one tablet taken under the tongue. Classic symptoms indicating the nitro is working include a burning under the tongue and a headache. In five minutes, if the chest pain remains, a second tablet may be given and, if that doesn't work, a third, as long as the patient's blood pressure remains high enough. Nitro should not be given if the patient's systolic blood pressure has dropped below approximately 100. The medication might drop the blood pressure even more and precipitate shock. Because of the possibility of a drop in BP, always give nitro with the patient sitting down in a comfortable, stable position. As long as the patient's radial pulse remains strong, the blood pressure is probably high enough (SEE CHAPTER 3: PATIENT ASSESSMENT).

With rest and/or nitroglycerin, the pain of angina usually goes away leaving no permanent damage. In almost every case, however, you'll want to evacuate the patient, even when the patient appears to have fully recovered, in order for him or her to be evaluated by a physician. If you work as a trip leader, it will prove beneficial if 1) you've screened the person prior to the trip, 2) you've discussed the outcome should the person suffer an attack of angina on the trip, and 3) you've ensured the patient is carrying nitroglycerin. If the patient remains unchanged for 15 to 20 minutes, it is recommended to assume a myocardial infarction (SEE BELOW) and initiate an evacuation. e.g., get help to carry the patient out.

Acute Myocardial Infarction

A *myocardial infarction* or MI (often called a "heart attack") results when a clot blocks a narrowed coronary artery or reduces the blood flow through that artery enough to cause the permanent death of the heart muscle cells fed by that artery. Although heart attacks can be painless and referred to as "silent MIs," probably more than eight out of 10 patients complain of center-chest discomfort: crushing, squeezing pain, or heavy pressure. Pain may radiate to the shoulder, down the arm, and/or into the jaw, predominantly on the left side. Pain may wax and wane, but it does not go away. Rapid, shallow respirations are common, as are complaints of shortness of breath. Pulse may be rapid or slow, regular or irregular. Nausea, vomiting, weakness, and lightheadedness are common.

Skin usually turns pale and cool with heavy sweating, and cyanosis is possible. Patients often deny the possibility that this could be "the big one"—a heart attack—but expect high levels of anxiety.

**Signs and Symptoms
Myocardial Infarction:**

1. Sudden chest pain
2. Shortness of breath
3. Nausea
4. Vomiting
5. Weakness
6. Lightheadedness
7. Pale cool sweaty skin
8. Anxiety
9. Denial

Myocardial infarctions create several possibilities for the patient: 1) MIs can cause sudden death, or death within a couple of hours of the onset of signs and symptoms, depending on the extent of damage to the heart. CPR should be initiated in hopes of salvaging the patient who is breathless and pulseless. 2) If the left ventricle sustains extensive damage, the heart will fail to adequately pump blood to the body, perfusion drops, and cardiogenic shock follows. As many as eight out of 10 patients who develop shock from a heart attack die, usually within 24 hours. 3) MIs may cause congestive heart failure (SEE BELOW). 4) The patient can live a long healthy life if he or she takes steps to prevent further MIs.

For a patient suspected of having an MI, do all you can to maintain an open airway for the patient. In the wilderness there is little else to be done other than keeping the patient physically and emotionally calm, in a position of comfort, insulated from a cold environment. Activity could make the patient much worse. The patient would benefit, often very much, from a high flow of supplemental oxygen, which is rarely available in the wild outdoors. If the patient has been prescribed nitroglycerin, follow the directions for providing aid (see above). The patient requires immediate transport to a medical facility.

Note: Aspirin is an extremely effective antiplatelet agent, a means to prevent further blood clot formation. For that reason, patients having heart attacks may greatly reduce the damage done to their hearts by taking aspirin, as soon as possible. Aspirin, in other words, could save a life. Although the dosage remains somewhat controversial, research indicates the dose should be approximately 160 mg orally to start—one half a standard adult aspirin or two "baby" aspirin—and approximately 80 mg for each new day until you turn the patient over to definitive care. It's better if the aspirin is chewed, which means chewable aspirin would be a better choice for a first aid kit.

Congestive Heart Failure

Heart attack, coronary artery disease, and other forms of damage to the heart may result in a myocardium no longer able to meet the demands for blood that a body makes. A weak myocardium may result in *congestive heart failure* (CHF), a somewhat complex process in which blood and tissue fluids congest (collect excessively) due to the heart's inadequacy.

Failure of the right side of the heart, the side that takes blood from the body and pumps it to the lungs, creates congestion in the periphery of the body, usually most noted in swollen ankles. More seriously, failure of the left side of the heart, the side that takes blood from the lungs and pumps it to the body, creates congestion in the lungs, pulmonary edema, which can rapidly turn into a threat to life. The most important indications are difficulty breathing and the terror such difficulty produces. A patient typically refuses to lie flat, preferring to sit upright, a position that makes it easier to breathe. Pulse will be elevated. Skin may be cyanotic. He or she may cough productively, revealing pink sputum. Death may follow.

**Signs and Symptoms
Congestive Heart Failure:**

1. Difficulty breathing
2. Rapid breathing
3. Anxiety
4. Rapid pulse
5. Cyanosis
6. Productive cough
7. Swollen legs and ankles

Assist the patient in sitting upright. It can prevent some blood from congesting in the lungs. Other than that, your emergency care will be limited to the techniques you use for a patient experiencing a heart attack.

General Treatment Guidelines

1. Maintain an open airway.

2. Keep the patient inactive, physically and emotionally calm, in a position of comfort.

3. Deliver a high flow of supplemental oxygen, if available.

4. Assist in the maintenance of body core temperature.

5. Assist the patient in following the instructions for prescription medications, if applicable.

6. Give aspirin.

7. Initiate a rapid evacuation.

Evacuation Guidelines

A patient suffering from angina should be, in almost every case, evacuated. A patient assessed with myocardial infarction and/or congestive heart failure should be evacuated as soon as possible by a means of transport that requires no exercise by the patient.

Conclusion

Although your assessment reveals Bob has a history of angina and has been prescribed nitroglycerin tablets, he forgot his medication, left it behind at the lodge. You reassure your patient. Digging your emergency foamlite pad and extra clothing from your pack, and stamping out a quick seat in a nearby snow bank, you make Bob as comfortable as possible. As the rest of the group gathers, you announce today's trip will be cut short. Within 10 minutes, Bob has greatly improved. With you carrying your patient's light day pack, the group tramps slowly back to the lodge where you intend to suggest a medical form be filled out by all clients prior to future trips.

Chapter 24:   Respiratory Emergencies

You should be able to:

1. *Describe the signs and symptoms of the most common respiratory emergencies including chronic obstructive pulmonary disease, asthma, pneumonia, pulmonary embolism, and hyperventilation syndrome.*

2. *Describe the treatment for the most common respiratory emergencies.*

It could happen to you

The trail into the Great Smoky Mountains rises toward a cloudless sky, and the summer heat mingles with humidity high enough to drown a small child. While you lead the group of back-packers up the steep path, your co-instructor brings up the rear. Somewhere in the middle of the group, unseen by you or your co-instructor, a voice lifts in a cry for help.

Hurrying back down, you come face to face with the other instructor over the torso of one of the young women on the trip. Although it's only the second day of the hike, you've already decided the woman on the ground, Jen, is strong willed, with an unusual drive to prove herself. You are worried.

"What happened?" you ask the cluster of clients.

"She just collapsed," says one.

"She hit her head," says another.

"I think she's dying," suggests a third.

Jen lies on her side, knees drawn up, curved almost into the shape of a crescent moon. Her upper arms are held tight to her body. Her hands, twisted into odd spasms near her chin, are curled back toward her forearms. Her skin looks pale. Sweat moistens her face. She breathes very rapid and shallow, apparently desperate for air.

Introduction

Comprised of five large and spongy lobes, the lungs are made of millions of air sacs—between 150 and 300 million—called alveoli, which are, essentially, spaces between small airways, called bronchioles, and an extraordinarily dense arrangement of tiny blood vessels, called pulmonary capillaries. The elastic walls of the air sacs are only one cell thick, and here oxygen passes through to enter the blood and bind onto oxygen-depleted red blood cells, and carbon dioxide leaves the blood to be breathed out on the next exhale. Without a steady diffusion of these gasses, oxygen in and carbon dioxide out, life fails to go on. There is simply no more important action for a First Responder than ensuring the patient keeps breathing, and few, if any, medical emergencies cause the patient, and rescuers, more distress than *dyspnea*—air hunger resulting in difficulty breathing.

Types Of Respiratory Emergencies

Chronic Obstructive Pulmonary Disease

The term *chronic obstructive pulmonary disease*, or COPD, covers a collection of diseases sharing the common symptoms of airway obstruction in the small to medium airways, excessive secretions, and/or constriction of the bronchial tubes. Many years of cigarette smoking is the cause of most COPD, with air pollution, genetic factors, and some occupational exposures, e.g., coal dust, sometimes playing a role. Because it takes so many years of inhaling "bad stuff" to produce the signs and symptoms of COPD, patients are seldom less than 50 years old. The most widespread of chronic obstructive pulmonary diseases are, by far, *chronic bronchitis* and emphysema—and most COPD patients have components of both diseases.

Chronic bronchitis is assessed after a patient has had at least two successive years of a productive cough lasting at least three months per year. The cough develops because, to be brief, the patient has inhaled so much smoke he or she has damaged the ciliated cells of the bronchial tubes. The cilia—hairlike processes—normally sweep excess mucus produced by the bronchial tubes up and out. Once damaged, excess mucus collects more and more in the tubes, forcing patients to cough continually to clear their airway. Ventilatory effort becomes less efficient, and more and more carbon dioxide is retained. In later stages, patients with chronic bronchitis may assume a mild but permanent cyanotic complexion.

Although virtually unheard of in a wilderness context, you may one day find yourself facing a patient with chronic bronchitis who needs assistance due to unusual respiratory distress. Almost undoubtedly the patient will relate the nature of the problem, having been diagnosed years before. The patient requires definitive medical care. Your transport should be rapid. Allow the patient to assume a position that makes it most comfortable for her or him to breathe. If possible, start a flow of supplemental oxygen high enough to meet the patient's needs.

Emphysema results from destruction of the alveoli, destruction that is irreversible. In a normal lung, the appearance of alveoli might be compared to a microscopic bunch of grapes. After years of inhaling a harmful substance, once again cigarette smoke the prime damaging agent, the alveoli of the emphysematous patient have eroded into rounded spheres, sort of like one larger grape instead of a bunch of smaller ones. Deterioration of the alveoli means a loss of surface area for gas exchange, which means less and less efficient breathing. The alveoli also start to collapse. In order to keep them as open as possible, the patient tends to sit up straight and breathe with chest muscles which eventually deforms the chest into a more circular shape instead of the normal oval shape. The chest shape of advanced emphysema is known as a "barrel chest." In attempts to breathe easier, emphysema patients often purse their lips to exhale against resistance, a technique that creates back pressure in the lungs which helps keep the alveoli from collapsing. Emphysema leaves the patient physically wasted and in a constant state of fatigue.

The patient may require emergency care when, for some reason, the ability to breathe suddenly decreases. Field treatment is the same as for chronic bronchitis (SEE ABOVE).

Note: People making their initial trip to high altitude may for the first time discover that they have COPD since they were not suffering at sea level.

Asthma

Asthma is often considered an obstructive pulmonary disease because it does involve airway swelling, increased mucus (very sticky mucus) production, and spasms of the lower airway, all of which lead to difficulty breathing. Asthma, however, is a "reactive airway disease." Instead of a disease that deteriorates the ability to breathe, a patient with asthma has an airway that reacts to something by narrowing. Millions suffer from asthma, and an estimated 5,000 will die in the coming year in the United States.

Asthma can be divided into two types: EXTERNAL (extrinsic, allergic asthma) is a reaction to substances such as dust, pollen, spores, mold, or animal dander. INTERNAL (intrinsic, non-allergic asthma) is a reaction to internal stress caused by such things as infection, cold air, emotion, or exercise. Asthma is not contagious, and not curable. No one knows why some people have asthma, but heredity seems to play a part.

Sufferers with a relatively mild form of asthma usually care for themselves, often with an over-the-counter inhaler, e.g., Primatene®. Primatene® inhalers release epinephrine in a mist, dilating the airway. Moderate asthma calls for more effective inhaled drugs, such as albuterol or ipatropium bromide (Atrovent®). A few severe asthmatics may be taking an oral drug to help control their disease. If an asthmatic is taking steroids, e.g., prednisone, for management of the disease, he or she should not be venturing into the wilderness.

Asthma attacks narrow a section of the airway, often leaving the patient able to inhale with relative ease, or actively suck air in past the closure, but not exhale with ease, or passively blow air out past the closure. This is sometimes called an "air trapping" syndrome. Breathing during an attack produces wheezes, sometimes audible to the naked ear, almost always audible through a stethoscope, as the patient moves air past the partial closure of the airway.

It is of great importance to identify and treat an asthma attack early in hopes of keeping it on the mild to moderate side.

The patient experiencing a moderate attack may need your help to shorten the attack. Treat-ment includes calm encouragement of the patient to relax and breathe with control. The patient may require assistance finding and using her or his inhaler. The inhaler should be held with the mouthpiece on the bottom, shaken, and placed between the lips. The patient should exhale before the bottle is depressed into the mouthpiece, releasing the mist. As the mist is released, it needs to be inhaled. The mist must be sucked deep into the airway to work. After inhaling, the patient should hold her or his breath for five to 10 seconds before exhaling.

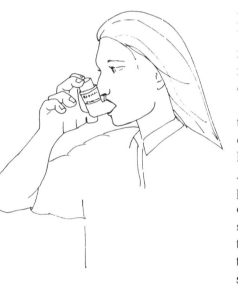

Figure 24-1:
Patient inhaling medication

The patient experiencing a severe attack may need your help to survive. Severe attacks usually prevent the patient from speaking except in one- or two-word clusters: "I (gasp) can't (gasp) breathe (gasp)." The lungs that were full of diffuse wheezes may have now gone silent. If the patient seems extremely tired, or can tell you he or she is "Tired" or "Too exhausted to breathe," respiratory collapse is imminent. When the patient cannot inhale and/or the inhaler is not working, an injection of epinephrine is usually the only life-saving treatment. The dose is the same as for anaphylaxis, and "bee sting kits" may be used (SEE CHAPTER 28: ALLERGIC REACTIONS AND ANAPHYLAXIS). When the patient can breathe, a high flow of supplemental oxygen would be of great benefit.

Status asthmaticus is a prolonged asthma attack unrelieved by conventional treatment. Only rapid transport to definitive medical care offers the patient a chance at life.

Care of asthma patients, after the attack, includes giving copious amounts of drinking water to keep the patient well hydrated. Adequate hydration helps the patient move the sticky mucus out of the airway. An asthmatic should carry medications at all times, especially on wilderness trips. Twice as much as necessary should be carried into the wilderness, one set of medications carried by the patient, and one set carried by someone else. On water-based trips, each set of medications should be carried in separate boats. If one set is lost or ruined, the second set will remain.

Pneumonia

Pneumonia is an infection in the lungs caused by a wide variety of agents including bacteria, viruses, protozoa, and fungi. The disease process can cause swelling and fluid collection in the lungs, leading to difficulty breathing. Unlike COPD, pneumonia is often curable. Unfortunately and despite antibiotic therapy, it will still be the fifth or sixth leading cause of death in the United States this year.

A patient most in need of emergency care will probably have an infection, most likely bacterial, that produces any or all of six classic signs and symptoms: shortness of breath (the most important), chest pain, chills, fever, increased sputum production, and a productive cough—which may produce sputum interestingly colored from yellowish to greenish, even brownish.

Requiring specific antibiotic treatment, the patient should be speedily transported to definitive medical care, preferably while breathing a high flow of supplemental oxygen. In the wilderness, the patient may be treated with antibiotics. e.g., erythromycin, during evacuation. As a group leader, you would do well to ask a physician for recommendations and a prescription. The patient may be given *antipyretic* (anti-fever) drugs, and should be kept well hydrated. Encourage the patient to breathe deeply from time to time, and to cough up the sputum collecting in his or her upper airway.

Pulmonary Embolism

An *embolism* is an obstruction in a blood vessel caused by a foreign substance or a blood clot, most often a blood clot. When the obstruction occurs in an artery of the lungs, the result is a pulmonary embolism, an emergency that will end the lives of an estimated 40,000 or more in the United States in the next year.

In approximately three out of four patients, the embolus formation takes place in a deep vein in the legs before it breaks loose and flows into the lungs. High altitude climbers are susceptible if they're dehydrated and tent-bound for an extended period of time, such as during a storm. A patient with a history of a recent illness or surgery that kept him or her bedridden may be susceptible. Smokers are more at risk than non-smokers. Oral contraceptives, especially taken by women over 40, predispose women to a pulmonary embolism. Trauma to the legs is also a risk factor.

The patient complains of the sudden onset of difficulty breathing. The patient may be apprehensive and complain of chest pain and a cough. About one patient in four will develop hemoptysis (the coughing up of blood). A high flow of supplemental oxygen and rapid transport to a medical facility are the only treatments available for use by the First Responder.

Hyperventilation Syndrome

Not a disease, *hyperventilation*—breathing unusually fast and/or deep—is a human response to some type of stress to the body, such as illness, emotion, exercise, pain, a sudden dip in icy water, etc. To treat hyperventilation, therefore, you have to assess and treat the cause of hyperventilation.

First and foremost in the assessment of a hyperventilating patient is determining if there are any immediate threats to life, a result of the initial survey. Finding none, you should move to the focused assessment, which may shed light on why the patient is breathing fast. A cause discovered and treated should reduce the hyperventilations.

Hyperventilation syndrome, here defined as breathing fast without another cause, occurs relatively often in otherwise healthy patients as a result of psychological stress. The patient, like most hyperventilating patients, will have a high level of anxiety or panic. Rapid breathing blows off carbon dioxide, altering the pH of blood, raising it, a condition called respiratory alkalosis. Alkalosis may cause numbness and tingling in the mouth, fingers, and toes. Alkalosis may cause carpopedal spasms, muscular spasms in the hands and feet. Rapid breathing may cause the slow onset of chest pain from overtaxed chest muscles. Lightheadedness and dizziness are not uncommon. Skin color may vary from pale to flushed. These physiological responses to hyperventilation do nothing the calm the psychologically stressed patient. Prolonged hyperventilation will cause constriction of the blood vessels in the brain, which may lead to fainting. Consciousness will return when the patient's carbon dioxide level returns to normal.

As soon as you know the patient's life is not threatened, you should begin to help the patient regain control of breathing. Stay calm. Clear the immediate area of other people. State clearly to the patient that he or she feels terrible *because of* fast breathing. Ask the patient to breathe slower. Ask the patient to breath-hold for three seconds, longer if possible, and you do the counting. Ask the patient to breathe through the nose. Ask the patient to breathe along with you in a slow, calm manner. Be supportive in your attitude and words. Do not ask the patient to breathe into a bag. It does not work faster than calming the patient down. It may cause more anxiety for the patient. When the patient returns to normal breathing, and the signs and symptoms go away, recovery is complete.

Evacuation Guidelines

Any patient treated for a medical emergency involving difficulty breathing should be evacuated as soon as possible with the exception of a patient successfully treated for mild to moderate asthma and hyperventilation syndrome.

Conclusion

At Jen's side in the Great Smoky Mountains, you do an initial assessment and discover no threats to your patient. Your focused assessment uncovers no apparent injuries. The carpopedal spasms indicate the possibility of hyperventilation syndrome.

Asking your co-instructor to move the group back and give you "lots of breathing room," you speak quietly and confidently to Jen, asking her to hold her breath for a count of three. She ignores you. You speak more firmly, telling her she feels sick because she's breathing so fast. She ignores you. Once again, you repeat your instructions. She stops breathing.

Already on her side, you assure Jen's airway is clear and open. It seems like forever, but she starts to breathe again. Her respiratory rate immediately starts to increase. You speak to her, going over your instructions one more time. Now she hears, and tries to control her breathing. It takes about 30 minutes before Jen seems to be completely in control again, not an unreasonable amount of time to recover from hyperventilation syndrome.

Several hours pass before she feels like her old self.

Jen, you learn, was pushing herself very hard to keep up, breathing hard and fast, suffering from the heat and humidity. She began to feel dizzy. Numbness crept into her lips and tongue. Fearing some kind of serious ailment, she began to breathe even faster. She collapsed to the ground, unable to continue.

You decide to slow the pace of the group, stopping more often for rest breaks. Jen, you are confident, will be able to finish the trip.

Chapter 25:   *Neurologic Emergencies*

You should be able to:

1. *Describe the assessment and emergency care of an unconscious patient.*

2. *Describe the signs and symptoms of the most common neurologic emergencies including cerebrovascular accident and seizure.*

3. *Describe the treatment of the most common neurologic emergencies including cerebrovascular accident and seizure.*

It could happen to you

In Oregon, one of Smith Rock's almost 1,000 named routes is perfect for introducing young students to rock climbing. From a secure anchor at the top, you belay the men and women up the face. From below, your co-instructor coaches them over the trickier moves. It is a warm, bright fall day, full of sunshine, devoid of clouds.

With all the students happily at the top, you tie a static line to a second bombproof anchor, and begin to teach rappelling. The general excitement among the students is apparently not shared by Ben. Ben, who has recovered, reported his physician, from a severe traumatic head injury that required surgical intervention, ascended slowly, requiring extra encouragement to finally make it.

When Ben's turn comes to descend, you check his harness and knots, and he steps back to the edge of the cliff. His nervousness alarms you, and you suggest he consider walking down the easy path to the bottom. Ben declines. He wants to overcome his fear.

As Ben leans out over the rock face, his body stiffens. You calmly remind him to relax and trust the rope. You put tension on the belay rope to remind him you're there providing security. Instead of relaxing, he grows more stiff, his eyes roll up in his head showing nothing to you but white. Ben's feet slip off the edge, and his body begins to jerk in violent convulsions.

Introduction

The brain, the spinal cord, and the peripheral nerves, known collectively as the neurological system—or nervous system—may be further divided into two distinct physiological components: 1) The central nervous system (CNS), the brain and spinal cord, and 2) the peripheral nervous system (PNS), all the other nerves. As far as performance goes, the brain—in charge of thought, vital body functions, and emotion—uses the rest of the nervous system to send its messages to all parts of the body.

Although a critical aspect of life, the PNS receives little emergency care. You should be able to recognize early signs of damage to the PNS, e.g., loss of CSM, but other than reducing a dislocation or an angulated fracture, First Responders primarily document PNS changes and report them to physicians. On the other rescuing hand, you will gear much of your medical efforts at preserving and protecting the CNS.

Basic Anatomy Of The Brain

The cerebrum, the largest part of the brain, is divided into right and left hemispheres, the right side controlling the right side of the head and the left side of the body, the left side of the brain controlling the left side of the head and the right side of the body. The cerebrum houses the speech center near the middle of the brain, the vision center in the back of the brain, and the hearing centers on both sides. In the front of the brain, creativity, abstract thought, and personality traits are housed. Voluntary movement and skilled movement are controlled by the areas of the brain near the top.

A spongy bundle of nerves weighing an average of only three pounds, the brain receives approximately 20 percent of the body's supply of blood and oxygen. Despite being made of so many nerve cells, the brain itself, interestingly, cannot feel pain, heat, or even touch, but deprive it of blood and oxygen for more than a few moments and brain cells begin to die. Unlike other cells of the body, nerve cells are never repaired.

Unconscious States

"Unconsciousness" ranks among the more ambiguous terms. The patient could be simply daydreaming, unaware of the immediate happenings, on one end of unconsciousness, and completely unresponsive—U on the AVPU scale (SEE CHAPTER 3: PATIENT ASSESSMENT)—on the other end. Determining the level of consciousness is an early part of all patient assessments. For patients with an altered level of consciousness, you should do your best to determine the reason for unconsciousness, especially when the patient lies in a wilderness environment, far from definitive care.

Common causes of unconscious states or, to say it another way, things that commonly cause the brain To STOP are:

To: Toxins, e.g., alcohol, co poisoning

S: Sugar, not enough

T: Temperature, too much or too little

O: Oxygen deprivation

P: Pressure, too much

AEIOU TIPS: another helpful mnemonic for determining, with more specificity, why a patient is unconscious (or has changes in mental status)

Allergies: Did an allergic reaction cause unconsciousness? Refer to Chapter 28: Allergic Reactions and Anaphylaxis.

Epilepsy: Did a seizure cause unconsciousness? See below.

Insulin: Did a diabetic reaction cause unconsciousness? Refer to Chapter 26: Diabetic Emergencies.

Overdose: Did an overdose, e.g., alcohol, legal or illegal drugs, cause unconsciousness?

Underdose: Did an underdose, e.g., oxygen, cause unconsciousness?

Trauma: Did a traumatic injury, e.g., a blow to the head, cause a pressure increase leading to unconsciousness? Refer to Chapter 9: Head Injuries.

Infection: Did a bodywide infection cause unconsciousness?

Psychological: Did a psychologically traumatic event cause unconsciousness? Is the patient faking unconsciousness?

Stroke: Did a stroke cause unconsciousness? See below.

The immediate emergency care, however, for all unconscious patients, despite the cause, is generally the same: 1) Protect the airway. 2) Protect the spine unless you can clear it (see Chapter 8: Spine Injuries). 2) Perform a thorough patient assessment. 3) Protect the patient from the environment. 4) Roll the patient into the recovery position (to help maintain the airway). 5) Monitor the patient. 6) Plan and carry out an evacuation. Specific treatment will depend, of course, on the cause of unconsciousness.

Types Of Neurologic Emergencies

Cerebrovascular Accident

A *cerebrovascular accident* (CVA)—also called a stroke—is an interruption of normal blood flow to a part of the brain. The interruption could be caused by a blood clot forming in a cerebral artery, an embolus circulating into the brain from another part of the body to form a clot, or a hemorrhage from a cerebral artery. As a rescuer, you won't know the type of stroke, but you don't need to: The signs and symptoms are all similar, as is the treatment.

Although not impossible in younger patients, strokes are far more likely in older patients with a history atherosclerotic disease (SEE CHAPTER 23: CARDIAC EMERGENCIES).

Signs and symptoms vary depending on the part of the brain affected by the interruption in blood flow. Alterations in mental status are common—often described by ambiguous terms such as confused, stuporous, semiconscious, unconscious—and may leave the patient unable to adequately manage his or her own airway. An open airway, as always, demands priority attention. Don't be surprised by a conscious patient who has lost the ability to speak, or who has slurred speech, or who complains of loss of memory. Breathing irregularities are not uncommon. Changes in heart rate and blood pressure give no accurate assessment clues for a CVA, but if you find a slowing heart rate accompanied by a rising blood pressure, suspect increasing ICP. Indications of

increasing ICP are ominous signs found late in the patient's deterioration (SEE CHAPTER 9: HEAD INJURIES). Facial paralysis or facial drooping may be apparent, usually one-sided. *Hemiparesis* or *hemiplegia* (weakness or paralysis affecting one side of the body) is likely. Loss of reactivity in one pupil—the pupil of the eye on the side opposite from the weakened side—is not uncommon. Blurred or decreased vision in one eye may be a complaint. Incontinence may occur.

The signs and symptoms may last for less than 24 hours, in which case the patient suffered a *transient ischemic attack* (TIA), also known as a "temporary stroke."

Note: You may be able to create a communication system with a CVA patient by asking him or her questions with "yes" and "no" for answers. Encourage the patient to communicate with, perhaps, a nod or shake of the head, or an eye-blink (one blink for "yes," two blinks for "no"). Most patients will feel great relief if you are able to establish some form of communication.

As far as treatment goes, the First Responder is somewhat limited. Emotional reassurance is of great importance, even if you think the patient can't hear or understand you. The fact is they often can. Allow the patient to assume a position of comfort unless the patient is unable to do so. Patients unable to assume a position of comfort should be placed on the affected side, the weak or paralyzed side, to protect

the airway. A high flow of supplemental oxygen should be started, if available. Evacuation should be immediate.

Seizures

Suddenly, there is a great discharge of uncontrolled electrical activity in the cerebral cortex, the outer layer of the cerebrum, the "peach pit" part of the brain. There is an episode of involuntary behavior, which may or may not be associated with an altered mental state. Your patient has had a *seizure*.

Although more than 20 different types of seizures have been identified, they can be classified as being either partial or generalized. For simplicity, *partial seizures* may be described as seizures affecting a localized part of the brain, typically causing no loss of consciousness. Violent or jerking motions, if present, will be limited to a single extremity. The patient may stare blindly, wander aimlessly, repeat a simple motor movement such as lip smacking, etc. No emergency care is required other than careful monitoring of the patient to make sure the seizure does not progress and/or the patient does not endanger himself of herself.

Generalized seizures, on the other hand, involve widespread firing of cerebral neurons. Not all generalized seizures cause tonic-clonic activity, but, when they do, it is the most dramatic form of seizure. The patient assumes a tonic (rigid) posture. The patient's head may turn to one side or be forced backwards. Within less than a minute, typically, the patient enters the clonic (jerking) phase, rapid thrashing around, striking the head and extremities on whatever happens to be in the way. Collapse and unconsciousness usually occur after the tonic/clonic phase. The patient may bite his or her tongue, drool, lose bowel and/or bladder control. Breathing may sound like snoring, or may stop. Skin turns pale or cyanotic. The seizure may last two minutes, but should not last more than five minutes. Following the seizure is a *postictal* period, a period of confusion, disorientation, drowsiness, fatigue.

Some patients describe an aura prior to their seizure, a "funny" feeling, a sick feeling, an odd taste or smell. Patients experiencing auras know they're going to have a seizure.

Although known sufferers are commonly referred to as epileptics, it is more correct to say the patient suffers a seizure disorder. The problem, however, may be caused acutely by head injury, heat stroke, high altitude cerebral edema, diabetes, fever, brain tumor, infection, eclampsia, alcohol or drug withdrawal, and assorted other overstimulations of the brain. Diagnosed patients often take drugs to suppress seizures, e.g., Dilantin®. The overstimulation of wilderness activities has been known to encourage seizures, even in people taking preventive drugs.

A seizure must run its course once it has begun. You can't stop it, but you can protect the patient during the episode. Do not restrain the patient. Move objects away that might cause damage if hit. Cushion under the head with a shirt or parka. The patient cannot swallow his or her tongue, so *do not try to put anything into the mouth.* Many seizure sufferers are harmed by misdirected aid.

If consciousness does not return immediately after the event, roll the patient gently into a stable side position to maintain an adequate airway. A high flow of supplemental oxygen, if available, should be started. Take some notes on what happened: Time, focal areas if you noticed any, length of seizure, triggering events if known. Stay calm, and comfort the patient once a normal level of consciousness returns. Protect the patient's dignity. Allow time and privacy for changing of clothes, etc., if required. Most often, the patient will not remember the event. Don't let the patient drink or move around at first. Check for injuries that could have occurred.

The greatest danger to a seizure patient is *status epilepticus*, a persistent seizure or series of seizures with no time for adequate breathing, a true emergency. If this goes on for too long, permanent damage or death may result. The patient needs medical intervention immediately, but, unfor-

tunately, there is little or nothing to be done in the wilderness for this person other than rapid evacuation.

A person diagnosed with a condition that causes seizures does not need to be immediately evacuated, as long as he or she is dealing with the situation, and the intended wilderness pursuits do not jeopardize his or her life. Patients with first time seizures, or seizures for unknown reasons, should be evacuated for medical attention, but there is seldom reason for a rapid evacuation. Once a seizure has occurred, thoughtful consideration should be given to continuation of the wilderness trip, and seizures for some known reasons, such as heat stroke, high altitude cerebral edema, etc., do merit a rapid evacuation.

A question often arises: Should known seizure sufferers risk participating in an extended wilderness venture? Because there is increased risk to the person and, possibly, to the group, it is recommended that the person be seizure free for at least one year. Seizure suppressing drugs, prescribed to the patient, should be carried in twice the amount thought needed. A full set of drugs should be carried by someone other than the patient, in case of loss or ruin of one set.

Evacuation Guidelines

In almost all cases, a patient with a significantly altered mental status due to illness should be evacuated. A patient assessed with a stroke or TIA should be evacuated as soon as possible. A patient suffering a seizure should be evacuated in most cases, especially if the seizure is a first time occurrence.

Conclusion

At Smith Rock in Oregon, you are empowered by a rush of adrenaline, and you pull Ben to the top of the cliff via the belay rope. Dragging him quickly away from the edge, you pad beneath his head with a coil of the rope. In less than two minutes, his seizure subsides.

Ben seems confused and drowsy. You roll him into a stable side position, and proceed with a patient assessment that reveals no injuries. Drool drains from Ben's mouth, and he has wet his pants. You ask the members of the group that remain nearby to descend and return with Ben's day pack.

By the time the other students return, Ben has regained a relatively normal level of consciousness. He changes into clean shorts. Keeping a watchful eye on Ben, you lead the group back to the foot of the cliff and prepare for the ride home.

Chapter 26:   Diabetic Emergencies

You should be able to:

1. Describe the diabetic emergencies of hypoglycemia and hyperglycemia.

2. Describe the treatment for these diabetic emergencies.

3. Describe the precautions diabetics should take prior to and during a wilderness trip.

It could happen to you

The man you have guided on numerous flyfishing trips along the Madison River of Montana is not himself tonight—very much not himself. Typically a quiet and thoughtful gentleman, this evening, the second of the trip, he sits near the fire complaining irritably about the slowness of your meal preparations, about the weather, about his lack of success that day. His speech is slurred, and you wonder, momentarily, if he is no longer a non-drinker of alcoholic beverages. He fidgets constantly.

You put your hand on his shoulder and ask, "Are you OK?"

He slaps your hand away.

Up close, you notice your client of several seasons has begun to drool. His skin has turned cool and clammy. His body shakes slightly. His breathing is shallow.

Introduction

Your body runs on sugar, a form of sugar called glucose, to be more precise. You manufacture glucose from the foods you eat. Some body parts (muscles, fat, liver) store glucose in various forms in case of future needs. Other parts, especially your brain, cannot store a significant amount of glucose. To meet the critical demands of the brain, you carry glucose in your blood at all times. Glucose passes freely across the blood-brain barrier. The rest of your body's cells cannot utilize glucose without the presence of insulin, a hormone produced in your pancreas. Insulin is required to move glucose out of the bloodstream and through cell walls.

If you have *diabetes mellitus*, your pancreas forms an insufficient amount of insulin. Sometimes the insufficiency of insulin production is complete, and diabetics have to inject it into their body on a daily basis. This is often referred to as *Type I diabetes*, or insulin-dependent diabetes, or juvenile diabetes since it typically begins in childhood. *Type II diabetes*, often called adult-onset diabetes, is diagnosed in patients who have partial insulin production and/or have a defect that prevents them from using the insulin they produce.

Depending on the extent of the problem, Type II diabetics can control their disease with diet, exercise, and/or an oral medication. With care, both types of the disease can be regulated well enough for extended wilderness trips.

If you are an insulin-dependent diabetic, you monitor your blood glucose level daily, usually twice a day with a glucometer, to discover the amount and form of insulin you'll inject. Dangerous conditions may occur if the blood glucose of insulin-dependent diabetics reaches low levels (hypoglycemia) or high levels (hyperglycemia).

Hypoglycemia

Signs and Symptoms Hypoglycemia:
1. Rapid onset of confusion
2. Irritability
3. Combativeness
4. Personality changes
5. Hunger
6. Normal or rapid pulse
7. Normal or shallow breathing
8. Pale, sweaty skin
9. Loss of coordination
10. Headache
11. Tremors
12. Slurred speech
13. Weakness
14. Dizziness
15. Possible seizures

Hypoglycemia (low blood glucose), or *insulin shock*, can occur when a diabetic exercises too much, eats too little, or takes too much insulin. Severe cold weather and severe emotional strain may bring on insulin shock. Glucose moves out of the bloodstream and into cells faster than it is being ingested or produced. Due to the brain's critical dependence on glucose, normal brain function cannot be maintained. An altered level of consciousness characterized by confusion, irritability, and perhaps combativeness is typical. Note these mental status changes could be the same demonstrated by patients with increasing ICP, heat stroke, or other emergencies where the brain is affected. Permanent brain damage, even death may result in a brief period of time. Hunger is common. Other signs may include a rapid pulse and pale, sweaty skin, and loss of coordination. Symptoms may include headache, dizziness, and weakness. Seizures are possible. Onset of signs and symptoms is typically rapid, within minutes to less than an hour.

Note: "Hypoglycemia" may also be a diagnosis made after a series of laboratory tests that reveal a condition in which blood glucose is persistently lower than normal. This is not diabetes, and the patient should have been given precise dietary and exercise instructions concerning the management of his or her glucose levels. The body is amazingly adept at maintaining a normal level of glucose, even after extended periods of exercise, and true hypoglycemia is a rare condition.

Hyperglycemia

Signs and Symptoms Hyperglycemia:
1. Slow onset of confusion and irritability
2. Hunger
3. Thirst
4. Frequent urination
5. Rapid, weak pulse
6. Rapid respirations
7. Sweet, fruity breath
8. Flushed, dry, warm skin
9. Headache
10. Nausea and vomiting

Hyperglycemia (high blood glucose) can be the outcome when a diabetic gets too little exercise, eats too much, or takes too little insulin. Too little insulin and too much blood glucose produces an increase of acids in the body. These acids are a result of the body's breakdown of tissues to use for energy since it cannot use the glucose. Too much acid and the diabetic will progress to *diabetic ketoacidosis* (DKA). DKA is a possibility in the wilderness when the diabetic loses his or her insulin. Infection and stress may also be factors in DKA. There is no immediate danger since the brain has an adequate supply of glucose, but, untreated, serious problems, even death, may occur. Three of the classic signals of DKA are thirst, hunger, and frequent urination. Other signs include warm, dry, flushed skin, and a rapid heart rate. Respirations with a "fruity," acetone odor may be deep and faster than normal. Irritability and confusion are common. Symptoms may include headache, nausea, and vomiting. Sweet breath odor and an altered level of consciousness have led rescuers to mistake DKA for intoxication. Do not assume a patient is drunk. Although hyperglycemia is sometimes referred to as "diabetic coma," the patient is seldom found in a coma. Onset is typically slow, over 12 to 48 hours.

Treatment

Hypoglycemia (insulin shock) is a true emergency that can cause death in minutes if untreated. Hypoglycemia must be field treated immediately with sugared drinks, sweet foods, glucose tablets or jellies. A diabetic patient may be carrying injectable *glucagon*, a hormone that increases the concentration of glucose in the blood, helping raise low blood glucose levels to normal. The patient may need help administering glucagon.

If the patient is unconscious and unable to take foods or drinks, glucose gel or glucosey substances, e.g., syrup, honey, can be rubbed into the gums. To prevent aspiration, the patient should be placed on his or her side before anything is placed in the mouth. It often takes a lot of glucose to do the job. Be constantly alert to the maintenance of the patient's airway.

For an unresponsive patient, the American Diabetes Association recommends:

1. Inject glucagon.
2. Do NOT inject insulin.
3. Do NOT give food or fluids until consciousness returns.

When enough glucose has been absorbed by the body of the hypoglycemic patient, he or she will return to a healthy level of consciousness. If you're unsure whether your patient is hypoglycemic or hyperglycemic, give glucose. It won't hurt the hyperglycemic, and it will save the hypoglycemic.

Hyperglycemic patients seldom require emergency care because the patient recognizes the onset of the problem and self-treats. Ask if the patient has checked his or her glucose level with a glucometer. A patient with an understanding of the disease will often know what dose of insulin is needed for elevated glucose levels, and the problem can be corrected over time. If you are treating a hyperglycemic patient, maintaining hydration is of critical importance because the patient is usually dehydrated already. For the patient who has lost her or his insulin, hyperglycemia is on the way, and only a trip out for more insulin or a trip in by someone else bringing insulin will prevent an emergency.

Note: As people with diabetes age, their circulation becomes inefficient in the small blood vessels. They heal slower and are more prone to infection from soft tissue injuries. Great care should be taken in the management of their open wounds.

Prevention

If you are a leader on a wilderness trip, and the group has one or more members with diabetes, there are precautions you can take to reduce the chance of a diabetic emergency to a minimum:

1. Ask anyone with diabetes to be free of "crashes," the need for emergency care, for at least one year, an indication that he or she understands the illness and how to cope with it.

2. Ask anyone with diabetes to practice on overnight and weekend trips before undertaking longer wilderness adventures. The person with diabetes must be able to make adjustments due to the changes he or she will experience in normal routine, changes such as exercise level, variations in diet, cold stress, and possible illnesses, e.g., diarrhea or vomiting.

3. Remind anyone with diabetes to stay in shape, a high level of physical fitness being an extremely important factor.

4. Refresh your memory concerning diabetic emergencies, and know how to give injections.

5. Remind anyone with diabetes to stay well hydrated.

6. Carry a readily available carbohydrate source, such as glucose tablets or gel, and make sure everybody traveling with you knows where the glucose is and how to best help get it into the patient if the need arises.

7. Ask anyone with diabetes to carry twice as much insulin, glucagon, and syringes as he or she thinks will be needed. Divide the supplies so that it's not all in one pack or canoe bag, just in case a set of supplies is lost.

8. Remember insulin must be carried near the body in extremes of cold to prevent freezing.

9. Remember to protect insulin from overheating in hot climates.

10. Learn how to use the glucometer. Suggest that anyone with diabetes check his or her blood

glucose often the first few days of the trip. If readings are high, suggest reducing the amount of carbohydrates being taken in before increasing the insulin dose.

11. Suggest that anyone with diabetes limit the use of concentrated sources of simple glucoses. For snacks, suggest nutrient-dense foods such as nuts and dried fruits.

12. Remind anyone with diabetes to not skip meals.

13. Work with anyone with diabetes to plan each day the night before, including wake-up time, activities, and meals. Sleeping late can be adjusted for by merely pushing all meals back. Adjust for late dinners by switching the bedtime snack with the regular dinner time or by reducing the morning insulin dose and taking an evening injection of regular insulin just prior to the evening meal.

Evacuation Guidelines

Evacuation of a hypoglycemic patient depends on whether or not the patient returns to a normal condition, and whether or not the patient wishes to remain in the field. If treatment of the hyperglycemic patient is not working, the patient requires evacuation to a medical facility.

Conclusion

Aware of your client's diabetic condition, you recognize the onset of hypoglycemia. Grabbing a full water bottle, you throw in a handful of presweetened Kool-Aid and add a couple of teaspoons of sugar. The man eagerly accepts the bottle and shakily drinks until the container is empty. As your patient begins to calm down and return to normal, you serve dinner—the fine trout you caught today. The evening discussion reveals not only that your client has been exercising much more strenuously that usual, but he also skipped lunch today in his eagerness to catch fish. He vows to be more careful tomorrow.

Chapter 27: Poisoning Emergencies

You should be able to:

1. Describe the ways in which poison can get into the human body.

2. Describe the treatment for the most common wilderness poisoning emergencies.

It could happen to you

Unseasonable snow keeps you and your partner, Daryl, huddled in the tent where you've been for more than 24 hours, waiting for a break in the weather in order to continue your ascent of Mount Rainier. Hunger and thirst lead to firing up the stove under the vestibule, but a harsh wind convinces you to move it inside where water now simmers, melting the snow you periodically dump into the pot.

At first you leave the tent's door about one-third open, but rushes of icy air insist the opening be closed. Eventually you're zipped up inside the tent without adequate ventilation. You develop a mild headache, pain that resolves when you step outside for a few minutes to urinate.

Back in the tent, and several cups of tea and a freeze-dried dinner later, your mild headache returns and reaches toward throbbing proportions, and your stomach has you thinking your culinary efforts might resurface on the tent floor. Daryl, complaining of head pain earlier, now seems irritable and increasingly confused. He periodically gasps for air, grumbling that he can't seem to get a full breath.

Introduction

Any substance you ingest, inhale, absorb through your skin, or get injected into your body that causes a malfunction in normal biological processes is called a *poison*. Most deaths from poisoning occur in homes to small children who eat something "bad." Absorbed poisons seldom occur outside of industrial or farming settings where strong chemicals are used. In the wilderness, fatal poisonings are rare. When they do happen, it is usually the result of cooking in an inadequately ventilated tent or snow cave that lets carbon monoxide build up, ingesting a poisonous plant, usu- ally a deadly fungus, or receiving the bite or sting of a venomous creature (SEE CHAPTER 21: NORTH AMERICAN BITES AND STINGS). In cases of serious poisonings, proper intervention by the Wilderness First Responder may save a life.

Ingested Poisons

Mushrooms

Out of 85,556 documented, questionable mushroom ingestions reported to the American Association of Poison Control Centers in a recent 11 year period, only 14 resulted in fatalities. Almost all the deaths were in adults who mistakenly ingested poisonous 'shrooms for dinner or for a hallucinogenic high.

The mushroom most likely to kill? The *Amanita* species (*Death Cap, Death Angel, Destroying Angel*)—responsible for 90-95 percent of all human deaths by mushrooms and containing cyclopeptide amatoxins—can produce fatal liver and kidney failure in two to three days. Typically growing under deciduous trees in the United States, *Amanitas* show a yellowish to white cap four to 16 cm in diameter and a thick stalk five to 18 cm long with a large bulb at the base. The gills under the cap are usually easily visible and white to green in color.

Onset of gastrointestinal distress—severe nausea, vomiting, abdominal cramps, diarrhea—with *Amanita*, and with all potentially death-causing mushrooms, usually falls in the six-to-12 hour range. As a general rule, remember this: If symptoms develop within approximately two hours of ingestion, it is unlikely that the mushroom is one of the potentially fatal varieties. In other words, if stomach discomfort soon follows mushroom munching, the chance of serious mushroom poisoning is extremely slim.

Here's the main point so far: By the time signs and symptoms show up in serious mushroom poisonings, it's too late to do anything except hurry to a hospital where supportive care might save the life of the patient. That means if you think someone has eaten a bad 'shroom, *start treatment quickly*. If you're in doubt, *start treatment quickly*. You don't want to wait for signs and symptoms. Each moment that passes lets more and more poison be absorbed into your patient's system (SEE BELOW TREATMENT FOR INGESTED POISONS).

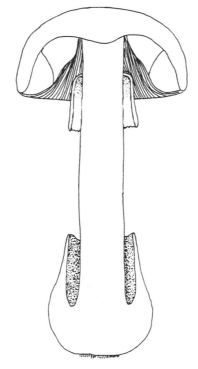

Figure 27-1:
Cross section of Death cap

Jimsonweed

Hallucinations and deaths in the wilderness have been attributed to a pot of tea—a tea brewed voluntarily by the patient from Jimsonweed, *Datura stramo-nium*, a plant that grows all over North America, sometimes known in differing locales as stinkweed, thorn apple, Indian apple, angel's trumpet, sacred datura, and belladonna. The genus *Datura* is responsible for a large percentage of plant poisonings that show up each year in hospitals of the United States.

Of the 25 species of *Datura* growing worldwide, most are shrubs that grow close to the ground. A few are treelike and reach a height exceeding 35 feet. But common to all are trumpet-shaped flowers in shades of red, pink, yellow, or, by far most familiar, white. Native cultures of the New World used *Datura* to treat venomous snakebites, insect bites and spider bites, asthma, sore throat, nasal congestion and bruises. But most often it has been, and still is, used to produce a state of euphoria. It is intentional ingestions by seekers of a hallucination that produce most modern poisonings. The leaves, roots, stems, seeds and fruit contain a combination of alkaloids including atropine and scopolamine. These alkaloids are anticholinergics, affecting the nervous system, and in proper doses are very useful. Scopolamine is the active ingredient in transdermal patches, the little sticky things that go behind your ear to alleviate motion sickness. In large doses the chemicals produce delirium, fast heart rates, dilated pupils and fever. In larger doses anticholinergics may produce coma, seizure, respiratory failure, and death.

Water Hemlock

Water hemlock is considered the most violently poisonous plant in the northern temperate regions of earth. Growing predominantly along waterways, hemlocks are tall perennial herbs, members of the carrot family. The entire plant is poisonous from the flat-topped clusters of small white flowers, down past the narrow, toothed, pointed leaves to the roots that exude a gummy yellow juice when cut. One mouthful of root will kill a large adult. Cicutoxin, the poison in hemlock, attacks the central nervous system, causing tremors, spasms, convulsions, paralysis and, often, death. On the way to death, extreme stomach pain, diarrhea and vomiting are common.

Solanums

An interesting group of plants, containing around 1500 species, is the genus *Solanum*. This genus includes the deadly nightshade (*S. nigrum*), climbing nightshade (*S. dulcumara*), Jerusalem cherry (*S. pseudocapsicum*), the potato (*S. tuberosum*), and the eggplant (*S. melongena*). Each of these has caused poisoning in humans. The poison is a group of alkaloids lumped together under the name solanine. It occurs in different parts of different *Solanums*. The vines, for instance, of the potato and eggplant contain large amounts of solanine, but the ripened fruit is perfectly wonderful to eat. Green potatoes and immature eggplants contain substantial amounts of solanine and should, of course, be avoided. Symptoms include nausea and vomiting, fever, weakness and, sometimes, paralysis.

Seeds

Other sources of plant poisonings not suspected by those people who regularly eat them include the seeds of the apple, apricot, plum, peach, and cherry. These seeds contain amygdalin, a cyanogenic glycoside. When broken down in the digestive tract, the seeds release cyanide. Although it is extremely rare for someone to eat enough of the seeds to cause harm, fatal ingestions have been well-documented.

Note: Not all ingested poisons in the wilderness are plant poisons. Students, especially young students, on outdoor programs may intentionally or unintentionally ingest harmful levels of medications from their own or the group first aid kit. Acetaminophen, e.g., Tylenol, for example, can be toxic to the liver when taken in large doses. Ibuprofen, e.g., Advil, can be destructive of the kidneys when taken in large doses over a long period of time.

Treatment: Ingested Poisons

It would be nice to have a Wilderness Poison Control Center to call. The people there could provide immediate and exact information to guide you. In their absence, you are left with some management principles.

Limiting the absorption of the poison from the gastrointestinal tract is the prime goal of field management. There are three practical methods of doing this in the wilderness: 1) diluting the poison with as much water as the patient will drink, 2) inducing vomiting, and 3) binding the toxin with activated charcoal.

If vomiting can be induced early, within one hour, it may be very beneficial, especially when a mushroom poisoning is suspected. Emetics are vomiting-inducers. A lightweight emetic for your first aid kit is a small bottle of syrup of ipecac. An adult (about 10 years old or older) gets two tablespoons with eight-to-16 ounces of water. Younger people get one tablespoon with the same amount of water. Do not sit facing them. The vomit tends to come suddenly and forcefully, and may repeat several times. If they haven't vomited in 20 minutes, repeat the dose.

Without ipecac, stimulation of the gag reflex may work to induce vomiting. Lean the patient forward, gently reach into their mouth with a finger, and tickle the back of their throat.

Do NOT Induce Vomiting if the:

1. Patient is losing consciousness.

2. Patient has a seizure disorder or heart problems.

3. Patient has swallowed corrosive acids or bases which can increase damage as they come up.

4. Patient has swallowed petroleum products which can cause serious pneumonia if even a small amount is breathed into the lungs.

Note: It is unlikely you'll be carrying many chemicals in the back-country. But in case of ingestion of corrosive chemicals or petroleum products, get the patient to drink a liter bottle of water. Diluting the poison will reduce its effects. If someone takes an accidental swallow of white gas, the petroleum product you brought for the stove, do not induce vomiting. White gas ingestion can typically be managed with dilution and without any harm to the patient.

Activated charcoal is post-combustion carbon residue treated to increase absorbency. With most poisons, even if your care will be short-term, binding the toxins with charcoal is even a better treatment than inducing vomiting. Why? By the time you realize you have a poisoned patient, much of the toxin has already passed out of the stomach, and there are no contraindications for the use of activated charcoal. Charcoal may also be administered post-vomiting. The usual dose is 50-100 grams for adults, and 20-50 grams for children. Although it is odorless and tasteless, swallowing the slurry of fine black powder may prove a chore. It can be added to flavored drinks (e.g., fruit drinks), but it should not be mixed with milk or milk products. Activated charcoal can be found in almost any pharmacy without a prescription, and some brands include Sorbitol®, a "sweetener," and rate as slightly more palatable. Sorbitol® also enhances the speed with which the contents of the bowel pass, reducing the time the poison has to be absorbed. Making a slurry from the white ashes of a camp-fire has been suggested, and might prove of some use.

If the patient goes unconscious, evacuation to a medical facility is probably what is going to save a life. Keep the patient on her or his side during the evacuation to maintain the airway.

Prevention

Many of these and other poisonous plants grow abundantly in wilderness places where they occur naturally or have escaped captivity and gone wild. The potential for harm is created when the cardinal rule of wild edibles is forgotten: *Absolutely positive identification of wild edibles must precede consumption.*

Inhaled Poisons

Carbon monoxide

Carbon monoxide (CO) poisonings account for approximately one-half the deaths by poison in the United States every year. This invisible, odorless, and tasteless gas creates one of the few serious poison threats on wilderness ventures.

Outdoor stoves burn inefficiently in an enclosed space with inadequate oxygen. Higher altitudes increase the chance of poor combustion of the fuel being burned, and CO poisoning may be mistaken for altitude illness (SEE CHAPTER 18: ALTITUDE ILLNESSES). The result of incomplete combustion of any organic fuel (gasoline, kerosene, natural gas, charcoal, wood) is carbon monoxide. Once inhaled, CO enters the blood of the patient where it is more than 200 times more bondable than O2 to the hemoglobin of red blood cells. Hemoglobin normally car-ries oxygen to the cells of the body. With CO attached, hemoglobin can't carry as much oxygen and can't release what is attached as efficiently. The brain and heart, the organs most in need of a constant flow of oxygen, begin to deteriorate. Tissue death can occur rapidly, and lead to the death of the organism, e.g., you and/or your tent partner.

As the amount of attached carbon monoxide increases in the body to approximately 20 percent of the maximum potential, the patient develops a terrible headache, nausea, vomiting, and a loss manual dexterity. At 30 percent, the level of consciousness descends into irritability, impaired judgment, and confusion. It will be increasingly difficult for the patient to get a full breath, and he or she will grow drowsy. At 40 to 60 percent, the patient lapses into a coma. Levels above 60 percent are usually fatal. The "cherry-red skin" often associated with the terminal stage of CO poisoning is, in truth, very rarely seen. Death typically results from heart failure. Death by CO is not a pleasant drift into slumber depicted in some movies.

In the field the treatment is simple: Move the patient to fresh air. If the patient has been exposed to low concentrations of CO (or high concentrations for a short time), he or she will probably recover completely in a few hours. The half-life of carbon monoxide attached to hemoglobin runs around 5.5 hours. If the concentrations have been high, the patient will not get better and may die even removed from the source of the gas. A high concentration of supplemental oxygen is the most important treatment for severe CO poisoning. Rapid evacuation to a high pressure (hyperbaric) chamber may prove beneficial. Although controversial, use of a Gamov Bag will not harm the patient, and may prove of some benefit. Patients unconscious from co poisoning will need to have their airway maintained during the evacuation.

Treatment: Inhaled Poisons

For any inhaled poison, including the intentional inhalation of poisons, e.g., glue, for a hallucinogenic high:

1. Remove the patient from exposure to the poison.

2. Administer a high flow of supplemental oxygen, if available.

3. Hyperbaric chamber therapy for patients of serious co poisoning.

Prevention

Do not burn any organic fuel in a tent, snow cave, or any other shelter unless the shelter is well ventilated.

General Treatment Guidelines

In general, with any suspicion of a poisoned patient, ask early about nausea and vomiting, abdominal cramps, diarrhea, loss of visual acuity, muscle cramps, or anything else unusual. Especially indicative of serious poisonings are changes in the level of consciousness of the patient and changes in the respiratory drive of the patient. All vital signs should be monitored with alertness to changes that indicate shock.

The historical evidence you gather may be extremely helpful in assessing and dealing with the problem:

1. What was ingested, inhaled, absorbed, or injected?

2. How much?

3. When?

4. Who? Age, Sex, Body Size.

5. With ingested poisons, when did the patient last eat? What else is in the stomach?

6. If more than one person suffers, what possible poison do they have in common?

7. Was contact with the poison accidental or intentional?

Evacuation Guidelines

Any patient suspected of having contacted a potentially lethal dose of a poison should be evacuated as soon as possible. Rapid evacuation is critical for patients with changes in level of consciousness and changes in respiratory drive.

Conclusion

Suddenly the light of realization shines on your tent on Mount Rainier: carbon monoxide poisoning. You turn off the stove and open wide the tent door. A blast of cold air sends a shiver down your back. After approximately 20 minutes, you notice the ill effects are beginning to wear off.

Daryl, whose exposure to the gas was constant, is no worse—but no better either. To attempt a descent in this storm, which has strengthened in intensity, is ridiculous. There's nothing to do other than keep the tent ventilated and hope for the best.

Daryl drifts in and out of slumber during the evening, fall-ing fast asleep sometime well after dark. His breathing, you are overjoyed to note, becomes more and more regular and easy. Early the next morning he awakes, not exactly feeling great, but definitely well along the road to full recovery.

Chapter 28: Allergic Reactions And Anaphylaxis

You should be able to:

1. Describe an allergic reaction.
2. Describe the treatment for an allergic reaction.
3. Describe an anaphylactic reaction.
4. Describe the importance and methods of using epinephrine in treating anaphylaxis.

It could happen to you

A fine spring day, plants blooming in a riot of color, and your group of budding naturalists are busy identifying flowers near Crested Butte, Colorado. The alpine meadow, bordered by a deep creek, is a picture of serenity until a scream pierces the air. You see one of your students running across the meadow engulfed in a swarm of bees that angrily spit from a disturbed nest. The student runs to the creek and immerses herself to escape. By the time you reach the water most of the bees have given up. You dodge the last few buzzers to reach her side. She sobs hysterically from pain and fright. You coax her onto shore, noticing at least a couple of dozen red raised welts from the stings.

The next few minutes pass so quickly you can hardly believe what is happening. Before your eyes her face begins to redden and swell. Suddenly she complains not of pain but of increasing difficulty catching her breath. Her breathing grows ragged and gasping. She can only choke out one and two words sentences. Less than five minutes after you help her from the creek, she collapses on the ground, her skin flushed, her tongue protruding slightly from her mouth.

Introduction

An *allergic reaction*, for the purposes of this book, is an acquired hypersensitivity to a substance that causes no reaction in the great majority of humans. The allergy-causing substance is called an *allergen*. Someone with an allergy has, essentially, an immune system disorder, a disorder that develops after an individual has been exposed to the allergen. You have to contact the allergen at least once to develop the hypersensitivity. It is important to remember that virtually anything that can be swallowed, rubbed on the skin, injected through the skin, or inhaled can result in an allergic reaction.

Types of allergic reactions range from relatively mild and delayed to immediate and severe. Reactions can be unpleasant, frightening, and in the most severe case of immediate reaction, potentially fatal. This most severe allergic reaction is termed anaphylaxis.

Allergens that commonly cause anaphylaxis include foods, medications taken either orally or by injection, and animal bites and stings, especially insect stings. Specific anaphylaxis-producing allergens include:

Foods: Shellfish and other seafood, nuts, berries, preservatives and food additives, e.g., MSG.

Medications: Penicillin and other antibiotics, aspirin and other anti-inflammatory drugs, anesthetics.

Animals: Hymenoptera (bees, hornets, wasps, yellow jackets, fire ants), jellyfish, spiders, caterpillars.

There are hormone and nerve transmitted reactions to the foreign substances that cause allergic reactions once they're inside an allergic person, including a massive release of histamines, a substance stored in cells and released in response to injury. In the case of an allergic reaction, the injury is the invasion of the foreign substance. Massive histamine release causes, among other reactions, increased dilation of capillaries, which could lead to shock in a severe reaction, and constriction of the smooth muscles of the bronchial tubes, which could lead to asphyxiation in a severe reaction.

Allergic Reactions

There are three types of immediate reactions which are termed 1) local, 2) general (systemic), and 3) anaphylaxis. These reactions can occur rapidly, within seconds, following exposure, or they may take several hours to develop (see Chapter 31: Common Simple Wilderness Medical Problems).

An immediate local reaction—a red, swollen area—encountered in the wilderness is generally from stings or puncture wounds that induce an allergic substance under the skin. In the case of a bee sting, the stinger should be removed as soon as possible. Cold packs or cold compresses may alleviate some of the pain. The immediate use of a non-prescription antihistamine, such as diphenhydramine, e.g., Benadryl®, may be helpful in minimizing the allergic reaction.

Immediate generalized reactions can come from any source, e.g., food ingestion, stings, and result in increased allergic symptoms (nasal and chest congestion, itchy eyes), *bronchospasm* (spasms in the muscles of the bronchi), *urticaria* (hives), and *angioedema* (swelling of the mucous membranes of the lips, mouth, or other parts of the respiratory system). These general reactions usually do not result in true anaphylaxis, but they can be quite severe and cause difficulty breathing that is potentially dangerous. Late generalized allergic reactions can occur starting six hours after exposure, but serious reactions causing difficulty breathing have not been known to develop after one hour.

Anaphylaxis

Anaphylaxis is a true, life-threatening emergency. It begins like a general reaction but rapidly results in respiratory and/or circulatory collapse. Breathing difficulties (from airway constriction) and anaphylactic shock (from rapidly dilating blood vessels) that result in a true anaphylactic reaction require rapid field treatment. The onset of the signs and symptoms of anaphylaxis typically occur within minutes of a bite or sting and within 30 to 60 minutes of ingestion of an allergen.

Signs & Symptoms of Anaphylaxis:
Anaphylaxis may involve any combination of reactions in the following body systems:

Integumentary system (Skin): Flushing, itching, burning, and swelling, especially of the face. Cyanosis of the lips. Swelling of the tongue. Hives that itch severely.

Circulatory system: Weak, rapid pulse. Drop in blood pressure.

Respiratory system: Painful tightness in the chest. Upper airway obstruction. Difficulty breathing. Coughing. Wheezing.

Neurological system: Restlessness. Lightheadedness. Convulsions. Confusion. Loss of consciousness.

Gastrointestinal system: Nausea. Vomiting. Abdominal cramps. Diarrhea.

Note: Fainting after a bite or sting may not be due to true shock from anaphylaxis, but rather from hyperventilation (SEE CHAPTER 24: RESPIRATORY EMERGENCIES). The WFR must be able to differentiate these two events and treat both appropriately.

Treatment

If you suspect a person susceptible to anaphylaxis has been exposed to a known allergen, give an oral antihistamine as soon as possible, a treatment that might forestall the anaphylactic reaction.

Since deaths due to anaphylaxis occur primarily from loss of airway and general circulatory collapse—shock—and since most fatalities occur within minutes to an hour of onset of symptoms, the ability to respond immediately typically means the difference between life and death. The ability to reverse fatal anaphylaxis requires the administration of epinephrine.

There are two ways in which the WFR can assist with the administration of epinephrine: 1) As many of the severe reactions involve bronchospasm and pulmonary congestion of a typical asthmatic nature, the use of inhaled epinephrine, e.g., Primatene®, to relax the airway can be life-saving. This is a non-prescription medication. Unfortunately, inhaled epinephrine won't work if the patient can't inhale, and it does not help significantly

in the case of cardiovascular collapse in severe anaphylaxis.
2) The most specific and valuable treatment is the use of injectable epinephrine which works to alleviate both bronchospasm and anaphylactic shock. This prescription product is available in kit form and the WFR should a) be aware of how to help the patient administer this medication if it is available, and b) consider acquiring a prescription and written protocols for its use from a physician prior to a wilderness journey.

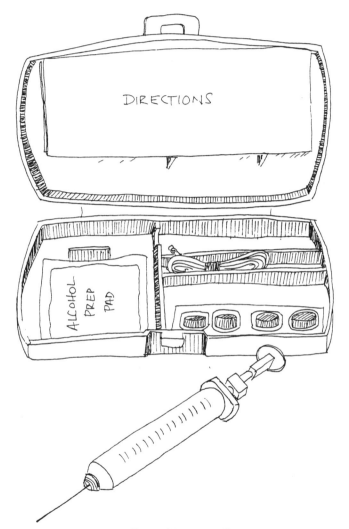

Figure 28-1: Ana-Kit

The two kit systems currently available are the EpiPen® with one (1) 0.3 ml bolus of epinephrine per injection (and EpiPen Jr®, for young children, with one 0.15 ml bolus per injection), and the Ana-Kit® or Ana-Guard® (with two 0.3 ml injections possible). Many persons with a history of insect sting allergy will have one of these kits prescribed for their use by their physician.

Note: With either EpiPen® or Ana-Kit®/Ana-Guard®, you must take great care to prevent injecting yourself in a finger or hand. The vasoconstricting effect of epinephrine is strong enough to cause loss of small, low circulation areas, especially a fingertip.

Use of EpiPen®

The EpiPen® is an auto-injection system. Using the EpiPen® involves three simple steps: 1) Pull off the safety cap. 2) Place the tip on the outer thigh, preferably against the skin, but it can be used through thin clothing. 3) With older units, push the unit against the thigh until it clicks, and hold it in place for approximately 10 seconds. With new units, press the top of the unit until it clicks, and hold it in place for approximately 10 seconds. It is very important to hold the unit in place until all the epinephrine has been injected.

Use of Ana-Kit®/Ana-Guard®

The Ana-Kit® and Ana-Guard® are manual injection systems utilizing the same type of syringe. The Ana-Kit® contains additional items including oral antihistamine tablets. The Ana-Guard® includes only the syringe. Using the syringe involves: 1) Removal of the red rubber needle cover. 2) Holding the syringe upright and pushing the plunger until it stops to expel air and excess epinephrine. 3) Rotating the plunger one quarter turn until the crossbar aligns with the slot in the barrel of the syringe. 4) Inserting the needle straight into the muscle of the upper thigh or upper arm. 5) Pushing the plunger steadily, but not quickly, until it stops. 6) Removing the needle from the muscle and protecting it in case the second injection is needed. The syringe barrel has graduations so that smaller doses may be measured for young children. By rotating the plunger once again, the second 0.3 ml injection may be administered.

Note: Sometimes one injection is not enough, and rebound or recurrent reactions can occur up to 24 hours after the original incident. A second injection should be given in five minutes if the condition of the patient worsens, and in 15 minutes if the condition of the patient does not improve. Some physicians recommend up to three total doses, and some recommend more. It is recommended that the Wilderness First Responder should have at least three injections of epinephrine at his or her disposal.

After Epinephrine

The patient will frequently have blanching of the skin around the injection site. This is a normal response to the local vasoconstriction caused by this medication.

The response to the administration of epinephrine in a normal healthy person is the development of *tachycardia* (increased heart rate). The anaphylactic patient will already have tachycardia, and the use of epinephrine will generally lower this rapid heart rate as it reverses the vasodilatation and bronchospasm of anaphylaxis.

Epinephrine is rapidly inactivated in the body and will become sub-therapeutic (too inactivated to be effective) within 20 minutes. Repeat dosage may be required, if symptoms worsen, every five to 20 minutes as necessary to maintain a stable patient.

Oxygen is the second most useful drug in treating anaphylaxis as hypoxia (too little oxygen) can rapidly cause cardiovascular collapse during this crises. If supplemental oxygen is available, immediately start a low flow via face mask or nasal cannula for both psychological as well as physiological support. In cases of severe respiratory distress, increase the flow to high (SEE APPENDIX B: OXYGEN AND MECHANICAL AIDS TO BREATHING).

The Ana-Kit® includes tablets of an oral antihistamine which should be given as soon as the patient can accept the tablets and swallow. Many over-the-counter antihistamines, e.g., diphenhydramine, may be in a wilderness medical kits and should be given. The recommended dose of diphenhydramine is 50 to 100 mg to start, and approximately 50 mg every four to six hours until the patient is turned over to definitive medical care. Since the heart muscle is very sensitive to histamine, the use of the above antihistamines may play a stronger role in the early treatment of anaphylaxis than was once thought.

There are other prescription medications the patient, or someone in the party, may be carrying which can be useful in treating anaphylaxis. Albuterol, e.g., Ventolin®, Proventil®, prescribed to treat asthma, may be given in two puffs inhaled every three hours to help with the respiratory component of anaphylaxis. Some asthmatic patients have access to an ipatropium (Atrovent®) inhaler, which can be life-saving, especially in recurring episodes of difficulty breathing. The treatment dosage may have to be fairly high, 15 to 30 puffs per four hour period for maximum results. This is a larger dose than an asthmatic person has generally been instructed to use by his or her physician. Under normal circumstances, you would never use a prescription medication for someone other than the person to whom it is prescribed, but, in this case, you are taking unusual steps in hopes of saving a life.

In case of cardiac arrest, CPR should be initiated, although artificial ventilations may be difficult until the bronchospasm relaxes.

Evacuation Guidelines

Any patient who has been treated for anaphylaxis should be evacuated from the wilderness as soon as safely possible in order to be evaluated by a physician. During the evacuation, the patient should be kept on an oral antihistamine, such as diphenhydramine. The recommended dose for over-the-counter diphenhydramine is 25 to 50 mg every four hours.

Conclusion

In the meadow near Crested Butte, you think back to your patient's medical form, recalling she reported once having a "bad reaction" to a bee sting. Recognizing an anaphylactic reaction in your budding naturalist, you grab the medical kit from the top of your pack. Your own labored breathing includes sighs of hopeful relief based on the foresight that allowed you to acquire a prescription for injectable epinephrine and written protocols for its use from your physician. Uncapping the Ana-Guard's syringe, you carefully plunge the needle into your patient's upper arm. Injecting the drug, you remove the needle, protecting the syringe in case you'll need the second injection. Within 30 seconds, your patient begins to breathe easier, returning slowly to a normal level of consciousness. When she is able to accept a water bottle and drink, you give her 50 mg of Benadryl, two 25 mg tablets. You begin plans for an immediate evacuation.

William W. Forgey, MD, contributed his expertise to this chapter.

Chapter 29: Abdominal Emergencies

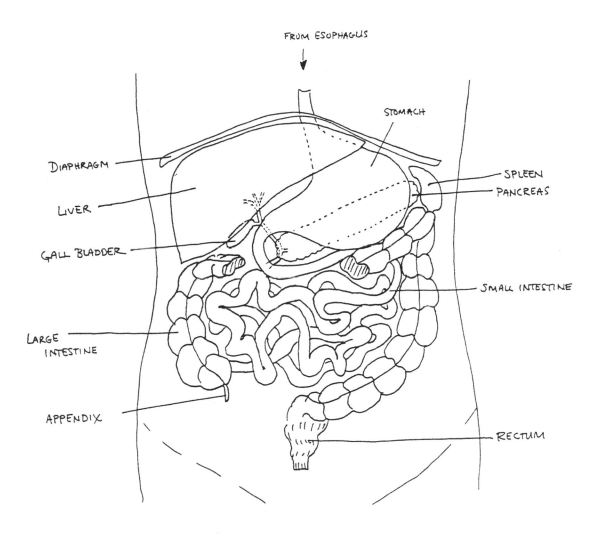

FROM ESOPHAGUS

STOMACH

DIAPHRAGM

LIVER

SPLEEN

PANCREAS

GALL BLADDER

SMALL INTESTINE

LARGE INTESTINE

APPENDIX

RECTUM

Figure 29-1: The Digestive System

You should be able to:

1. *Demonstrate an assessment of an acute abdomen.*

2. *Describe the treatment for a patient with acute abdominal pain.*

3. *List the guidelines for deciding when to evacuate a patient with acute abdominal pain.*

It could happen to you

Jake begins to complain of abdominal discomfort about nine o'clock on a sunny morning during a backpacking trip in the Superstition Mountains of Arizona. You give him a quick assessment which reveals the discomfort is general to his mid-abdominal area, nothing of significance, and he completes the day's hike. By evening, however, his discomfort has increased, and he complains of nausea. Before dinner he vomits, and reports some relief of pain.

Jake declines food, saying he isn't hungry, and soon complains the pain is back and worse than before. The pain now centers in his lower right quadrant, pain he describes as a "dull ache with pressure, a sharp pain when I breath deep, and a sharp pain when you push on it." He calls the pain a five on a scale of one-to-10 in general, but it increases to a seven when palpated.

By nine o'clock in the evening, as the rest of the group begins to think about sacking out, Jake is found lying on the ground in a fetal position, groaning in pain, unable to straighten out because, he grunts, "it hurts too bad."

Introduction

The abdomen contains the liver and spleen, the digestive, urinary, and reproductive systems, and the major blood vessels supplying the lower extremities. For anatomical reference, all of these body parts lie in one of four abdominal quadrants (SEE CHAPTER 11: ABDOMINAL EMERGENCIES). Numerous medical problems can develop in this region of the body, but, for convenience, they can be divided into four categories:

Hemorrhage: An ectopic pregnancy, for example, may cause life threatening bleeding if the ectopic pregnancy ruptures (SEE CHAPTER 33: OBSTETRICAL EMERGENCIES). Puncture wounds and blunt trauma are covered in Chapter 11.

Perforation: An ulcer, for example, may "eat" a hole through the stomach or intestinal wall allowing contents to spill into the abdomen.

Infection: Any organ of the abdomen may get inflamed or infected, appendicitis being a common example. The lining of the abdomen itself may suffer inflammation, a problem called peritonitis.

Obstruction: The tube-like pathways of the abdomen may become blocked with kidney stones, gallstones, fecal impactions, and twisting of the intestines being the most common blockages.

You may have a "good guess" about the problem existing in the abdomen of the patient, but you will not know for sure until a physician has examined the patient and, even then, you may not know. Some abdominal pain goes away without leaving substantial clues to its cause. In all cases of acute abdominal pain, the primary responsibilities of the Wilderness First Responder are 1) assess if the condition is serious, calling for an evacuation of the patient, and 2) properly care for the patient up to and, perhaps, during the evacuation.

General Abdominal Illness Assessment

1. Observe the patient's body position when you first approach. A patient who lies still with legs drawn up into a fetal position is often assuming a posture that minimizes serious pain.

2. When assessing abdominal pain, you must inspect the abdomen. Make the patient as comfortable as possible, warm and insulated from the ground, and remove enough clothing to see the entire abdomen.

3. Look at the abdomen with the patient lying in a supine (face up) position. A normal abdomen is gently rounded and symmetrical. Look for distention and/or an irregularly shaped abdomen, both of which may indicate a serious illness.

4. Palpate the abdomen with flat fingers. Press gently in all four quadrants of the abdomen. Watch for a pain response. Normal abdomens are soft and not tender to palpation. Feel for rigid muscles, lumps, and pain specific to a local spot, and guarding by the patient, all of which may be signs of serious illness. Check for rebound pain, pain that increases when you release the pressure of palpation, another indication the illness could be serious. Your palpation of the abdomen is a key assessment tool.

5. Ask the patient about his or her condition. Has this ever happened before? The OPQRST questions may be very helpful:

O-Onset: Did the pain come on suddenly or gradually? Some problems bring sudden pain, some gradual pain, and knowing which can help you guess what the problem may be.

P-Provokes, Palliates: Does anything make the pain worse or better? Pain increased by movement is not always but may be more serious.

Q-Quality: How does the patient describe the pain? Although descriptions can be misleading, many patients describe non-serious pain as dull, cramping pain.

R-Radiate, Refers, Region: Where is the pain, and does it radiate or refer to another region? Specific pain can help you guess what part of the body has a problem.

T-Time: How long has the pain been there? Prolonged pain, greater than 12 to 24 hours, is a key sign of serious illness.

6. Listen with an ear or stethoscope pressed against each of the four quadrants. This takes time. In two or three minutes, within each quadrant, bowel sounds (gurgling noises) should be heard. Absence of noise means something is not working right.

7. Ask about nausea and vomiting. Although nausea and vomiting are common (SEE CHAPTER 31: COMMON SIMPLE WILDERNESS MEDICAL PROBLEMS), pain associated with prolonged nausea and vomiting, could indicate a serious problem.

8. Ask about diarrhea and constipation. When was the patient's last bowel movement. Diarrhea and constipation are seldom indications of a serious abdominal illness, but both can become serious problems if they continue for several days (SEE CHAPTER 31: COMMON SIMPLE WILDERNESS MEDICAL PROBLEMS).

9. Ask about blood which may appear in the urine, stool, or vomit. Mild *gastritis* (inflammation of the stomach) may produce a bit of blood in vomit, and anal fissures or hemorrhoids may cause some bright or brown blood in stools. This type of bleeding is typically not serious, but the patient should be monitored closely. Dark blood in vomit, appearing somewhat like coffee grounds, and dark blood in stools, appearing something like tar, and frank bleeding from the mouth or rectum are serious signs.

10. Check for a fever. A fever of 102 degrees F (35 degrees C) or higher, especially if it comes on fast, could indicate a serious infection.

11. Monitor the vital signs for indications of shock.

Types Of Abdominal Emergencies

Appendicitis

The appendix is a pouch of the intestine most commonly located in the lower right quadrant. *Appendicitis* is an inflammation of the appendix with numerous causes. Due to the obstruction, mucus builds within the appendix causing pressure, swelling, and infection. The highest incidence of appendicitis occurs between the ages of 10 and 30.

The problem typically begins as mid-abdomen discomfort that grows worse over six to 24 hours, localizing in the right lower quadrant (RLQ). Rebound pain usually develops in the RLQ. Movement usually aggravates the pain once it is localized. Loss of appetite is very common. Nausea, vomiting, and a low grade fever (less than 102 degrees F and 35 degrees C) are also common. If the appendix ruptures, peritonitis will develop, which may lead to septic shock. Appendicitis is a serious illness, and often difficult to diagnose. You do not want to miss at least recognizing the patient has a serious illness.

The patient should be rapidly but gently evacuated in a position of comfort. Food should be avoided, but small sips of fluid may be given to avoid dehydration.

Fecal Impaction

A *fecal impaction* results when hardened feces form a blockage in the descending colon preventing the passage of fecal material. The patient usually reports a history of constipation. In the wilderness, constipation is often caused by a lack of ease defecating outdoors and/or dehydration (SEE CHAPTER 31: COMMON SIMPLE WILDERNESS MEDICAL PROBLEMS). Gradually increasing pain in the left lower quadrant (LLQ) builds to severe cramping. You might be able to palpate a mass in the LLQ, and the lower abdomen may be distended. Nausea and vomiting often occur. If untreated, the condition can lead to bowel obstruction, dead bowel, a perforation, and on to septic shock. A high level of hydration is an important aspect of treatment. Sometimes a bowel movement can be stimulated by giving the patient a large drink of cold water, followed immediately by a cup of hot liquid such as coffee or tea. Sometimes a caffeinated drink such as coffee alone will do the job. In the case of a true impaction, you will have to resort to manual disimpaction, going up the rectum with a well-gloved finger to dislodge and remove the mass.

Food Poisoning

Gastrointestinal distress caused by ingesting bacterially contaminated food is termed "food poisoning." Leftovers served later are common wilderness sources. "Stomach" cramps with diarrhea, nausea, and vomiting are common signs that appear one to 12 hours after ingesting the germs. The problem usually affects more than one person in a group of wilderness travelers, and the problem is typically self limiting. Patients should be kept well hydrated and monitored for changes. Antiemetic (anti-vomit) and anti-diarrheal drugs may be considered. Bloody diarrhea, a fever above 102 degrees F (35 degrees C), and the signs and symptoms of shock are reasons for evacuation.

Gallstones

Gallstones form in the gallbladder most often when bile contains more cholesterol than can be kept in solution. Pain usually comes on gradually in the right upper quadrant (RUQ) when the gallbladder becomes inflamed or when the stone tries to escape through the cystic duct, the duct carrying bile to the small intestine. The pain may radiate into the right shoulder, sometimes into the back. Nausea and vomiting are common. The pain often subsides in as little as a few hours, but the patient should be evacuated if the pain persists and either a fever and/or jaundice (yellowness of skin, yellowness of whites of the eyes) develops. Strong pain killers and adequate hydration are recommended.

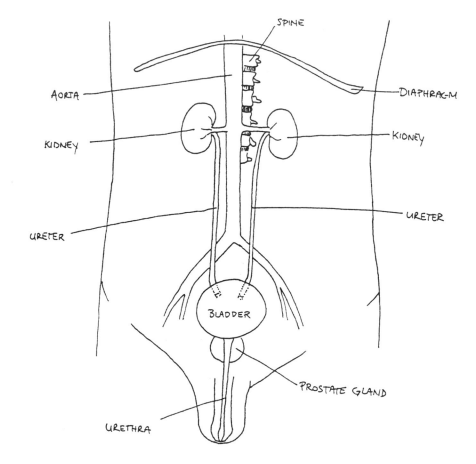

Figure 29-2: The urinary system

Gastroenteritis

Gastroenteritis, an inflammation of the gastrointestinal tract, is a common wilderness medical condition, most often generated by poor camp hygiene (see Chapter 30: Communicable Diseases). The patient complains of gradually increasing discomfort, usually diffuse in the abdomen, often worse in the lower quadrants. Cramps come and go, and diarrhea is common. Nausea and vomiting may be present, and, sometimes, a low grade fever. Malaise, a general feeling of discomfort or indisposition, is a common complaint. Seldom a serious problem, gastroenteritis typically resolves in a day or two, less often in as long as three days. Gastroenteritis, however, is a diagnoses of exclusion, and the most common misdiagnoses in patients with serious abdominal illness. Hydration is critical. Anti-diarrheal and/or anti-emetic drugs may be considered. Watch the patient closely for signs of serious illness: Fever rising above 101 to 102 degrees F, blood and mucus in stools, the signs and symptoms of shock.

Kidney Stones

Kidney stones are formed from minerals in urine. They can grow to an inch (2.5 cm) or more, and cause sudden, sharp, stabbing flank pain that radiates down into the lower abdomen and/or groin as they pass from the kidney and down the ureter. The pain tends to wash over the patient in excruciating waves, and no position of comfort can be found. Blood may appear in the urine, and nausea and vomiting are possible. The pain will last for 24 hours or more, and it will suddenly subside if the patient is able to pass the stone from his or her ureter into the bladder or out of the body through the urethra. A patient with a kidney stone will appreciate strong pain killers. Adequate hydration is of great importance. Any patient with a fever and a suspected kidney stone must be evacuated immediately.

Ulcers

An *ulcer* is an open sore or lesion developing, in this case, in the lining of the stomach or intestine. In the stomach, an ulcer hurts more when the patient eats and the production of stomach acid is stimulated. In the duodenum, the first section of the small intestine, the pain of an ulcer may be reduced when the patient eats, especially bland foods, but the burning discomfort returns in one to four hours after eating. Pain is typically described as "burning" in the mid-epigastric region (upper middle abdomen). Alcohol, caffeine, nicotine, aspirin, and non-steroidal anti-inflammatory drugs worsen the condition. A history of similar pain can often be described by the patient, and the pain usually resolves spontaneously in a few days. Watch the patient for signs and symptoms of a serious ulcer: unremitting pain; vomiting "coffee grounds"; dark, foul-smelling, tarry stools; weakness; fainting; shock. For patients with mild ulcers, antacids may provide relief of symptoms. Monitor the patient in the wilderness, and evacuate if serious signs and symptoms appear.

Evacuation Guidelines

Determining the exact cause, even the severity of abdominal pain in the wilderness is a baffling undertaking. For that reason, it is recommended to evacuate any patient with abdominal pain if:

1. The pain is associated with the signs and symptoms of shock.

2. The pain persists for longer than 12 to 24 hours.

3. The pain localizes, and especially if the pain involves guarding, tenderness, or abdominal rigidity.

4. Blood appears in the vomit, feces, or urine.

5. Nausea, vomiting, or diarrhea persist for longer than 24 to 72 hours.

6. The pain is associated with a fever above 102 degrees F (35 degrees C).

7. The pain is associated with signs and symptoms of pregnancy (SEE CHAPTER 33: OBSTETRICAL EMERGENCIES).

8. The patient is unable to eat or drink, unable to stay well hydrated.

Note: The more signs and symptoms of serious abdominal illness a patient develops, the more seriously ill the patient tends to be.

Conclusion

In the Superstition Mountains, you recognize Jake's signs and symptoms, especially the classic progression from generalized mid-abdomen pain to localized RLQ pain, as suggestive of appendicitis. The group, a strong and mature party, meets and decides a team will be formed to hike out with a SOAP note and an appeal for help, but, for safety, the team will not leave until first light. You make Jake as comfortable as possible, staying by his side during the night, offering sips of cool water frequently.

With dawn almost more of a suggestion than a reality, a team of three leaves for the roadhead.

By early afternoon, the thwop-thwop of a helicopter brings you to your feet. Later that day, Jake's appendix lies in a stainless steel pan in a hospital's operating room.

Chapter 30:   Communicable Diseases

You should be able to:

1. *Describe the ways germs are communicated to humans.*

2. *Describe ways to prevent the spread of communicable diseases.*

3. *Describe the basic principles of camp hygiene.*

It could happen to you

The tortured turns and twists of the Badlands of South Dakota have always held a mystical attraction for you, and near one of the area's trails you're setting camp. The group of eight you lead is young. For many, these past five days have been an initiation into laboring under a backpack and sleeping on the ground. You've been as busy as a homeless beaver teaching these kids to pitch tents, cook meals, and leave no trace. Although your stomach feels a little upset, tonight, with the group better trained, you're hoping for a more relaxing evening.

Your hopes are dashed when two thirteen-year-olds come to you with complaints of "bad stomachaches." Your investigation reveals they both have been suffering from diarrhea. As you question them, a third student, overhearing the conversation, admits to the same problem: Diarrhea and "bad cramps." You are encouraging hydration and rest when, with a sigh, you realize you've got to excuse yourself for a trip to the bushes. Into your cathole goes the first of what will be numerous explosive bowel movements.

Introduction

As an outdoorsperson you might think the great majority of "germs"—a scientific term representing all the microscopic things that might infect a human and cause disease—lurk in the wilderness waiting for a suitable host to pass near enough for an attack. Not so. In fact, generally speaking, the contrary is true: Most germs hitch a free ride into the wilderness with you or some other unwary bipedal primate. As more and more *Homo sapiens* show up more and more often in wilderness areas, the presence of humans, even if only for a short while, builds a community of disease possibilities.

Germs are *pathogens*, microorganisms that cause at least some "pathos" (suffering) as part of their nature. Some pathogens are more pathological than others, and some hosts are more susceptible. Hence the degree of pathos is a product of the attributes of the "bug" and the host. Some humans, you will have noticed, tend to be continuously ill while others seem to be superhumanly immune. Despite your personal level of immunity, however, you should be determined to prevent the spread of pathogens at all times.

Agents Of Infection

Unseen and ubiquitous, microorganisms live among us and on us and in us. Some are beneficial. Pathogens are divided, generally, into four classifications: viruses, bacteria, fungi, and parasites.

Viruses cannot exist for long outside of living tissue, and must penetrate human cell walls to multiply and cause disease. They are unimaginably tiny, and account for the respiratory infections that are responsible for approximately one-half of all acute illnesses. Major viruses include influenza, the common cold, mumps, and measles. Some viruses set up housekeeping in the central nervous system and cause forms of meningitis and encephalitis. Herpes simplex virus type-1 causes cold sores, and herpes simplex virus type-2 causes genital lesions. The Epstein-Barr virus produces infectious mononucleosis. Varicellar-zoster causes chicken pox that may later appear as shingles. Viruses cause hepatitis and AIDS.

Bacteria grow independently without need for a host cell. Staphylococcus aureus lives on the surface of human skin and is responsible for nasty things like wound infections, abscesses, bacterial pneumonia, and some food poisonings. Some bacteria grow in chains, called streptococci, and cause problems such as strep throat, scarlet fever, rheumatic fever, and acute sinusitis. Clostridium tetani lives in soil and causes tetanus. Many bacteria live helpfully in a normal GI tract, but this group also includes Escherichia coli which causes urinary tract infections and Salmonella which causes typhoid fever, and both produce diarrheal illness. Shigella, causes dysentery, and another group, the Mycobacteria, cause tuberculosis and leprosy.

Fungi are primitive life-forms that feed on living plants, decaying organic matter—and animal tissue. Fungal infections are usually bothersome but relatively mild, such as athlete's foot (SEE CHAPTER 31: COMMON SIMPLE WILDERNESS MEDICAL PROBLEMS). In the immunosuppressed, however, a fungal infection can be overwhelming and fatal.

Examples of *parasites* that cause disease in humans are protozoa that include the mosquito-borne *Plasmodia* of malaria, and the water-borne *Giardia lamblia* of giardiasis and *Cryptosporidium* of cryptosporidiosis.

Communication Of Disease

Germs can be transmitted in a variety of ways, but all communication falls into one of two broad classifications: Direct and indirect. Direct transmission means the person carrying the germs passes them directly to another person. Contact with blood and other body fluids may pass germs directly. Coughs and sneezes, inhaled by a nearby person, are methods of direct transmission. Sexual activities offer an opportunity for direct contact. Germs may be picked up directly through cuts or other open wounds. Indirect transmission methods include those in which the germs are passed without direct contact with another person. Eating contaminated food and drinking contaminated water are examples of indirect transmission. Bites from infected insects may pass pathogens indirectly. Sharing a water bottle, a towel, or an eating utensil provides a means of indirect contact with germs.

Specific Diseases

Norwalk Virus

Norwalk virus, named for Norwalk, Ohio, where it was first isolated, makes more people sick than any other food-related virus. It's passed easily from one sufferer to another by hand and mouth, and rolls into high gear 24 to 48 hours after contact has been made. Though it lasts about a week, the problems of vomiting and diarrhea are relatively mild, rarely requiring a doctor's care.

Hepatitis A

Hepatitis A virus can be swallowed with some fecal-contaminated foods and water. Undercooked shellfish from water polluted with human wastes has been a common source of hep A. It can spread through sharing water bottles and utensils, improperly washing hands (fecal-oral route) and intimate contact between people. Stomach pain, nausea, vomiting, fatigue and loss of appetite show up 15 to 50 days after ingestion. Severe cases may cause jaundice (yellowing of the skin and whites of the eyes) and dark urine. Hepatitis B produces similar but more severe symptoms, but it's transmitted primarily by blood contact.

AIDS

AIDS stands for Acquired Immune Deficiency Syndrome, a sincerely life-threatening infection that destroys the body's ability to fight off other types of infections. AIDS is the final, completely fatal stage of a continuum of problems caused by the Human Immunodeficiency Virus (HIV). Once the HIV is in human blood, they develop antibodies to the virus which will show up in a blood test. Seropositivity (testing positive for a certain antibody) usually shows up four to six weeks after HIV infection. It is communicated by blood-and-body fluid transmission. Saliva, tears, sweat, urine, semen, vaginal secretions and stool can all carry the HIV, but only blood and semen have been known to transmit the virus.

Patients who have been infected but have not yet developed the antibodies are considered to be in the first stage of the continuum. Stage two patients have the antibodies but no symptoms of the disease. Once signs and symptoms appear, the patient may still not be technically classi-

fied as an AIDS sufferer. For a while, this stage was called the AIDS-related complex (ARC).

Regardless of the stage of the disease, the HIV-infected patient can pass the virus.

Bacillus Cereus

Bacillus cereus lives as a bacterial spore (a dry seed-like structure) in grains and spices, and germinates when the food is moist and when contaminated cooked food is improperly stored. Stomach pain, nausea and vomiting, sometimes mild diarrhea, usually occur within eight to 16 hours of ingestion. The problem almost always self-limits in less than 24 hours.

Staphylococcus Aureus

Staphylococcus aureus may drop off of contaminated hands into breakfast, lunch and dinner. *S. aureus* multiplies with great speed in protein-rich foods at warm temperatures. Rather than an infectious disease, the bacteria produce a toxin. The reaction that erupts suddenly 30 minutes to six hours after you've eaten produces cramps, vomiting, diarrhea, headache, sweats and chills. Although the problem may last one to two days, medical treatment is seldom required unless you let yourself get seriously dehydrated.

Shigella

Shigella most often gets into you from food and water contaminated with fecal matter, usually from the hands of he or she who last handled the food and water. Shigellosis causes dysentery (bloody, mucus-ridden diarrhea), fever, bad stomach

cramps, and a search for a doctor. Illness will probably appear less than four days after ingestion, but some cases have shown up seven days later.

Salmonella

Salmonella are bacteria common in eggs and poorly processed dairy products. Within an average of 12 to 24 hours, sometimes faster, symptoms appear: stomach pain, diarrhea, nausea, vomiting, headache, chills, weakness, thirst. Fever may be present. Although cases have been known to become severe, most people recover by drinking lots of fluids and waiting in distress.

Campylobacter Jejuni

Campylobacter jejuni contaminates meats primarily, especially chicken, although some types are common in backcountry water and fecal matter. The likelihood of contacting the bacteria increases if you handle raw or eat undercooked flesh. An average of four to seven days passes after ingestion before you get stomach pain and bloody diarrhea. The problem may last two to seven days. Find a doctor.

Clostridium Perfingens

Clostridium perfringens are bacteria found in meat usually stored at too warm a temperature before serving. Eight to 22 hours later abdominal cramps, nausea and diarrhea may make you think it's all over. Vomiting, headache, fever and chills are rare with *C. perfringens*. Symptoms usually go away harmlessly within 36 hours.

Giardia

Giardia lamblia parasites swim or float around as cysts in many wilderness water sources and spread through fecal contamination by humans and other animals. Giardiasis ranks as the most common water-borne illness in the United States. Unpleasant, but typically benign, the illness usually causes more than a week of diarrhea with bloating, flatulence and stomach cramps. Symptoms take about 10 days to show up, but the parasites may hang around inside for weeks before you feel sick. Some patients never develop the typical signs and symptoms of giardiasis. They have periodic mild cramping and bloating, but they never explode with diarrhea. Some carriers of *Giardia lamblia* are asymptomatic.

Cryptosporidium

Cryptosporidium protozoa, although transmittable via food and body contact, are primarily water-borne parasites. They get in the water from feces of infected animals, including humans. Explosive diarrhea and tummy cramps appear after an incubation period of four to 14 days, and usually self-limit, going away after five to 11 miserable days.

Prevention

The obvious bottom line in the prevention of rescue-related communicable diseases is universal body substance isolation (BSI) with all patients (see Chapter 3: Patient Assessment). It is safest to disregard thoughts of "This is a high risk person" and "This is a low risk person." Consider all patients as potential transmitters of infectious disease. Prevention requires, more than anything else, a change in behavior on the part of the rescuer.

1. Contact with blood poses the greatest risk, and disposable protective gloves should be carried in wilderness first aid kits, and used at any time you might contact blood or other body substances.

2. Wear protective glasses if splashing of body fluids may occur.

3. Use a pocket mask with a one-way valve when performing rescue breathing.

4. Wash your hands for at least 10 seconds with soap and water immediately *after* contact with blood or other body fluids, even if you have worn gloves.

5. Boil soiled first aid gear and reusable bandages and let them air dry, or soak them for at least 30 seconds in one-to-ten solution of household bleach.

6. Double-bag in plastic all soiled bandages and dressings if they cannot be completely burned in an environmentally safe, hot fire. Properly dispose of all double-bagged contaminated items after leaving the wilderness.

7. Keep your vaccinations, e.g., hepatitis B, tetanus, up to date.

Hand Washing

Skin, the outer layer, is an overlapping armor of dead cells that protect the living cells beneath. Under a microscope, this outer layer looks like the surface of the Colorado Plateau from 30,000 feet: canyons and mesas, cracks and fissures. Resident microbes are wedged firmly into the low spots. Some of these microbes are friendly, serving to keep skin slightly acid and resistant to other microbial life-forms like fungi. Others, such as *S.*
aureus, can make you severely sick. In addition to the residents, transient germs come and go as fortune dictates. They can accumulate rapidly after bowel movements, and they congregate most thickly under fingernails and in the deeper fissures of fingertips. Hands are the single most important "tool" in communicating illness. *Hand washing is the single most important method of preventing the spread of disease.*

Hand washing, even with detergents, does not remove all the flora living on hands, but it does significantly reduce the chance of contamination. For your information, science recommends the following eight-step hand washing technique for maximum cleanliness:

1. Wet hands with hot flowing water (100 to 120 degrees F/38 to 49 degrees C).

2. Soap up until a good lather is attained.

3. Work the lather all over the surface of the hand concentrating on fingernails and tips.

4. Clean under fingernails.

5. Rinse thoroughly with hot water (very important).

6. Re-soap and re-lather.

7. Re-rinse.

8. Dry (very important).

In most cases, hot water is a rare wilderness commodity. You can still get clean hands with this modified wilderness technique which substitutes germicidal soap for hot water. In tests, adequate hand sanitation was achieved with as little as one half-liter of water.

1. Wet hands thoroughly.

2. Add a small amount of germicidal soap, e.g., Betadine Scrub®, Hibiclens®.

3. Work lather up, especially fingertips.

4. Clean under fingernails (and keep your nails trimmed).

5. Rinse thoroughly.

6. Repeat soap, lather, and rinse.

7. Dry.

Sure, it's a bother—but so is getting sick, especially when the sickness migrates through a group. Even plain old hand washing beats no hand washing.

Camp Hygiene

Some germs are waiting in the wilderness, e.g., the bacteria that causes tetanus, the protozoa that causes giardiasis, but far more, as mentioned earlier, are carried into the wild places by humans. Germs are typically passed around a group by very casual means. More people get sick in the wild outdoors from poor camp hygiene than for any other reason.

Trash

In the plus column, the amount of litter has steadily decreased in wilderness areas over the last twenty years despite an increase in trash-producing people. The potential impact of trash ranks low as a health hazard, while the disposition of left-over food and, far more important, human waste products rank as the greatest risk.

Food For Thought

Leftovers result, most often, from cooking more than you can eat. Storage of cooked-but-uneaten food in the wilderness poses an almost insurmountable problem. Bacteria grows optimally at temperatures ranging from 45 to 140 degrees F (7 to 60 degrees C), and unhealthy populations of bacteria can be reached in a brief period of time. Reheating cooked food, although it kills bacteria, often leaves dangerous toxins produced by the bacteria at sickening levels. Your safest bet is to get rid of leftovers.

Buried food usually ends up being unburied by hungry animals. If campfires are appropriate, small amounts of dry food will burn to nothing, but wet food usually becomes an unsightly lump of ash unless the fire is extremely hot. Leftover food should be sealed in plastic bags and packed out.

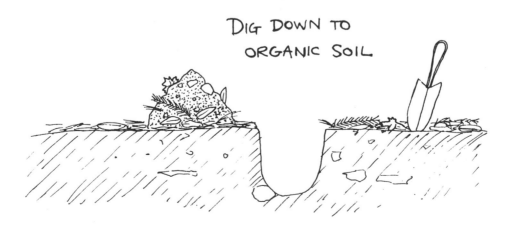

Figure 30-1: Cathole

Successful fisherfolk face the question of what to do with fish heads and guts. Scattering fish parts widely in secluded spots probably rates as the best disposal method in most cases.

Throwing the fish remains into cold wilderness water is a poor method of disposal since the parts will stay visible for a long time. Where hungry bear populations are dense, water disposal of

unused fish parts might still be the best idea. It could prevent parts of you from becoming the leftovers of a bear's meal.

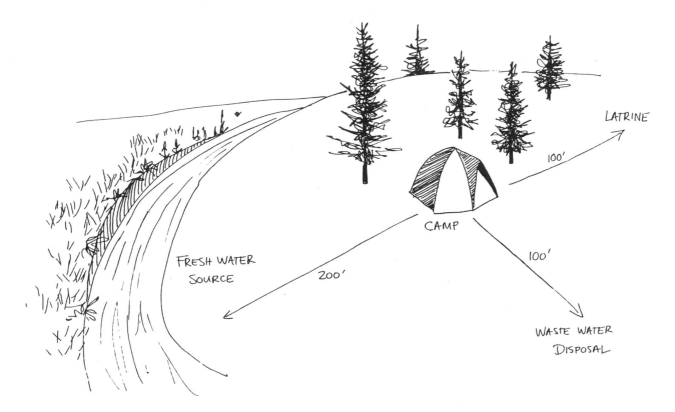

Figure 30-2: Camping Healthy

Another major source of food contamination in the wilderness is dirty utensils. Cooking and eating utensils should be boiled daily, and cleaned prior to use in the preparation and serving of food.

Wilderness food usually shows up in plastic bags, and food contamination can be further reduced by pouring the food out instead of reaching in for it.

Fecal Contamination

You can't realistically pack out everything you pack in, except in special circumstances (such as dragging frozen feces off

of winter trips), but you can, with an adequate poo-poo plan, reduce the risk of fecal contamination to an absolute minimum. Transmission of fecal-borne pathogens occurs in four ways: direct contact with the feces, indirect contact with hands that have directly contacted the feces, contact with insects that have contacted the feces, and drinking contaminated water. Human waste products breakdown to a harmless state as a result of two mechanisms: 1) Bacterial action in the presence of oxygen, moisture and warmth, and 2) sterilization from direct ultra-

violet radiation. Deposition of solid body wastes should include placement 1) to maximize decomposition, 2) to minimize the chance of something or someone finding it, and 3) to minimize the chance of water contamination. Latrines are out, except in established spots. They concentrate too much human waste in one place. They carry a high risk of water pollution. They invite insect and mammal investigation. They are unsightly, and they stink. If you are ever required to dig a latrine, make it at least a foot deep, and add soil after each deposit, and fill it in when the

The Wilderness First Responder

total excreta lies several inches below the surface.

For years, environmental and health-oriented wildland managers have recommended catholes as the best thing to do with your doo-doo. Preferably in a level spot, a cathole should be dug several inches into an organic layer of soil, where decomposing microorganisms live most abundantly. After you've dropped your droppings, stir them into the soil to speed decomposition. Cover the excrement with a couple of inches of soil, and disguise the spot to hide it from later passersby.

In some wilderness areas where the sun shines often and human traffic is light, feces will rot to harmlessness quickest if you use the smear technique, smearing or scattering your dung over the surface to maximize sun and air exposure. The smear technique has obvious drawbacks in well-used areas where, for one thing, waste won't decompose fast enough to eliminate health hazards. In those places it remains best to defecate in thoughtfully situated catholes.

Smears and catholes should be at least two hundred feet, or approximately seventy adult paces, from water, and placed where little chance of discovery exists.

Urine

Although urine is usually considered a sterile waste product, it can carry germs. To stay on the safe side, urinate on rocks or in non-vegetated spots far from water sources whenever possible.

Sanitation Around The Nation

Wilderness areas are not created equal. Some are especially wet, some dry, some cold, and some hot. Special sanitation considerations may be required in special environments to stop the spread of disease.

1. **Lakes and Rivers:** Moving well away from bodies of water and carefully selecting your poopsite will eliminate most of the health risks associated with water contamination. In some places, however, such as deep dry-country canyons, moving well away isn't possible. In those spots, the only safe alternative is packing it out. The most acceptable means to do this requires a sturdy sealable can and several heavy-duty garbage bags. Line the can, such as a large ammo box, with a couple of garbage bags folded out over the rim. Before and after each use, throw in some chemicals to reduce the smell and slow decomposition. (Rapid decomposition inside a plastic bag may produce a disgusting explosion.) Chlorox or quicklime will do. Toilet paper goes into the bag, too, but urine should be squirted elsewhere. Urine dilutes the added chemicals and greatly increases bag weight. Before packing the bag for the day's travel, squeeze out the air and tie it firmly closed.

On some wilderness waterways, travelers are encouraged to urinate directly into the water. In some areas, this practice is discouraged. Follow local recommendations.

2. **Deserts:** Human excrement won't decompose in sandy, predominantly inorganic desert soil. Instead, it filters down through the ground. For this reason, deposits should be made far from water sources, out of gullies and other obvious drainages, and off of slickrock. Insect contamination in dry regions is low, and smearing your personal manure rates as a healthier alternative than deeply burying it. Because it will remain visible for a long long time, discretion is the better part of desert defecations, and the best all-round choice in most areas is shallow burial. High near-surface temperatures will cook pathogens to death in short order.

3. **Above Timberline:** In the frozen north and in the fragile oft-frozen high country, decomposition goes slowly due foremost to the cold. Fecal monuments may stand for ages. The smear technique offers the fastest decomposition of human wastes. Sun can decontaminate, and rain and snow can wash away the smear. Once again, please choose a secluded spot well away from water sources.

4. **Snow:** Stools deposited in snow, no matter how far they're buried, will appear on the surface come springtime. For that reason, proper choice of burial sites remains of paramount importance.

Water Disinfection

Long gone are the days when you could drop your exhausted body to the ground beside a sparkling flow of wilderness water and plunge your face into the cold rush for a drink. Pathogens inhabit, to some degree, most of the world's water, and, unless you're willing to risk gut-ripping misery, it is of critical importance to carry some means of water disinfection on wilderness trips.

There are three proven ways to guarantee your wilderness water is safely disinfected:

1. Boiling: The rule is very simple: Once the water is hot enough to produce one rolling bubble, it is free of organisms that will cause illness, worldwide and up to at least 19,000 feet above sea level. The reason: All of the time it takes to bring water to a boil works toward the death of organisms in the water. By the time water *reaches* the boiling point it's safe. *Giardia lamblia* cysts, for instance, die at approximately 122 degrees F (50 degrees C). If you want to "feel" safer, let the water roll around at a boil for a couple of minutes. Boiling is cheap—the only cost is fuel—and effective, but it consumes time, and it's inconvenient if you run out of water on the trail.

2. Halogenation: As for chemicals that kill water-borne pathogens, both chlorine and iodine have been proven relatively effective, given enough of the chemical and enough time. Halogenation is effected by water temperature, the pH of the water, and the turbidity of the water. Halogens are generally more convenient and faster than boiling the water (when you consider lighting the stove or building the fire), but they cost more and can't be guaranteed to work as well as other means of water disinfection.

Chlorine and iodine, for instance, have not been proven fatal to *Cryptosporidium*. Halogens also tend to leave the water tasting crummy, a phenomenon reversible by adding flavoring, e.g., energy drink powders, *after* the disinfection process has been completed. If you flavor the water prior to complete disinfection, the added substances may disrupt the disinfection process. If you use halogens, the safest bet is to buy a commercial product and carefully follow the directions on the label.

3. Filtration: Water filters physically strain out some of the organisms and contaminants in water that could cause disease. Structurally, there are two basic kinds of filters: 1) Surface or membrane filters are thin perforated sheets that block impurities. 2) Depth filters are made of thick and porous materials that trap impurities as the water is forced through. The effectiveness of filters vary greatly from one that removes only relatively large particles such as *Giardia lamblia* to one that removes virtually everything removable. Viruses are too small to be filtered out, but some filters kill viruses with iodine from resins on the filter as the water passes through. Mechanically, once again, there are two basic types: 1) Pump-feed filters that require manual force to push the water through the filter. 2) Gravity-feed filters that just

hang there while water drips via gravity through the system.

Filtered water looks "clean," but the purity of the water depends on the specific filter. Read the claims of a filter carefully before your purchase. They are available in a wide variety of costs, shapes and sizes. Filtration, in general, costs more but offers the quickest route to safe water.

Principles Of Camp Hygiene

1. Wash your hands with a biodegradable soap after a bowel movement and before food preparation.

2. Do not share handkerchiefs, toothbrushes, lip balm, water bottles, eating utensils, etc. If you can't finish your candy bar or your lunch, dispose of the leftovers properly instead of passing your germs to someone else.

3. Keep your hands out of food bags, e.g., trail mix bags, and your personal utensils out of group cooking pots and pans.

4. Keep all sick people out of the "kitchen."

5. Daily wash with a biodegradable soap, rinse with hot water, and dry all community and personal kitchen gear.

6. Do not eat leftovers unless they have cooled off quickly and remained cold as in a winter environment. If you eat leftovers, thoroughly reheat them for at least 30 minutes.

7. Disinfect all drinking water.

Conclusion

By morning in the Badlands of South Dakota you notice a little blood in your diarrhea. Questioning the group reveals a report of bloody diarrhea in several other patients. There is nothing to do—for the sick members of the group or yourself—except stay hydrated and hike out.

A drive to the nearest hospital and series of lab tests later, and a doctor tells you there is *Campylobacter*, a bacteria, in the stool samples. Sometimes found in wilderness water sources, someone probably failed to disinfect, or at least properly disinfect, a bottle of water. How did it get passed around the group? You will never know.

The doctor says the problems typically resolve eventually in these cases, but she recommends an antibiotic, and writes prescriptions. You will carry the prescriptions to the parents, and you will, you promise yourself, pay more attention to camp hygiene in the future.

You should be able to:

1. *Describe the most common simple wilderness medical problems.*

2. *Describe the proper wilderness care of the most common simple problems.*

Introduction

When a Wilderness First Responder reaches for his or her first aid kit, the injury or illness to be treated, most of the time, is a minor and simple one—a small wound, a headache, a stomach-ache, sunburn. It is important for the WFR to be well acquainted with common simple problems because 1) proper management can ease suffering and speed healing, 2) proper management often keeps a simple problem from becoming more complex, and 3) recognizing when a simple problem is no longer simple allows the WFR to better care for and to arrange an evacuation for patients who require definitive medical treatment.

Types Of Common Simple Medical Problems

Blisters

The fluid-filled bubble of a blister is a mild partial thickness burn caused by friction. The friction produces a separation of the tough outer layer of skin from the sensitive inner layer. Only where skin is hardened is it thick enough for this to happen: heels, soles, palms. Loose skin just wears away with friction leaving an abrasion.

The space between the outer layer of the blister (the roof) and the inner layer (the base) fills with fluid drawn from the circulatory system to protect the damaged area while it heals. Gravity encourages this to happen, causing foot blisters to swell rapidly. Wet skin blisters much more quickly than dry skin, and warm skin more quickly than cool skin— and what skin is more moist and hot than feet in heavy boots after a long walk?

Blisters would probably heal best if the patient sat with his or her feet propped up for a few days, but that doesn't happen. He or she keeps moving. You don't want the blisters to pop inside a dirty sock inside a dirty boot, so the best wilderness medicine is to drain the blister in a controlled setting. Besides, the patient feels better when the bubble is deflated. Clean around the site thoroughly with soap and water, or alcohol, if either is available. Or wash as best you can with just water. In a flame, sterilize the tip of a knife, or use a sterile scalpel. Carefully slice the blister open and let it drain until the fluid is gone. Leaving the roof intact will let it feel better and mend quicker. If the roof has already been rubbed away when you discover the injury, treat the wound initially as you would any other: Clean it and keep it clean to prevent infection.

After draining, you want to reduce the friction on that area as much as possible while keeping the foot in action. Many techniques and products are available for treating a deflated blister. A simple and proven technique involves creating a moleskin or molefoam "donut" to surround the blister site, then filling the hole of the "donut" with a glob of gooey antiseptic. Any antimicrobial ointment will work well. A liberal application of tincture of benzoin compound on the skin before the moleskin will greatly increase its stick-to-it-ness. A second patch of moleskin or a strip of tape over the filled donut will keep the ointment in place. A product called 2nd Skin® works as well or better to reduce friction over a deflated blister. 2nd Skin® can be used to fill a "donut" or placed over the deflation site and held in place with moleskin or tape.

You may never need these directions if you take precautions to prevent blisters from forming. Of critical importance is the fit of boots. It doesn't matter how expensively feet are shod if the fit is poor. Fit boots with the socks that will be worn in them. Boots that are the right size and

are well broken in go a long way toward preventing blisters.

Keeping feet cool and dry is also important. Take frequent breaks with boots off. Wear a thin liner sock that wicks moisture away from feet and into a thicker outer sock. Some folks report success from applications of antiperspirants to their feet. Most people think it makes their feet sticky which increases friction. Some foot powders help reduce moisture and friction, but they also tend to cake up and require frequent applications.

If a "hot spot"—a sore, red spot—develops at a prime blister

site, stop and cover the area with tape or moleskin or 2nd Skin® *before* the blister has a chance to form. Moleskin will conform to the shape of feet better if you cut it into strips or ovals first instead of laying down a wide piece that inevitably refuses to go flat. Once again, tincture of benzoin compound applied first will help keep the tape or moleskin from peeling off when feet start sweating. Without tape or moleskin, benzoin alone can be applied to the skin to prevent blisters. Benzoin hardens protectively over the outer layer of skin.

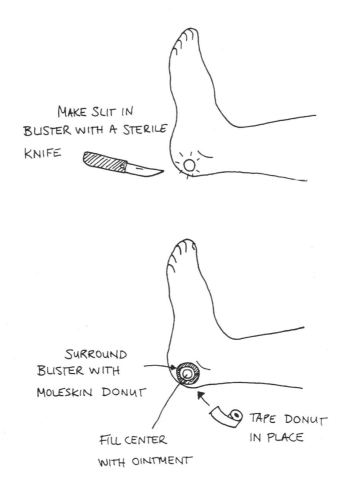

Figure 31-1: Blister treatment

Colds, Coughs, Sore Throats

"Rhino" comes from the Greek word for nose, and *rhinoviruses* are a group of viruses, of which there are probably more than 100, that cause the common cold, an illness that seems to affect the nose as much or more than anything else. Although you can only grow ill from a specific rhinovirus once, there are enough to offer numerous chances to get sick every year. To make matters worse, viruses other than rhinoviruses can cause a cold.

A cold begins with sneezing and clear mucus running from the nose, followed by congestion (the stuffy nose) and perhaps a bit of scratchiness in the throat. The patient may complain of a mild headache and fatigue, but, overall, there isn't too much suffering. Symptoms usually last four to nine days, fading away without complications.

The patient needs rest and plenty of water. An antihistamine, e.g., diphenhydramine (Benadryl®, 25-50 mg), two or three times a day, usually eases the symptoms. Pseudoephedrine (Sudafed®) often helps without causing the drowsiness that an antihistamine typically causes. Acetaminophen or aspirin may also help.

Droplets carrying the virus are easily passed by coughing, sneezing, and hand-to-hand contact, allowing a cold to sweep through a group that doesn't practice good camp hygiene (SEE CHAPTER 30: COMMUNICABLE DISEASES).

If the patient develops a profuse green or yellow nasal discharge, he or she may have sinusitis (a sinus infection). Rest and hydration are important, and warm compresses on the face may help, but a broad spectrum antibiotic, e.g., Amoxicillin, usually offers the patient the greatest benefit.

Most wilderness coughs are the result of mechanical irritation of the throat, irritation caused by rapid breathing, e.g., panting in high, dry air. Hydration and rest usually ease the cough, and sucking on a throat lozenge or a piece of hard candy tends to help. A patient coughing up green, yellow, or rust-colored phlegm is indicating he or she has bronchitis or pneumonia (SEE CHAPTER 24: RESPIRATORY EMERGENCIES). Both require treatment with antibiotics. Coughing is best controlled by increasing oral fluids and a cough suppressant, e.g., Robitussin DM®. If the patient has a high fever, severe shortness of breath, vomiting, and/or if the cough last more than a week, an evacuation should be organized.

Sore throats of a mild variety are not uncommon complaints with viral infections, especially if the patient has been coughing. A severe sore throat, however, a throat so sore it hurts to swallow and associated with a fever and a beefy red pharynx, perhaps splotched with patches of white, indicates strep throat, a serious bacterial infection requiring antibiotic therapy. Strep throat is not associated with coughs and stuffy noses.

Constipation

Constipation is infrequent and/or difficult movement of the bowels usually created by either a fluid level too low to lubricate the tract, a fiber level too low to keep things rolling along, and/or a poor attitude concerning squatting over a cathole. Constipation can be encouraged by poor exercise habits.

Treatment should start with forcing fluids. Encourage the patient to eat lots of whole grains, fruits (dried is okay), and vegetables. Peanut butter, cheese, and high-fat foods should be avoided. If one is prone to the problem, add a stool softener—preferably a suppository, e.g., Dulcolax®—to your first aid kit.

Stimulating the gastrocolic reflex will sometimes work to relieve constipation. Have the patient drink water, at least a half a liter, followed by a cup of hot coffee or tea.

Someone who hasn't had a bowel movement in three days typically feels uncomfortable. A patient without a movement in five days could be developing serious problems from the toxins building up in the intestinal tract. Check for a fecal impaction (SEE CHAPTER 29: ABDOMINAL EMERGENCIES). It might be necessary to go in with a lubricated, gloved index finger to break up the impaction and pull it out. Disgusting as it may sound, it might prove life-saving.

Prevention of constipation is a combination, essentially, of drinking plenty of water (try for at least three liters per day) and eating healthy. A wilderness leader can encourage those who have psychological trouble going without a porcelain toilet by creating a relaxed attitude toward "pooping the woods." You may suggest the patient pick a secluded spot with a scenic view and a minimum of tickling grasses—and practice.

Dental Problems

The heart of a tooth is the soft, inner *pulp* which contains blood vessels and nerves that support the outer, hard *dentin* and *enamel*. The part of the tooth you see rising above the *gingiva* (gums) is called the *crown*. The part you don't see that fits into the socket in the jaw is called the *root*.

A lost filling probably creates the most common dental emergency. The discomfort is often elicited when cold, sweets, or the tongue hits where the filling or crown has fallen out. If the pulp becomes inflamed—*pulpitis*—the pain can be much more than a discomfort. Gently clean the area—rinsing and brushing—to remove any food that may be trapped in the tooth. You can dip a cotton pellet in *eugenol* (oil of cloves) and swab out the vacancy to help relieve pain. To ensure longer lasting results, mix a little zinc oxide powder with a few drops of oil of cloves and stir the stuff until it becomes a paste. Push the paste into the hole. Even better, carry a tube of Cavit® in your first aid kit. A squeeze of the tube sends a bit of pre-mixed paste onto your finger. Roll it into a ball and place it where the filling or crown used to be. Have the patient bite the Cavit® gently into shape. The Cavit® will harden into an excellent temporary filling that must be periodically replaced, typically every two to three days. Sugarless gum (chewed to softness), ski wax, or candle wax can sometimes be successfully used to plug the hole where a filling or crown fell out. All of these temporary fillings will eventually wash out, requiring you to monitor each regularly.

If a crown comes off a tooth, clean the crown and coat it with a little oil of cloves. Place it back on the tooth to see if it can be fitted properly. Remove it again, and put a dab of Cavit® on the bottom of the crown. Set it immediately back in place, and bite it gently into position.

A *broken tooth* that doesn't expose the pulp is merely a nuisance that can wait until the wilderness venture is over, but a broken tooth that exposes the pulp can be a source of infinite pain. A tiny piece of a crushed aspirin placed directly on the pulp will "cauterize" the pulp, a technique that produces fierce pain followed by blessed relief. Do not put an aspirin on the gum next to an aching tooth. This will cause an acid burn of the gum which can be severe. The void left by a broken tooth may possibly be filled with Cavit® or another temporary filling. When the pulp is exposed, the patient should see a dentist as soon as possible, preferably within 48 hours.

Severe dental pain can result from trauma or infection. If the tooth is knocked out, pick it up by the top, not the root. Rinse it off, but do not scrub it. Your best chance of saving the fang is by pushing it gently back into the hole from whence it came. If this procedure is going to be successful, it must be attempted soon after the tooth is knocked out, within about 10 to 15 minutes or at least within 30 minutes, after which swelling will prevent the effort from working. If it hurts the patient too much, or refuses to go back in, don't force it. Wrap it in sterile gauze, and have the patient hold it in his or her mouth if possible, or keep it in a container of cold water. If evacuation is very fast, less than an hour, the tooth may be replaced by a dentist. With longer evacuations, a dental surgeon will be required to either reattach the tooth surgically or, more commonly, replace the missing tooth with an artificial one. If a blow to the mouth has simply loosened a tooth, don't wiggle it until it firms up or a dentist is found. Eugenol applied to the gum around the tooth often eases the pain.

Infection is indicated by a lot of swelling of the gum and cheek around an aching tooth, and may indicate a *periodontal abscess*. Gas and pus can be trapped inside the gum, causing extreme pain. If the swelling from infection reaches a major stage, the gum may form an elevated bulge that can turn blue. The patient needs antibiotics, and a dentist. Ice packs on the jaw will help alleviate pain. If evacuation is not possible, you might have to consider lancing the abscess. Have the patient brush, floss, and rinse out her or his mouth. A gentle and careful slice horizontally through the abscess with a sterile point will allow the pressure to release, after which the patient needs to repeatedly rinse out his or her mouth, flushing disinfected water through the open abscess. The rinsing process should be repeated several times a day until healing appears complete and/or the patient is evacuated. Lancing is dangerous and not advisable except in radical circumstances. Likewise, attempting to pull a tooth out of an infected socket is dangerous.

Both can cause significant bleeding. Ask your physician for information concerning antibiotic treatment for a dental infection.

Any bleeding inside the mouth, for any reason, can be given direct pressure. You can do this with a gauze pad you have bitten to hold in place. A moistened tea bag (non-herbal) can be used instead of gauze, and may work better. The tannic acid in tea initiates the formation of clotting. Avoid irritating the wound which can renew the bleeding.

Irritants are smoking, extremely hot food, chewing on the "bad" side, and sucking on the wound site.

To prevent dental emergencies, see your dentist regularly, and at least 30 days before an extended trip, giving yourself time to have any discovered problems fixed. Routine oral hygiene includes brushing with a soft nylon bristle toothbrush. Try to eat apples, carrots, or celery regularly. These fibrous fruits and vegetables after a meal help

scrape teeth clean. And don't forget to floss, cleaning where the brush can't reach.

A friendly dentist, outdoors person or not, should be willing to help you in finding and learning how to use the first aid items specific to dental problems. Some excellent commercial wilderness dental kits are available.

Considerations for a wilderness dental kit include: eugenol (oil of cloves), zinc oxide powder, cotton pellets, tea bags, aspirin, and Cavit®.

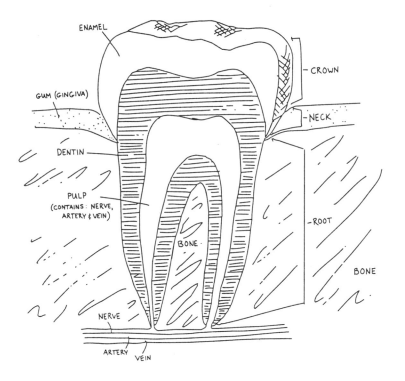

Figure 31-2: Basic anatomy of the tooth

Diarrhea

"Frequent passage of unformed watery bowel movements," as described by *Tabor's Medical Dictionary*, diarrhea falls into two broad types: invasive and non-invasive. From bacterial sources, invasive diarrhea, sometimes called "dysentery," attacks the lower intestinal wall causing

inflammation, abscesses, and ulcers that may lead to mucus and blood (often "black blood" from the action of digestive juices) in the stools, high fever, "stomach" cramps from the depths of hell, and significant amounts of body fluid rushing from the patient's nether region. Serious debilitation, even death,

can occur from the resulting dehydration and from the spread of the bacteria to other parts of the body. Non-invasive diarrhea grows from colonies of microscopic evil-doers that set up housekeeping on, but do not invade, intestinal walls. Toxins released by the colonies cause cramps, nausea, vomiting, and massive gushes of fluid from the patient's lower intestinal tract. Non-invasive diarrhea carries a high risk for dehydration.

Diarrheal illnesses come and go with the vagaries of what one voluntarily and involuntarily ingests; erupt from numerous sources that include bacteria, viruses, and protozoas (SEE CHAPTER 30: COMMUNICABLE DISEASES); and last as briefly as a relatively blessed six hours or as long as a destructive three weeks or more. "Traveler's diarrhea," to note in passing, is not a specific disease but a syndrome. Although *E. coli* gets the nod as the cause of the largest number of traveler's diarrheas, many of the water-borne or food-borne germs may be the source.

Whatever the causative agent, a diarrheal illness can be mild, moderate, or severe depending on the frequency of the rush to the bushes, the pain of cramping, the wateriness of the bowel movement, and the vileness of the gas, the latter being often a matter of personal opinion. All cases, however, have in common the departure of water from humanity's hindmost orifice—sometimes oceans of fluid, up to 25 liters in 24 hours in the most severe cases. And it's not just water your body spills onto the ground. An impressive amount of electrolytes. e.g., potassium, sodium, can be lost during an episode of diarrhea.

Initially, the field management of all diarrheal illnesses looks the same: Replace the lost water. Clear liquids are the best choice, liquids such as plain water, broths, herbal teas, fruit juices you can see through. If the illness continues and dehydration

threatens, the patient will grow weaker with bouts of lightheadedness and dizziness, and he or she will require additional electrolytes. You can pack Oral Rehydration Salts in your first aid kit, or whip up a mixture in your water bottle. To one liter of water add one teaspoon of salt and eight teaspoons of sugar. If you've got baking soda, throw in a pinch, but you can get by without it. Mix well. Approximately one-third of the solution should be taken every hour along with all the plain water one can manage to get down. Look for clear urine, the most reliable field sign of a well hydrated person.

Pepto-Bismol® not only relieves some of the torture of diarrhea, but also, according to controlled studies, provides reasonable protection *against* traveler's diarrhea. Imodium®, another and stronger over-the-counter drug, reduces the cramps of diarrhea and the frequency and volume of stools. With a prescription, Lomotil® probably ranks as most seen at the scene of diarrhea. If you've been giving anti-diarrheal drugs for 48 hours and the diarrhea persists, you should stop the drugs and start considering an evacuation of the patient.

Note: Anti-diarrheal drugs should not be used if you think you have dysentery. Severe diarrhea, bloody stools, high fever, and tenacious vomiting are indications of something inside you that your body eagerly wants to get out. In case of dysentery, you should not be stopping the flow, and you should be looking for a physician.

In the best interest of the patient, stick to liquids for persistent and voluminous diarrhea. If and when the problem subsides in the field, provide bland foods such as bread, crackers, cereals, rice, potatoes, lentils, pasta, and bananas. Avoid alcohol, caffeine, spices, fruits, hard cheeses and other fat-laden foods.

Ear Problems

That flap of flesh, the external ear, directs sound down a canal to the eardrum, the tympanic membrane, where the vibrations are transmitted to the three little bones of the middle ear. A tube, the eustachian tube, leads from the middle ear to the nose, balancing the pressure and allowing you the interesting pastime of pinching your nose and blowing to make your ears pop as pressure changes. The little bones pass the vibrations on to the snail-shaped cochlea of the inner ear, which breaks the sound up before sending it along nerve pathways to the brain for decoding.

An injury to the ear will probably be external damage that is obvious and treated as any soft tissue injury is handled (SEE CHAPTER 15: SOFT TISSUE INJURIES), or a ruptured eardrum, or a foreign object stuck up the ear canal. Damage to the eardrum can be caused by a blow to the side of the head, a change in pressure while diving underwater (SEE CHAPTER 22: DIVING EMERGENCIES), or a nearby explosion (possible in a lightning strike). The patient will complain of pain, ringing or whistling in the ear, or loss of hearing, and maybe a loss of coordination (an upsetting phenomenon called vertigo).

Keep the ear covered to reduce the chance of infection. Evacuation will depend on the level of pain and discomfort the patient is experiencing.

A foreign object lodged in the ear can be carefully removed with forceps if the object is visible. Otherwise objects lodged in the ear should be removed by a physician, unless it is an insect. Insects can be drowned with water, alcohol, or vegetable or mineral oils. Once dead, the insect will ooze out with the oil or drop out later. The insect can be encouraged to fall out by irrigating the ear canal with warm water from an irrigation syringe.

Ear infections can develop in the outer, middle, or inner ear. An outer ear infection, called *otitis externa* or "swimmer's ear," is typically caused by swimming in contaminated water and/or by periods of high humidity that encourage bacterial or fungal growth in the ear canal. The patient complains of ear pain which undergoes a marked increase if you tug on the external ear. The ear canal should be flushed with a dilute solution of alcohol or vinegar, approximately four parts water to one part alcohol or vinegar, and the ear should be kept as dry as possible. If the condition worsens, it may be *otitis media*, middle ear infection. Middle ear infections should be treated with appropriate antibiotics which means an evacuation will provide the best care.

Eye Injuries

The eyeball is truly round, but only a small slice shows to the outside world. A jelly-like fluid called *vitreous humor* fills the ball. A bulge, the cornea, sits on the front of the eyeball and is filled with salty fluid called *aqueous humor*. Between the bulge and the ball lies the lens. Over the lens is a special muscle, the iris, that has an adjustable opening, the pupil. Working together, they focus images on a layer of sensitive cells, the retina, covering the back of the eye. Translated into electrical signals and carried by the optic nerves from each eye to the back of the brain, the image is decoded into thought. Since the images are translated from the back of the brain, sometimes a blow to the back of the head causes visual disturbances.

Nature has determined to protect our eyes in several ways. The outside of the ball, except over the cornea, is covered with a tough membrane called the *sclera*, the "white" of the eye. A thin, mucous membrane, the *conjunctiva*, covers the exposed part of the eye and the inner side of the eyelid. Together these see-through "skins" are much hardier than the skin that covers the rest of our bodies. *Lacrimal* (tear) glands keep the eye moist, washing out most of the dust and debris. The eyelids add protection and help keep the surface of the eye clean when you blink. A bony socket, the orbit, surrounds everything and forms a protective shield. It is lined with fatty "shock absorbers," a final barrier against physical abuse. Still, it is possible to injure the eye.

The most common problem is when something is in your eye that doesn't belong: debris, hair, insects. The discomfort can be enormous, but usually the patient's own tearing mechanism will wash the eye clean before any serious damage occurs. Healthy first aid is simply to avoid rubbing the eye and immediately washing it out with a lot of clean water. Lay the patient down while a steady stream of water is poured on the bridge of the nose. Rapid blinking encourages the flushing process.

There is nothing harmful about removing large chunks of debris from an eye, as long as force is never used. If the matter does not come loose with the aid of a soft tissue or additional rinsing, leave it alone, cover the eye with a folded gauze pad or sterile eye patch, and get to a doctor. Also, do not try to remove anything stuck to the surface of the cornea.

Occasionally the eye will feel irritated after the matter has been removed, making it painful to blink. Most likely, the eye has suffered an abrasion. Rinse the eye again, and if still uncomfortable, patch it shut. Take an anti-inflammatory analgesic like ibuprofen. Ophthalmic ointment or drops will often provide relief. For irritation that is unrelieved in 24 hours, head for a doctor.

The classic "black eye" is a result of rapid swelling and discoloration following a blow. The whites may also turn an alarming red. But don't worry. A cold compress will reduce the pain and swelling. Within 12 to 24 hours the eye will look relatively normal in size. It can take a week to 10 days for the black to fade.

Reasons to see a doctor after a punch in the eye include persistent blurred vision, double vision, extraordinary sensitivity to light, and discharge of something other than tears.

An eyeball impaled with a sharp object is a serious injury, not a simple problem. If the object is still there, do not try to remove it. Keep the patient lying down to prevent gravity from pulling the critically important vitreous humor out. Stabilizing what has pierced the eye is necessary. One way to do this is to make a "donut" out of a rolled handkerchief or triangular bandage. Place it gently around the eye, adding a cup over the donut so nothing can catch or jar the object. Tape it all securely in place, and patch the other eye shut as well. If the good eye looks around nervously, the bad eye will try to follow it, possibly causing more damage. The patient should be evacuated to a hospital reclining at approximately 45 degrees to prevent undue pressure from rising within the eye when the patient lies fully reclined.

A cut in the lid produces a lot of blood. Relax, and check the eyeball for damage. If it has been cut, the patient must be kept still and lying down, with both eyes patched. Otherwise, cover the wound with a light, sterile dressing. Although the slice may be quite small, a scar on the eyelid can be a discomfort for the rest of your life. Doctors can stitch the wound neatly with little or no noticeable scarring.

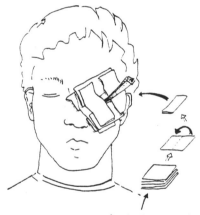

4x4" STERILE GAUZE PADS

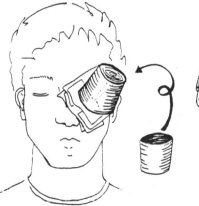

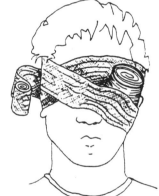

Figure 31-3: Stabilization of object in eye

Fishhooks

There are three ways to remove an imbedded fishhook: the good, the bad, and the ugly.

The good way is the *string jerk technique*: Loop a length of string, approximately 12 inches long, around the curve of the hook, and wrap the ends around your index finger. Push down on the eye and shank of the hook with your free hand to disengage the barb. Align the string with the long axis of the fishhook, then give it a jerk. The hook will come out easily and almost always without pain.

The bad way in the *push-through and snip-off technique*: Wash the skin around the wound with antiseptic solution, then numb it with ice or another source of local anesthesia. With pliers, grasp the fishhook and push the point through the skin. Snip off the barb, then back the hook out.

The *ugly technique* involves gently slicing through the skin with a sterile scalpel until the barb is released. This technique is not recommended except in extreme situations.

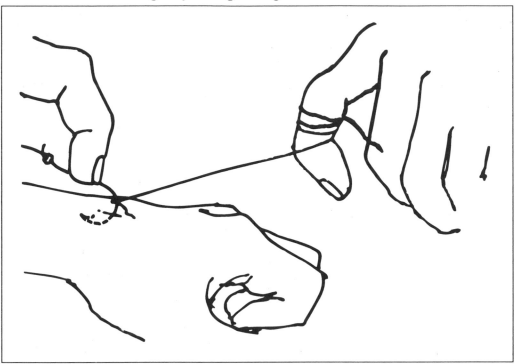

Figure 31-4: Fishhook removal

Fungal Infections of the Skin

The fungi that cause skin infections are known as dermatophytes ("skin plants"), and they live on keratin, a hard protein in skin, hair, and nails. "Ringworm," a popular name for several fungal infections, takes its name from the leading edge of the inflammation which is wavy and worm-like, sometimes circular. Ringworm of the foot bears the name of *tinea pedis* or athlete's foot; of the groin, *tinea curis* or jock itch; of the skin in general, *tinea corporis*; of the scalp, *tinea capitis*; of the bearded area in men, *tinea barbae*. Most cases are passed human-to-human or furry animal-to-human. Dermatophytes like it warm, wet, and dark, and are encouraged by poor skin hygiene, skin chafed by tight clothing, and skin puffy from long exposure to moisture.

Highly contagious, the best place to pick up a foot fungus is off the floor of a locker room or public shower after a workout, which is how athlete's foot got its popular name. But be not deceived, you don't have to be athletic—you don't even have to pass a gym on the way to work. The fungi can be involuntarily harvested, sometimes, from the soil outside your tent. For some unknown reason, it grows on men twice as often as women. The fungus prefers the bottom of feet and between the toes. Starting with mild scaling, athlete's foot progresses to burning pain and irresistible itching, the kind of itching that makes you want to scratch the hide off your toes. Skin will crack, and blister, and smell. The inflammation can spread up the sides and onto the top of the foot. Almost half the sufferers of athlete's foot claim the problem comes and goes for years. The reason for recurring *tinea pedis* is failure to treat it correctly. Treat it right by 1) starting treatment as soon as the signs and symptoms appear, 2) keeping feet as clean and dry as possible, 3) applying an anti-fungal cream, lotion, or spray—such as Tinactin Antifungal® or Lotrimin AF®—twice a day, and 4) the part people most often fail to do, keep up the treatment for four weeks even if you think you've got it whipped before four weeks end. Giving feet some direct sunlight every day might also help curtail the growth of fungus. If the itch and smell persist for more than four weeks of treatment, you really should have a doctor take a look.

Most foot fungi can be stopped before they blossom. Feet should be washed and dried well every day, if possible, especially in warm, humid climates. Socks should be thoroughly dry before being put on. Boots should be allowed to dry out at night. If a patient seems prone to athlete's foot, suggest the use of Lotrimin AF® athlete's foot powder or Tinactin® antifungal deodorant spray every 24 hours. A dose a day keeps the fungus away.

The treatment of any fungal infection of the skin is basically the same: Change the moist, dark environment that bred the infection. Stay as clean and dry as possible. Wear loose fitting clothing. Apply antifungal lotions or sprays. Apply a thin layer of one percent hydrocortisone cream a couple of times a day for intense itching. Expose the infected skin to fresh air and sunshine a couple of times a day.

Hay Fever

It begins as an itch in the nose—gradually or abruptly—just after the onset of the pollen season. It spreads, like ants fanning out from a disturbed anthill on multitudes of tiny feet, to the eyes and the roof of the mouth and the back of the throat. Eyes begin to water, and the patient begins to sneeze. Hacking cough, headache, rash, loss of appetite, lack of sleep, depression, irritability may all describe the patient. There might be a feeling of tightness in the chest and a whistling sound, a wheeze, when the patient takes a breath. This is an allergy.

An allergy is an acquired hypersensitivity to a substance that most people do not react to. You can be allergic to just about anything, but most seasonal allergies are caused by inhaling windborne pollens. In spring allergies are often caused by tree pollen, e.g., oak, elm, maple, alder, birch, cottonwood. In summer it's likely to be grass pollens, e.g., Bermuda, Johnson, timothy, or weed pollens, e.g., ragweed. Fall allergies may result from weeds and, occasionally, airborne fungus spores. Fungi sometimes cause allergic reactions in winter. All of these allergies are often lumped under the general category of "hay fever."

When an allergy-producing substance (an allergen) gets into your body, it stimulates the release of several chemicals. The primary chemical released is histamine. In a non-allergic person, histamine performs a valuable function, a part of the healthy immunological response to something that doesn't belong inside you. Nobody knows why, but instead of producing the right amount of histamine, allergy sufferers overproduce histamine. Overproduction of histamine is the most significant cause of the signs and symptoms of an allergy.

Is there relief? About 95 percent of all allergy-relief medications contain the same ingredients, and they can be divided into two categories: antihistamines and decongestants. It doesn't matter what you take, as long as it works for you.

Antihistamines work by blocking the body's normal response to histamines. That usually makes the symptoms ease off. All of the over-the-counter antihistamines also tend to cause drowsiness. You can put the drowsiness to good use if you need a mild sleeping aid, but it can be dangerous if you're hiking a rough trail in steep terrain and debilitating if you're trying to cast a fly precisely. Now available over-the-counter, clemastine (sold as Tavist-D®) does not cause drowsiness in many people who take it.

Decongestants work by decreasing blood flow to nasal tissue, shrinking mucous membranes, and opening up your airway. Sometimes a decongestant will put your nerves on edge, so try it out during the day before taking it at bedtime. Use with caution if you have high blood pressure, heart disease, thyroid disease or diabetes.

If you know you have a tendency to react with wheezing and chest tightness, you should carry an over-the-counter pocket inhaler. The inhaler contains a drug, usually epinephrine, that dilates constricted bronchial tubes. Squirt the mist into your mouth while you're inhaling, and your airway opens up almost immediately (SEE CHAPTER 28: ALLERGIC REACTIONS AND ANAPHYLAXIS).

Another way to fight allergies is to visit a physician who specializes in the problem. First the doctor figures out what an individual is specifically allergic to. There could be a vaccination program ("allergy shots") to cure the particular sensitivity. Allergy shots do not pump medications into the body. They are, instead, small doses of what an individual is allergic to, given over a long period of time, until that person develops a natural immunity to the allergen.

Headache

Brains, just to stay physiologically factual, are immune to pain. It's the nerve rich membranes that surround the brain, collectively called the meninges, that detect some sort of abnormality in the "gray matter" and proclaim the news via pain. "Headache" is a generic term meaning anything from mild discomfort to agonizing debility. The message carried by the pain could be as insignificant as "Slow down and rest" or as critical as "You will soon be dropping pack forever in that Great Campsite in the Sky."

Long a medical mystery (and still to some degree today), headaches have been blamed on such things as wimpishness, psychological disorders, repressed emotions, demons, mother-in-laws, red wine, old cheese, and bad karma. Some of that blame may be valid. More than two dozen types of headaches have been identified by experts including pain related to diet, stress, heredity, and personality traits. What you should know for sure includes 1) what to do for the pain, 2) how to prevent the pain, and 3) when to consult a physician.

In the wild outdoors, head pain can usually be traced to one of three sources, or a combination of two of the three.

Most headaches are a familiar companion: A dull ache in the forehead or sides of the head, often associated with muscular tightness in the back of the neck. It may feel as if your hat's too small when you aren't wearing one. A painkiller, a long drink from the water bottle, maybe a short nap, and the pain takes a hike. Beginning treatment as soon as you feel the headache developing, in most cases, keeps the discomfort on the low end of the pain range. These episodes are called tension (or muscular contraction) headaches, probably the most common source of pain in the head for all people and usually the result of emotional and physical stress and exhaustion. Muscles in the head, and muscles in the neck and shoulders that attach to those reaching up over the head, squeeze down tight putting grief on nerves and blood vessels. These muscles often feel like someone tied them into a bowline-on-a-coil, and massaging the muscles provides some relief.

Tension headaches are nothing more than a nuisance. The chance of one can be reduced by maintaining a fair to middling level of physical fitness, making sure your pack fits well and rides comfortably, and talking a companion into carrying the heaviest gear. Since you'll sometimes wake up with a tension headache when you sleep uncomfortably, adequate sleeping pads and a flat tent site can be of benefit in prevention. Dehydration headaches may be even more common than tension headaches in the outdoors. Very few people give their bodies, and their brains, enough water to function at maximum

efficiency (SEE CHAPTER 17: HEAT-INDUCED EMERGENCIES). The first symptom of a drop in your optimal internal water level is usually a headache, your brain complaining of the inadequacy.

As with tension headaches, the problem rates initially as merely a nuisance. Prolonged dehydration, however, will eventually lead to the breakdown of important body parts. If a dehydration headache strikes, an hour of rest during which you slowly sip a quart of water should put you back in the pain-free zone.

Vascular headaches, the third source of pain, can be brought on by a variety of causes, any of which produce unusual dilation or constriction of blood vessels in the brain. Blood pounding through the vessels sometimes creates the throbbing often associated with a vascular headache. Hangover and hunger headaches are this type. Certain foods cause vascular headaches in susceptible people: alcoholic beverages, especially red wine, bananas, caffeine-rich drinks, chocolate, citrus fruits, onions, peanut butter, ripe cheese. Shifts in hormones can trigger these headaches with boys and girls affected about equally, but with adult women suffering more than twice as often as adult men.

Migraine, from a combo of French and Greek meaning "half a head," describes more vascular headaches than any other term. Hour after hour of severe pain usually dominates one side of the brain, with unwelcome accompaniment that may include blinding light in one eye, blurred vision, nausea and numbness or tingling in arms or legs. Migraine headaches are announced in one out of five patients by an aura such as flashing lights or pre-pain numbness. Although migraines can have numerous causes, some unknown, they strike women over men about seven out of 10 times, they appear to be hereditary, and they may be related to personality traits, perfectionist types being more likely to suffer.

Patients with migraine headaches sometimes find relief by pouring ice cold water over their heads, which apparently constricts swollen blood vessels in the brain. Strong drugs typically provide the only reliable source of pain mitigation, drugs prescribed by physicians.

Even worse than migraines are cluster headaches which most often occur in "clusters" of one to three headaches a day over a period of several days. The pain may feel as if someone has pounded a tent stake through your eye directly into your brain. Fortunately, the agony lasts an average of no more 45 minutes, but 45 minutes can be a long time to have an imaginary stake in your brain. The cause of this particular head pain remains unknown, but, in the plus column, four out of five patients report the pain eases off in minutes after they start breathing 100 percent supplemental oxygen.

Most headaches will be successfully treated with rest, at least a liter of water, and an over-the-counter painkiller. If headaches come on strong and sudden, like nothing the patient has ever felt before, persisting for 24 hours unrelieved by rest and medication, causing weakness, dizziness or other neurological manifestations, evacuation to a doctor as soon as possible is the best choice. Other indications of a serious headache include: 1) The patient also has a high fever. 2) The patient also has an unusually stiff neck. 3) The patient experiences a series of headaches growing steadily worse each time. 4) The patient's arms and legs are tingly, weak, numb or paralyzed. 5) The patient has an altered mental status.

Insect Bites

Mosquitoes and other biting insects have done as much or more to ruin a wilderness experience than anything else known to man or woman. You can apply an ice pack to minimize the swelling and itching in the first few minutes after a bite, or use a topical itch-reducing product, e.g., StingEze®. Use an antihistamine, e.g., diphenhydramine, 25-50 mg every six hours, for more intense reactions.

Prevention of insect bites is most easily handled with a repellent.

The most effective repellent is N, N, diethyl-methyl toluamide, known as DEET, but it is often smeared on in a much stronger concentration than is needed, especially in children. DEET is absorbed by the body, but only about 40 percent of the absorbed amount is excreted in urine. Where does the other half go? Use only the concentration needed to repel insects, and wash the skin where DEET was applied as soon as possible after exposure to insects has passed. DEET may be applied to clothing, such as collars, cuffs, and hats, in order to repel insects. For the skin of small children, many experts recommend using a non-DEET product, such as Natrapel®.

Permethrin, originally extracted from chrysanthemum flowers, is a potent insect neurotoxin currently synthesized for human use as an insect repellent. It's not really a repellent, it's an insect killer. Within minutes after contact with permethrin-treated clothing, the insect dies. It bonds strongly to the fibers of clothing and, depending on the concentration and application process, can withstand numerous washings, remaining active, in some cases, for years. Permethrin is colorless and odorless, and does no harm to vinyl, plastic, or other fabrics. It can be applied to mosquito netting on tents, to sleeping bags, even to window screens at home. It should *not* be applied to human skin. After many tests, the experts agree it apparently does no harm to humans, but it quickly loses its efficacy when applied to skin.

Loose clothing helps prevent bites from bugs that can reach their biting apparatus through tight clothing. Smoke keeps some insects away. In desperation, mud smeared on exposed skin prevents insects from biting.

Some insects, especially mosquitoes, feed primarily at dawn and dusk, and sometimes throughout the night. Use a tent with adequate insect netting to sleep safe from bites. Set camp in a high and dry place where winds may keep some insects away. Avoid low and wet areas where mosquitoes breed.

Motion Sickness

Three systems process information about body movement and position in space, providing a sense of body orientation: the visual system (the eyes), the vestibular system (three semicircular canals and two small bones in the inner ear), and a system of specialized nerve cells in the skin, muscles and joints that relay data on body position. Normally, these three systems work together, sending information to the brain to maintain a sense of equilibrium. When you're on a moving platform, however, on, for instance, a boat or airplane, you get mixed messages from these systems. Your eyes may say you're sitting still while the specialized nerve cells feel your tension and motion as you try to stay balanced. At the same time, the vestibular system reports side to side, back and forth, up and down movement. The confused brain sends out "sick" messages, and the stomach often responds with vomit.

A plethora of "home remedies" recommended for motion sickness have passed down many throats, remedies that include dill pickles and saltine crackers, stewed tomatoes and saltine crackers, horseradish with or without the crackers, and crackers all by themselves. They universally have had the same effect on most people: None. Some experts claim a stomach containing only liquids deals with motion easier than one full of solids. Others claim the opposite. If you've tried something and it works, keep using it. If motion sickness seems to persist, perhaps one of the following remedies will work.

Ask the patient to focus his or her eyes, whenever possible, on a distant stationary point. Something on the horizon would be appropriate, such as a mountain peak or a tall tree. A fixed point of

reference gives the brain help in sorting through the mess of messages. If the patient can go below on board a ship, don't let them. Below decks offers no point of reference.

Since motion is the culprit, attempt to avoid as much of it as possible. In a large boat, have the patient sit or stand near the center, head still, eyes straight ahead. On an airplane, suggest sitting over the wings where the ride rocks the least.

By lying semi-reclined, with eyes closed, taking deep calming breaths, and reducing the flow of messages to the brain, the patient might be able to put a stop to the ailment.

Chinese medicine claims acupressure on the *Nei-kuan* point will control nausea. The magic spot lies on the inside of both wrists, between the two tendons you can feel on the thumb side of the arm, just below the bones of the wrist itself. Pressure can be applied here with one finger for at least a full minute each on both wrists, or the patient can wear Sea-Bands®, a wrist-band available in many pharmacies that presses constantly on the Nei-kuan point.

Two capsules of powdered ginger root (500 mg each), taken 20 to 30 minutes before motion, prevent sickness for numerous sufferers. If you've got raw ginger root, grate one teaspoon, add it to four ounces of water and steep it for 10 minutes for the same result. Since a cup of ginger tea must be downed approximately every half hour in order to maintain a non-nauseous state, you might as well brew up a thermos full.

Antihistamines are medications that prevent motion sickness apparently by interrupting communications, the nerve impulses, between the vestibular system and the brain. Over-the-counter you can buy many antihistamines, but some have proven to be particularly effective for many people. A good bet is meclizine (Antivert®, Bonine®), a drug that should be taken once every 24 hours starting at least an hour *before* the rocking and rolling starts. The recommended dose is 25 to 50 mg. Meclizine may cause mild to moderate drowsiness and a dry mouth. Another antihistamine, one of the oldest and least expensive, is dimenhydrinate (Dramamine®) which must be taken every four to six hours (50 mg) starting at least an hour before you shove off or take off. Dimenhydrinate tends to cause extreme drowsiness, but, in the plus column, it comes in liquid form suitable for small children. Available with a prescription only, promethazine (Phenergan®, Mepergan®) works to prevent and, for some people, treat motion sickness, a bonus if the patient forgot to take a pill before she or he started feeling nauseous. It is recommended, however, to take 25 mg prior to motion. Promethazine, too, causes severe drowsiness in some folks. People report successes and failures with these drugs, and the only sure-fire way to know if one of the antihistamines will work for you is to try it.

Transderm Scop® (scopolamine), a patch placed behind the ear, was supposed to release small amounts of the drug over a period of three days right through your skin. When it was available, by prescription only, you could press the patch in place the night before a trip and expect no motion sickness. Currently off the market due to the patch's failure to reliably release the medication, Transderm Scop® is expected to be back some day in the arsenal of anti-seasickness medications.

Mouth Injuries

A profusion of blood vessels in the mouth leads to an abundance of bleeding from even very trivial wounds to that area. Active bleeding from mouth trauma almost always stops on its own, and immediate care of the patient should center on maintaining an open airway.

Mouth lacerations tend to look horrible for the first couple of days, but they also tend to heal nicely with little care. The patient should rinse his or her mouth with warm, salty water every two or three hours and after every meal until the wound is completely closed.

If the wound gapes open significantly, the wound should be packed open—wet to dry—(SEE CHAPTER 15: SOFT TISSUE INJURIES) and the patient should be evacuated from the wilderness for stitches, especially if the lips are involved. Gaping wounds to the mouth and lips that heal puckered are unsightly, in the way, and difficult to repair once they heal that way.

Nausea and Vomiting

Nausea and vomiting, a pair of ugly cousins, can have many causes, and they're common enough in the wilderness to more often leave you wondering why the patient feels sick than not. Infections somewhere in the gastrointestinal tract, lumped under the name gastroenteritis, typically viral, are a prevalent source. Then there's motion sickness (SEE ABOVE) and altitude illness (SEE CHAPTER 18: ALTITUDE ILLNESSES). Usually it is just the body's way of dealing with something that is upsetting the normal balance.

Protracted vomiting can lead to dehydration and electrolyte imbalances. You can give the patient an anti-emetic, such as prochlorperazine, e.g., Compazine® 25 mg suppository twice a day, or promethazine, e.g., Phenergan® 25 mg suppository every four to six hours as needed. Once the vomiting has stopped, ask the patient to drink plenty of clear liquids for the next 24 hours.

Nausea and vomiting may be signaling a serious injury, such as a head injury (SEE CHAPTER 9: HEAD INJURIES), or a serious medical emergency, such as a heart attack (SEE CHAPTER 23: CARDIAC EMERGENCIES) or an acute abdominal problem (SEE CHAPTER 11: ABDOMINAL EMERGENCIES), in which case an evacuation is indicated.

Nose Injuries

Nose injuries usually produce one or two similar manifestations: pain and blood. Keep the patient sitting up and leaning slightly forward, if possible, to prevent blood from entering the airway. If blood is visibly running out, pinch the fleshy part of the nostrils closed, using direct pressure to promote clotting. Try to prevent your patient from moving around for about a half hour after the bleeding stops, to give clotting a chance to complete. Instruct your patient to please restrain from nose picking, sneezing, and bending over and straining for the next couple of days.

Epistaxis (a nose bleed) is almost always anterior. A few, especially in people with chronic high blood pressure, may be posterior. The blood runs down the throat, and the patient may require a doctor's care to stop the bleeding. Decongestant nasal sprays usually help reduce bleeding.

Susceptible people are encouraged to have nose bleeds by dry weather. Applications of an ointment inside the nose can reduce the dryness, and prevent bleeds. The same stuff you use on dry lips will work if gently applied to the inside of the nose once or twice a day.

To avoid the possibility of serious damage, an object securely wedged inside a nose should be left in place until a physician can remove it.

Rapid swelling often makes it difficult to make an assessment of a broken nose. If you aren't sure, give the patient painkillers and apply cold packs for 20 to 30 minutes, three or four times a day. If the patient's level of discomfort is acceptable, it's okay to stay in the wilderness. When the nose is obviously broken, the same treatment is advisable, but consider evacuation to a medical facility as well. Your patient may wish to have a bit of surgery done so the nose eventually looks the same as before. There is no rush. The surgery will be just as successful if a week goes by first. In fact, some surgeons like to have the patient wait until the swelling goes down, since it's easier to tell where to realign the nose.

Poison Ivy, Oak, and Sumac

These poisonous plants grow in every state except Alaska and Hawaii, and can be a small shrub as well as a woody, ivy-like vine, with several different varieties east of the Rockies bearing the name "poison ivy." West of the Rockies you're more apt to encounter poison oak. Wet areas of the southeastern United States provide habitat for poison sumac. All three—ivy, oak, sumac—fall into the genus *Toxicodendron*. Although the leaves may be smooth-edged, or sawtooth-edged, or lobed, they do indeed *almost* always grow in threes with the middle leaf extending farther than the other two—excepting poison sumac which grows in a complex leaf of seven to 13 paired and pointed leaflets. The message here: Learn to identify the members of this genus that grow in your area because what all *Toxicodendrons* share in common, without any exceptions, is urushiol.

Urushiol, the usually colorless (sometimes light yellow) oil in these plants, is potent stuff. Two to 2.5 millionth of a gram will trigger a reaction in the very sensitive, and about 50 percent of all adults in the U. S. are very sensitive. Another 35 percent will have a reaction to higher concentrations of urushiol. The rest do not react, even to extremely high concentrations. No one knows why some people are tolerant of urushiol—perhaps an acquired immunity, perhaps a genetic blessing—but, without a doubt,

sensitivity to the oil is the single most common source of allergic skin reactions in the United States and perhaps the whole wide world.

When urushiol soaks into human skin, an allergic reaction takes place. Not everyone reacts exactly the same, but most people first develop redness where they contacted the oil. The redness often appears in streaks where the plant brushed the skin. There may be swelling. Blisters, sometimes large, sometimes small, erupt later, and discharge the fluid that fills them. The discharge eventually crusts over. The entire area itches with indescribable ferocity.

After contact, it takes varying amounts of time for the reaction to show up. On thicker areas of your body, such as hands and feet, the oil soaks in more slowly than on thinner areas. Still, if you're sensitive, you can see the bad stuff beginning to happen in two to six hours. Those of low sensitivity may not develop signs or symptoms for days to as long as two weeks. For most people, 12 to 48 hours brings assurance that the next 10 days to two weeks or more will be cursed with the misery of the reaction. Adding agony to misery, parts of your body that have reacted in the past could fire up again when a new body part reacts to a fresh contact.

Unpredictability in the way the rash emerges has created the myth that scratching the blisters open spreads the poison. Not so. The fluid in the blisters is harmless, but you can spread the oil easily when it gets on your hands, causing the rash to show up in places you know never touched a plant.

For stability, urushiol finds few equals, being found active in dried plants dating back more than 100 years. Hike through it. Store your boots for a couple of years. Slip back into your boots, and you could suddenly react to poison ivy. You can pick up the oil from your clothing, the bottom of your tent, your hiking staff, or the hair of your dog or cat. Neither dog nor cat, by the way, nor any other critter, seems to react to urushiol—humans only.

Good news: The oil is contained within the plants, not on the surface, which means casually brushing against an intact *Toxicodendron* will not spread urushiol on your skin. Bad news: The plant may not be intact, even though it appears so, for many reasons, such as a previous hiker stomping the plants, a bug chewing the plants, a strong wind whipping the leaves into a frenzy.

Speaking of wind, it will not carry the oil, so standing downwind of one of these poisonous plants is safe. When burned, smoke particles will take the oil aloft, allowing you the opportunity to break out all over, even, horror of horrors, in your airway if you breathe in the smoke.

An allergic reaction for all seasons, urushiol remains equally devastating throughout the year. Beware, therefore, even the brown stems and roots of winter, and the red leaves of fall if they're still attached to the stems. Plant juices return to stems and roots in the fall leaving dead poison ivy leaves littering the ground with virtually no urushiol in them. On the other itch-ridden hand, why take a chance. Avoid all contact.

Nothing cures the rash, but you'll assuredly want to try several methods of relieving the itch. Aspirin, non-steroidal anti-inflammatory drugs (such as ibuprofen), and oral antihistamines have no effect, although the antihistamine might enable you to sleep better. Topical lotions, creams, or sprays that contain antihistamines or anesthetics (words that usually end in "-caine") should be avoided since the additives have a tendency to make things worse. Topical corticosteroids sold over-the-counter are too weak to work well. Your physician may be able to prescribe a strong topical steroid that will work, if you start using it before the reaction has turned to blisters. Topical applications of plain old calamine lotion or soaking in a tepid bath with one cup Aveeno® oatmeal or two cups of linnet starch added usually reduces the itch. A cold wet compress sometimes brings relief, but, on the other end of the heat spectrum, many sufferers report substantial aid from standing in a hot shower for several minutes, then gently patting the water off the itchy area. But you don't need a shower. Simply soaking the affected body part/s in water as hot as tolerable often provides anti-itch relief for hours.

Home remedies abound with recipes for folk medications against the itch numbering over one hundred. If you've tried one, and it works for you, you should use it.

Unproven but often recommended—and, therefore, worthy of a few words—are two plants whose juices may ease the torment. Plantain, common and buckhorn, has leaves that release a pale green sap when crushed. Dabbed on the rash, plantain sap reportedly stops the itch for 24 to 48 hours. The second plant, jewelweed, has as many supporters as plantain. Once again, the juice from crushed plants is applied to the rash with what you pray will be helpful results. Jewelweed supporters also claim satisfaction from soaking in a bath tub of water to which the juice of approximately one pound of the plant has been added.

You should definitely forego self treatment and high-tail it to a doctor if you swell significantly, if your airway, face, or genitals are involved, or for any reaction that seems serious to you.

In addition to recognition and avoidance of the enemy, several actions may prevent the reaction. Of prime importance is washing as soon as possible after you realize you may have touched one of these poisonous plants. Lightning fast reflexes are not required since even the extremely sensitive have an estimated five to 10 minutes to wash off the urushiol before it soaks in enough to cause trouble. Those of low sensitivity may have two hours. Cold water, lots and lots of it, inactivates urushiol, so plunging into a nearby stream or lake, depending on your ability to swim, would be a reasonable act. If you have plenty of cold water available, especially within the first three minutes of contact, soap, say the experts, does not help. Avoid hot water which may spread the oil around more than off and/or open the pores so the oil soaks in faster.

Washing with soap and water after exposure to urushiol goes back to at least the 1930s, and soap is still recommended by many dermatologists after the three minute period ends. As to what kind of soap, the experts vary in exact recommendations, but detergents—such as dish and laundry—seem to work as well as anything. Of greater importance than what kind of soap is how you use it. Dermatologists seem to agree on this: Repeated rubbings, not scrubbings, with sufficient rinses in between.

Organic solvents such as alcohol and gasoline work even better than water, or soap and water. The preferred method is to dab repeatedly with several pieces of solvent-soaked cotton to pick up urushiol from the skin before giving your skin a good rub with fresh solvent-soaked cotton. Once the solvent dries, urushiol caught in the cotton will redeposit on your skin, so don't use the same piece of cotton for more than a few moments. The National Safely Council, opting on the side of extreme caution, recommends washing five to six times, followed by a wash of rubbing alcohol, followed by a clear water rinse. Solvents are especially useful for removing urushiol from gear.

When you wash your hands, be sure to clean under your fingernails.

Remember to wash any clothes that may be contaminated. Clothing may hold the oil, protecting your skin at first, but the oil will remain active for a long, long time, returning to haunt you with the aggravating itch if you don't wash that shirt thoroughly.

Going over-the-counter in the second half of the 1990s, two products carry U. S. Food and

Drug Administration approval as skin protectant barriers against urushiol: IvyBlock® and Work Shield®. Applied prior to exposure, these barrier creams trap the urushiol, allowing you to harmlessly wash off the cream and the oil after exposure. Work Shield® may also be used as a cleansing cream after your skin has contacted urushiol.

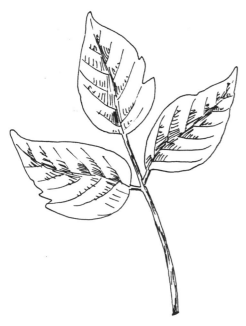

Figure 31-5: Poison Ivy

Snowblindness

Six to 12 hours after overexposure to the sun's ultraviolet radiation, to which eyes are especially susceptible as it bounces off snow, the eyes may feel painful, like an "eye full of sand." The patient often complains of blurred vision, and the eyes may appear red and swollen. The cornea of the eye has been sunburned, and it's very sensitive to light. Called snowblindness, the patient is not truly "blind," but practically so, because it hurts so much to open up the eyes. Cool, wet compresses may be applied for pain. A small amount of an

ophthalmic (eye) ointment may be applied several times a day for two to three days. Pull down the bottom lid of the eye and apply a thin line of ointment, and ask the patient to blink a few times, and then keep still with eyes shut until the ointment melts. If possible, remain in camp, allowing the patient to rest his or her eyes for 24 hours. Snowblindness almost always resolves harmlessly in 24 to 48 hours. If the problem doesn't resolve, an evacuation is recommended. Problems can be prevented by wearing sunglasses that block all, or almost all, UV light. On snow or water, sunglasses should fit well and have side-shields to block reflected light.

Splinters

Forceps (tweezers) are one of the handiest tools to keep in your first aid kit, and splinter removal is one of their best uses. Splinters and other small imbedded objects, e.g., cactus spines, should be removed as soon as possible. In addition to being irritating, an organic splinter, such as wood or other plant parts, may lead to an infection. If the end is visible, grasp it with the tweezers and pull it gently out. If the end is buried, probe with your fingers until you find the orientation of the splinter, and push it toward the opening of the wound until the end is graspable. With deeply buried splinters, you may need to cut superficially, preferably with a sterile scalpel from a well-equipped first aid kit, to expose the imbedded object. Clean and dress any wounds left after removal (SEE CHAPTER 15: SOFT TISSUE INJURIES).

Subungual Hematoma

Smashing a finger or toe may cause an accumulation of blood under the nail, an often painful accumulation called a *subungual hematoma*. You can relieve the pressure—and the pain—by drilling a tiny hole, allowing the blood to escape. Heat a sharp point, e.g., needle, safety pin, paper clip, scalpel, to red hotness and gently drill through the nail into the accumulation of blood.

Sunburn, Sun Allergies, Skin Cancer

Sunshine, essential for life, strikes the Earth in rays of varying wavelengths. Long rays (infrared) are unseen but felt as heat. Intermediate length rays are visible as light. Shorter rays (ultraviolet) are, also, invisible and are further divided into three groups: 1) ultraviolet A (UVA), beneficial in low doses but may increase the chance of cancer in high doses, 2) UVB, primarily responsible for sunburn and cancer, and 3) UVC, the shortest and most dangerous. UV rays contain enough energy to damage DNA in living skin and eye cells. DNA controls the ability of cells to heal and reproduce.

Melanoma, a form of skin cancer, occurs in the melanocytes, the cells of the skin that control pigmentation, and it occurs most often in people who are fair-skinned and freckled, people who sunburn easily. It's more common in women than men (no one knows why), and the average age at which melanoma strikes has been dropping dramatically. Ten years ago it was considered unusual to find skin cancer in anyone under 40. This year fully one-fourth of all melanomas will involve people in their 20s and 30s. In the last few years, skin cancer's association with exposure to ultraviolet light has been firmly established.

If caught early, malignant melanoma is virtually 100 percent curable. Physicians recommend a monthly skin check for the symptomatic ABCDs of skin cancer.

A for Asymmetry: One half of a mole or skin spot doesn't match the other half.

B for Border Irregularity: Ragged, notched, or blurred edges.

C for Color: Changes in color from black to brown to red, often with a combination of colors. Blue and white may appear.

D for Diameter: Any mole or spot that grows to more than one-fourth inch, about the size of the end of a pencil eraser.

About one-half of all melanomas arise from a previously existing mole, but they can also appear as a completely new spot on the skin. *Consult a physician if any mole or spot appears suddenly, looks scaly, becomes itchy, painful, or tender, or starts to ooze blood.*

Malignant melanoma is one of three common forms of skin cancer, but not the most common. That distinction belongs to *basal cell carcinoma*, with about one half million cases reported annually. Basal cells make up the base of the epidermis, the outermost covering of the body. UV radiation can cause these cells to reproduce too fast, producing a tumorous growth. Basal cell car-

cinoma usually starts as a slow-growing, small, shiny (or pearly) bump that becomes an open sore taking longer than three weeks to heal. They often bleed, crust over, and open to bleed again. The cancer may be an itchy or tender reddish patch that comes and goes. Sometimes it's a pale splotch, like a scar, and sometimes a circular growth with a raised border and depressed center.

Squamous cell carcinoma, the second most common skin cancer, accounts for about 100,000 cases each year. Like the other forms, it appears most often on the face, ears, hands and forearms. In the past 50 years, shoulders, back and chests on men, and the lower legs of women, have become increasingly popular sites for skin cancer due to deliberate exposure of those body parts to UV radiation.

Squamous cells make up most of the epidermis. When they become cancerous, they may look like basal cell cancer, but the problem can also appear as a wart that bleeds and crusts over, bleeds and crusts over. Cancerous squamous cells grow faster and metastasize more frequently than basal cell carcinoma.

The earliest sign of skin damage is sunburn. Even a glorious tan, which most people would enjoy, does not promote skin health. All tanning should be considered visible evidence of injury. That includes tans from tanning lamps.

Sunburn that continues to worsen several days after exposure may be a sun allergy. Sun allergies sometimes show up as severe sunburns, and, less often,

as a poison-ivy-like rash (SEE ABOVE).

Treatment should include avoidance of the damaging rays of the sun. Cool compresses will provide relief. Moisturizing lotions and creams, including aloe, help, as does aspirin, acetaminophen, or ibuprofen.

Sun-related skin problems, happily, are among the most preventable of wilderness illnesses and injuries. The first line of defense is worn. Tight-weave clothing blocks a large amount of UVR, especially if it stays reasonably dry. A full-brimmed hat will shade face and neck, and a floppy brim breaks up scattered UV better than a rigid brim.

Sunscreens dramatically reduce the chance of skin problems. Although most experts agree screens with an SPF of 15 sufficiently protect most skin, recent studies show that higher SPF numbers offer additional protection, especially in the first few hours of exposure. Sunscreens are maximally effective if smeared on when skin is warm, and allowed to soak in for about a half-hour before extreme exposure. People with very susceptible skin-types might do better to completely block UVR on exposed skin with an opaque substance such as zinc oxide.

Ultraviolet A bombards the earth at an almost constant rate throughout the day, but approximately 80 percent of UVB strikes between 10AM and 3PM. Plan to be in the sun early and late in the day for minimum exposure.

Smoke absorbs UVR, but clouds do not. Cool, overcast days in the summer are dangerous, because UVR penetrates the densest cloud cover, while heat-carrying infrared waves are filtered out. People feel cool, fail to take precautions, and often get severe sunburns.

Note: Wind will dry skin, removing the natural skin protection of urocanic acid. Wind does not truly burn skin, but it makes skin more susceptible to sunburn and irritates already sunburned skin, a problem often called "windburn."

Activities associated with water provide an excellent opportunity for a serious sunburn because sunlight bounces off the water's surface to attack exposed skin. The more directly the sun overhead, the more the reflectivity, and rough, choppy water is much more reflective than calm water. Snow, by the way, is also highly reflective, as much as 85 percent as reflective as water.

Altitude is another factor. For every 1000 feet above sea level, UVR increases around five to six percent.

Some medications, combined with sunshine, decrease the time it takes for UV light to damage skin: tetracyclines, antihistamines, sulfa drugs, diuretics, some oral contraceptives. Consult your physician or pharmacist.

UV light damages eyes as well as skin. The conjunctiva can swell from UV exposure, sun-induced cataracts can form from repeated exposure, and direct UVR will burn the retina. Wear sunglasses that absorb or reflect UV light.

Teach children well. According to the Skin Cancer Foundation, 80 percent of lifetime exposure to skin-damaging UV light occurs during the first 18-20 years of life.

Chapter 32:   *Gender-specific Emergencies*

You should be able to:

1. Describe the basic anatomy of male and female genitalia.

2. Describe medical problems specific to males and specific to females.

3. Explain the proper wilderness treatment of these specific problems.

Introduction

Injuries involving the genitalia can be embarrassing, frightening and, from time to time, life-threatening. A variety of illnesses can also affect the reproductive systems of males and females.

These emergencies range from epididymitis, urinary tract, and vaginal infections to the more serious testicular torsion and pelvic inflammatory disease. These problems have occurred on wilderness trips. The Wilderness First Responder should be able to assess, treat, and know when to evacuate a patient with injured or ill genitalia.

Guidelines For General Assessment

Both you and the patient will appreciate a private place to talk. The patient will benefit if you can maintain eye contact while being straightforward, respectful, and non-judgmental. Use proper medical terminology and/or terms that you both understand. Avoid jokes or slang. A member of the patient's sex should be present before and during any physical exam—especially where minors are involved—unless it is impossible.

Basic Anatomy Of The Male Genitalia

The penis and scrotum comprise the visible external male genitalia. The penis contains a canal, the *urethra*, which provides a route for urine expelled from the bladder and sperm expelled from the testes. The scrotum is a pouch-like structure located to either side of and beneath the penis. Two roundish glands called testes lie within the scrotum and are the site of sperm and testosterone production.

Sperm travels out of the testes via the *epididymis*, a comma-shaped organ that lies behind the testes. The epididymis is composed of approximately 20 feet of ducts. From the epididymis, sperm travel through the *ductus deferens*, a tube approximately 18 inches long, that loops into the pelvic cavity on its journey to the ejaculatory duct.

Male-specific Emergencies

Inguinal Hernia

Inguinal hernias are possible in women but far more common in men.

An *inguinal hernia* occurs when part of the intestine protrudes into the groin or scrotum. Weak abdominal muscles due to congenital malformations, trauma, aging, or any activity that increases intra-abdominal pressure such as coughing, straining, lifting, or vigorous exertion may cause a hernia.

The patient will complain of a lump or swelling in the groin and a sharp, steady pain. If the hernia becomes incarcerated (can't be reduced), the intestine may become blocked. The portion may then become strangulated, the blood supply cut off, with death of the bowel resulting. If the intestine is blocked, the lump in the groin will become more swollen and more tender, the patient may vomit and complain of wave-like abdominal cramps, the abdomen will become swollen, and the patient will not have any stools. If you monitor bowel sounds by periodically placing your ear on the abdomen, you will hear an increase in bowel sounds, then a decrease, and finally an absence of bowel sounds.

Attempt to reduce the hernia by lying the patient on his back with the head and chest lower than the abdomen. Apply moderate, steady, upward pressure on the hernia to reduce it. It may take 10 minutes or longer to reduce the hernia. Monitor the patient for the next 24 hours for signs of intestinal obstruction.

If you are unable to reduce the hernia or if the hernia reappears after reduction, the patient will need to be evacuated. If signs and symptoms of intestinal blockage or strangulation are present, evacuate the patient immediately. Do not give the patient anything to eat or drink unless dehydration becomes a problem during a long evacuation in which case small amounts of water at regular intervals may be given.

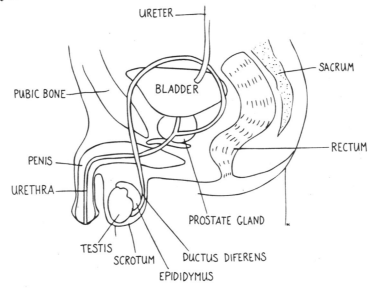

Figure 32-1: Male specific anatomy

Epididymitis

Epididymitis is an inflammation of the epididymis, a problem that can be caused by gonorrhea, syphilis, tuberculosis, mumps, prostatitis (inflammation of the prostate), or urethritis (inflammation of the urethra). Epididymitis is not caused by traumatic injury to the scrotum.

The patient suffers from pain in the scrotum, possibly accompanied by fever. The scrotum may be red and swollen. Epididymitis tends to come on slowly, perhaps over several days, unlike torsion of the testis which sometimes comes on rapidly (SEE BELOW).

The treatment is bedrest and support of the scrotum with a jock strap or whatever can be improvised to create support for the testicles. A non-steroidal anti-inflammatory drug (NSAID) such as ibuprofen may decrease the fever and pain. It is very difficult to differentiate epididymitis from torsion of the testes. Antibiotics are necessary, so the patient must be evacuated when epididymitis is a possibility.

Torsion of the Testis

Torsion of the testis is a twisting of the testis within the scrotum. Mechanisms for testicular torsion could be as dramatic as violent physical activity or as simple as rolling over in a sleeping bag. The ductus deferens and its accompanying blood vessels becomes twisted, decreasing the blood supply to the testis. If the blood supply is totally cut off, the testis dies. After 24 hours without blood supply, little hope of saving the testicle remains.

With many patients, the scrotum is suddenly and intensely full of pain, sometimes rendering the patient unable to move. The scrotum grows red and swollen, and the testis may appear slightly elevated on the affected side. The pain, however, can come on slowly, and the other "classic" signs and symptoms may be absent.

Cool compresses and pain medication will provide some relief. An improvised "jock strap," made, for example, from a triangular bandage, will elevate the scrotum and may increase blood flow to the testis. The patient who is unable to walk must be evacuated for treatment immediately. If evacuation will be delayed, attempt to rotate the affected testicle back into position. Since most testicles rotate "inward," a gentle rotation "out-

ward" may give immediate and blessed relief. The patient may wish to make the rotation himself. If it doesn't work, perhaps the testicle rotated in the opposite direction, so rotate the testicle two turns in the opposite direction. If you fail, the patient is no worse off than before the attempt was made. In either case, the patient suspected of suffering torsion of the testes should be evacuated as soon as possible.

Basic Anatomy Of The Female Genitalia

The female reproductive organs lie within the pelvic cavity. The vagina, or birth canal, is approximately three to four inches long. The vagina is continuously moistened by secretions that keep it clean and slightly acidic. At the top of the vagina is the *cervix*, a circle of tissue pierced by a small hole that opens into the uterus. The cervix thins and opens during labor to allow the baby to be expelled.

The *uterus* is about the size of a fist and is located between the bladder and rectum. Pregnancy begins when a fertilized egg implants in the tissue of the uterus. The uterus is an elastic organ that expands with the growing fetus.

On either side of the uterus are the *ovaries*, which lie approximately four or five inches below the waist. The ovaries produce eggs and the female sex hormones estrogen and progester-

one. Each month an ovum (egg) is released from one of the ovaries and travels down the fallopian tube to the uterus. The *fallopian tubes* are approximately four inches long and wrap around the ovaries but are not directly connected to them. When the egg is released from the ovary, the *fimbria* (finger-like structures at the end of the fallopian tube) make sweeping motions across the ovary, sucking the egg into the fallopian tube.

The Menstrual Cycle

At approximately 12 years of age, a woman starts her menstrual cycle, the monthly release of ova. Hormones regulate the cycle, which continues until menopause at approximately 50 years of age.

The endometrial tissue that lines the uterus undergoes hormone-regulated changes each month during menstruation. The average menstrual cycle is 28 days long, with day one being the

first day of the menstrual period. From days one through five the endometrial tissue sloughs off from the uterus and is expelled through the vagina. The usual discharge is four to six tablespoons of blood, tissue, and mucus. During days six through 16, the endometrial tissue regrows in preparation for implantation of an ovum, becoming thick and full of small blood vessels.

Ovulation occurs on day 14. The egg takes approximately six and a half days to reach the uterus. Days 17 through 26 the endometrium secretes substances to nourish the embryo. If conception has not occurred, the hormones progesterone and estrogen decrease, causing the uterine blood supply to decrease and the lining of the uterus to be shed (SEE CHAPTER 33: OBSTETRICAL EMERGENCIES).

Assessment Guidelines Specific to Women

Gather information about the patient's menstrual and sexual history. When was her last menstrual period? How long is her cycle? Does she use contraception? Has she had sexual intercourse in the past month, and what is normal for her? If she has had the problem before, how did she treat it? Ask open-ended questions. For example: "Tell me about your normal menstrual cycle." This type of questioning will usually allow you to gather more information.

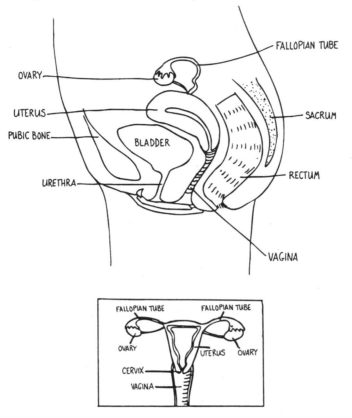

Figure 32-2: Female specific anatomy

Female-specific Emergencies

Abnormal Vaginal Bleeding

The most common female reproductive system-related problem is heavy menstrual bleeding. This is usually due to an imbalance in the amount of estrogen and progesterone that are produced by the ovaries, and commonly occurs at the times in a woman's life when her ovaries is gaining, or losing, their function: When she first starts having a period and prior to menopause. It also may occur under times of stress when she skips ovulating that month—an *anovulatory* cycle. When ovulation does not occur, the ovaries do not produce progesterone, and the uterine lining does not undergo its usual maturation phase. The endometrium is shed in an abnormal fashion and the menstrual flow will be abnormally heavy and irregular.

An anovulatory cycle, with its heavy, prolonged bleeding, is usually not associated with any of the usual cramping that occurs with the menstrual period, and this may be a clue as to the cause of the abnormal bleeding.

There is not much that can be done in the field except reassurance for the patient that the problem will likely be of limited duration. It is usually more of a nuisance than a serious medical problem, though it may be alarming for a young woman who is just starting to menstruate. She should seek medical attention if the problem persists, or is unusually heavy. If there is any chance the patient could be pregnant, suspect ectopic pregnancy and evacuate immediately (SEE CHAPTER 33: OBSTETRICAL EMERGENCIES).

Mittelschmerz

Some women experience cramping in the lower abdomen on the right or left side or in the back during the middle of the menstrual cycle when the ovary releases an egg. The pain is sometimes accompanied by bloody vaginal discharge. This is called *mittelschmerz* from the German *mittel* for "middle" and *schmerz* for "pain."

The pain may be sudden, sharp, and severe enough to be confused with appendicitis or ectopic pregnancy. Ask the patient where she is in her menstrual cycle. Has she ever had this pain before? Typically, a woman will have had similar cramping in the past. Any light bleeding or pain should cease within 36 hours. Her abdomen is soft. Women taking birth control pills do not ovulate, so they cannot have mittelschmerz.

Managing the symptoms with over-the-counter pain medications and general support of the patient is all that is usually required unless there is reason to suspect ectopic pregnancy (SEE CHAPTER 33: OBSTETRICAL EMERGENCIES). Monitor the patient closely for signs of another serious abdominal emergency (SEE CHAPTER 29: ABDOMINAL EMERGENCIES).

Dysmenorrhea

Dysmenorrhea is pain in association with menstruation. Possible causes include prostaglandins, which cause the uterus to cramp; endometritis, inflammation of the endometrium; pelvic inflammatory disease; or anatomic anomalies such as a displaced uterus.

Drugs such as ibuprofen reduce the pain as well as the volume of flow and the length of the period. Relaxation exercises such as yoga and massaging the lower back or abdomen help reduce pain. Applying heat to the abdomen or lower back may also help reduce pain. A change in diet may help. Decreasing the amount of salt, caffeine, and alcohol in the diet while increasing the B vitamins—especially B6, found in brewers yeast, peanuts, rice, sunflower seeds, and whole grains—can offer some relief during the acute phase of the cramps. Because exercise causes *endorphins* (natural opiates) to be released by the brain, many women find that cramps diminish when they participate in strenuous exercise.

Secondary Amenorrhea

Secondary *amenorrhea* is the absence of menstrual periods after a woman has had at least one period. Causes of secondary amenorrhea include pregnancy, ovarian tumors, intense athletic training, altitude, and stress (physical and emotional). In the past it was thought that excessive weight loss in female athletes, resulting in low body fat, was the cause of amenorrhea. It is now believed that stress (physical and emotional) may cause hormonal changes resulting in amenorrhea. Changes in the menstrual cycle are common on wilderness expeditions and may be normal adjustments to unfamiliar stresses.

Premenstrual Syndrome

Premenstrual syndrome (PMS) is a cluster of symptoms that occur prior to menstruation. PMS typically starts when a woman reaches her middle to late 20s and disappears in the late 30s to early 40s.

The most common symptoms are depression, anxiety, breast tenderness, and food cravings. Other symptoms include anger, anxiety, irritability, bloating, edema, headache, fatigue, and acne. Most researchers believe PMS is a physiological phenomenon, but the exact cause is still unknown.

Treatment includes decreasing stress, such as through yoga, meditation, and deep-breathing exercises. A high carbohydrate diet, low in caffeine and fat, decreases breast tenderness. Reducing salt consumption helps control edema; reducing alcohol helps alleviate depression; reducing nicotine and caffeine lessens anxiety. A physician may prescribe diuretics to decrease edema. Vitamin B6 supplements (25-50 mg to start) may help to decrease the bloating, moodiness, and depression that come with PMS. The dose should not exceed 200 mg a day. B6 is better absorbed by the body when taken along with or as part of a B complex vitamin.

Oral progesterone has been prescribed by physicians to treat PMS, but studies of its effectiveness are inconclusive. Daily aerobic exercise such as running or hiking helps ease all symptoms.

Vaginal Infections

The normal pH of the vagina is slightly acidic. An alteration in the pH may cause a vaginal infection to develop. Infections usually result from lowered body resistance due to stress (physical and emotional), a diet high in sugar, or taking birth control pills and/or antibiotics. A diabetic or prediabetic condition also increases the risk of infection. Cuts and abrasions from intercourse or tampons, not cleaning the perineal area (the area between the vagina and anus), or not changing underwear can lead to an infection.

There are three major types of vaginal infections: *yeast* (fungus), *bacterial vaginosis* (bacteria), and *Trichomonas* (a parasitic protozoan). For the purposes of field diagnosis, the symptoms are similar, and initial treatment is the same.

Signals of vaginal infection include excessive or malodorous discharge from the vagina with redness, soreness, or itching in the vaginal area. There may also be a burning sensation during urination.

Treatment should restore the acidity of the vagina. One approach is for the patient to douche with plain disinfected water or a solution of one to two tablespoons of vinegar in a liter of warm disinfected water. Vaginal douches can also be made from povidone-iodine (two tablespoons of 10 percent povidone-iodine per liter of water) or Zepharin chloride (1:1000 to 1:5000 strength). In the field, douching is accomplished by pouring the solution into the vagina while the patient lies on her back with hips elevated. This process may require two people. Ideally the patient should douche in the morning and evening at the onset of infection.

Women with a history of vaginal yeast infections may want to take an over-the-counter medication, e.g., Gyne-Lotrimin® or Monistat 7®, with them on extended expeditions. These are the most common medications used to treat yeast infections. Women with bacterial vaginosis or Trichomonas will require antibiotic treatment. Acetaminophen and warm, moist compresses should provide symptomatic relief from the pain. Itching, which may be severe, often responds to cool compresses and over-the-counter 0.5 percent hydrocortisone cream, e.g., Cort-Aid®. If these treatments don't provide relief within 48 hours, the patient should be evacuated. An untreated infection can develop into Pelvic Inflammatory Disease.

The best prevention for vaginal infections is education. To help prevent vaginal infections, women should take care 1) to clean the perineal area with plain water or a mild soap daily and to 2) wear cotton underpants and loose outer pants. Unlike cotton, nylon doesn't allow air to circulate, thus giving bacteria a moist place to grow. Women should avoid coffee, alcohol, and sugar, which can change the pH of the vagina.

Urinary Tract Infection

Urinary tract infections (UTIS) are relatively rare in men but common in women due to the relatively short length of the urethra through which pathogens are introduced causing the problem. The infection can affect the urethra, bladder, ureters, even the kidneys.

Urinary tract infections cause increased frequency or urgency of urination with decreased urine output and/or a burning sensation during urination. The patient usually complains of pain above the pubic bone and a heavy urine odor with the morning urination. Blood and/or pus may be present in the urine. Urinary tract infections can progress to kidney infections. If the kidneys are infected, the patient usually complains of pain in the small of the back where the ribs join the backbone, and usually complains of tenderness when that area is palpated. The patient may have a fever.

The best treatment for a UTI is antibiotics. Have the patient drink lots of water every day and empty the bladder often. A patient with a UTI should get as much rest as possible.

The perineal area should be cleaned with water or mild soap daily. Eating cranberries, plums, and prunes makes the urine slightly acidic, which improves the effectiveness of antibiotic therapy.

On extended expeditions, consider carrying antibiotics, such as Bactrim® or Keflex®, to treat urinary tract infections. Consult your physician for antibiotic specifics. Pyridium®, available over the counter, will help relieve the pain of urination, and should also be considered for first aid kits on extended wilderness trips. UTIS can be managed in the wilderness, but not kidney infections—therefore, if an infection persists for more than 48 hours despite the use of antibiotics, the patient should be evacuated.

Pelvic Inflammatory Disease

Pelvic Inflammatory Disease (PID), another common source of abdominal pain in women of child-bearing years, is an inflammation of the fallopian tubes, peritoneum, ovaries, and/or uterus. It is primarily caused by gonorrhea, Chlamydia, or enteric bacteria. PID is most often seen in women who are sexually active, who use an intrauterine device, and/or who have decreased immune defenses.

Because PID affects the reproductive organs bilaterally, the patient complains of diffuse pain in the middle of the lower abdomen. The pain begins gradually and develops into a constant ache. She may also complain of pain in the right upper quadrant due to a bacterial irritation of the tissues surrounding the liver. Lower back or leg pain may also occur.

Signs and symptoms include a fever, nausea, vomiting, anorexia, and abdominal bloating. Ask about a pus-filled, foul-smelling discharge from the vagina. She may complain of irregular bleeding, an increase in menstrual cramps, and pain or bleeding during or after intercourse. Some women develop acne-like rashes on the back, chest, neck, or face. Usually these signs and symptoms start within a week following the menstrual period.

The treatment for PID is evacuation to a physician for antibiotic therapy. Untreated PID can lead to peritonitis (inflammation of the lining of the abdomen), scarring of the fallopian tubes, and sterility.

Toxic Shock Syndrome

Toxic shock syndrome (TSS) is an infection caused by the bacterium *Staphylococcus aureus*. If the patient uses a synthetic tampon, versus the cotton variety, the fibers in the tampon may abrade the vaginal lining, allowing the bacteria to enter the vaginal tissues causing an infection. This particular bacteria is capable of producing a chemical, or toxin, which can result in death for the patient. TSS also occurs with the use of highly absorbent tampons left in place for prolonged periods of time— more than eight hours—which happens sometimes on long trips when supplies are short.

The onset of toxic shock syndrome is abrupt. The patient has a high fever, chills, muscle aches, a sunburn-like rash, abdominal pain, sore throat, vomiting, diarrhea, fatigue, dizziness, and/or fainting. In some people the onset may be gradual and the characteristic rash does not appear for one or two days. Mucous membranes are beet-red. The sunburn-like rash appears on the palms or all over the body. It typically peels, just like a sunburn, one to two weeks later.

Any woman who is menstruating, and has the above symptoms, should remove her tampon, drink lots of liquids to avoid dehydration, and seek medical attention as soon as possible. If shock is indicated, the patient should be treated for shock. Interestingly, although antibiotics have not been definitely proven to speed recovery, they are still considered a mandatory part of treatment.

To decrease the risk of TSS, women should change their tampons frequently and use pads at night and on light flow days. Pads and tampons should be carried out of the mountains or burned in a very hot fire. The staphylococcus organism is frequently found on the hands, and adequate hand washing prior to inserting a tampon is a must. If the patient has had TSS previously, there is a 30 percent chance of recurrence.

Pelvic Pain

Pelvic pain, a common complaint of women, is usually due to some abnormality in the reproductive organs, and may produce bleeding or a vaginal discharge. There is little to be done in the wilderness except for over-the-counter pain medication. Acetaminophen, e.g., Tylenol, is a good choice because aspirin and drugs like ibuprofen can increase the blood loss with some of the more serious conditions like ectopic pregnancy. Since some of these conditions can have severe consequences, and may be difficult to differentiate from some of the lesser problems, a woman with increasing pelvic pain, especially with symptoms of early pregnancy (SEE CHAPTER 33: OBSTETRICAL EMERGENCIES) should seek medical attention as soon as possible.

Linda Lindsey, RN, contributed her expertise to this chapter.

Chapter 33:   Obstetrical Emergencies

You should be able to:

1. *Describe the basic anatomy and physiology of pregnancy.*
2. *Describe a normal pregnancy.*
3. *Describe complications of pregnancy and treatment for those complications.*
4. *Describe the process of normal childbirth.*
5. *Describe the assistance a mother might need with her childbirth and with the proper care of her newborn infant.*
6. *Describe the treatment for women with common complications of labor and delivery.*

Introduction

Most obstetrical emergencies could be prevented if women followed the same recommendations for wilderness travel that they do for commercial airline travel: Avoid both during the last four to six weeks of pregnancy. Some women, however, leave on wilderness journeys not knowing they are pregnant—not a problem unless they experience an early and potentially life-threatening complication, such as an ectopic pregnancy—and some women in otherwise healthy pregnancies develop a later complication prior to the last four to six weeks of pregnancy.

Some women, furthermore, will go into labor early and find themselves a little farther from civilization than they had planned when the birth process starts. Most of these women will deliver normally with or without assistance. Occasionally, delivery will be complex and life-threatening to mom and baby, made so by one of several possible complications.

Although medical problems associated with pregnancy and birth are rare in wilderness situations, the Wilderness First Responder should be able to manage the emergency.

Basic Anatomy And Physiology Of Pregnancy

At *menarche*, the initial menstrual period, the hypothalamus begins stimulating the pituitary gland to release Follicle Stimulating Hormone (FSH) and Leutinizing Hormone (LH), which when produced in exactly the right quantity and timing, cause the ovaries to produce estrogen and to *ovulate*, release one egg each month. The estrogen that is released during the first half of the cycle causes the *endometrium*, the lining of the uterus, to thicken. Following ovulation the ovary that released the egg begins producing progester-one which causes the endometrium to mature, so as to be ready to receive a fertilized egg should intercourse occur at the proper time. A single sperm fertilizes the egg well up in the fallopian tube, and the developing embryo travels down to the uterus, where it sticks to the mature endometrial lining, and begins developing. If a woman does not become pregnant during a menstrual cycle, the falling levels of ovarian hormones causes the built-up uterine lining to be shed during menstruation, and the cycle starts all over again.

If conception does occur, and the embryo begins developing, there is still a high probability, about 25 percent, that the pregnancy will not continue. If that particular egg or sperm were nearing their normal life span of two to three days at the time of conception, then there is a strong likelihood that their genetic material may not divide and reproduce properly and, therefore, the fetus will not develop properly. In such cases the fetus will fail to develop beyond a few weeks, and a miscarriage will occur.

Normal Pregnancy

The *placenta* is a fairly complex organ. It may be thought of as a tissue that is similar to a tumor, one that invades into the wall of the mother's uterus to provide the blood supply from her side. It is constructed something like a lung, in that the mother's blood is brought in close contact with the baby's blood, with only a thin membrane in between. Oxygen, carbon dioxide, water, nutrients, and waste products cross over this membrane much in the same way that the same molecules cross the alveolus in the lung. The fetal heart provides all the blood flow to the fetus through the placenta, which is connected to the fetus by the *umbilical cord* containing two arteries and one large vein. A thin membrane, the *amniotic sack*, covers the developing fetus, placenta, and amniotic fluid. The amniotic fluid is essentially fetal urine, which is made from the excess fluid that crosses the placenta from the mother's circulation.

The fetus continues to develop normally through the usual 280 days (40 weeks) of pregnancy. The length of pregnancy is measured from the beginning of the woman's last, normal menstrual period, with conception occurring approximately two weeks later. A woman usually feels her baby move within the uterus at about 20 weeks for the first pregnancy, or a couple of weeks earlier if this is the second or subsequent pregnancy. At term, the fetus normally weighs from five to eight pounds, lies head down within the uterus, and is surrounded with about a liter of amniotic fluid. The ready-to-be-born infant, placenta, and amniotic fluid take up most of the space within the mother's abdomen.

Signs, Symptoms of Pregnancy

The first sign of pregnancy and the most common reason a woman thinks she might be pregnant is the absence of an anticipated menstrual period. If a period is two weeks late, and the woman has been sexually active, she generally feels no doubt about being pregnant. Additional early signals of pregnancy may include breast tenderness and enlargement, nausea which may be associated with vomiting, unusual fatigue (probably the most common symptom), and frequent urination. Some women will note abdominal enlargement unusually early in a pregnancy. Undeniable proof of pregnancy is delivery of a fetus.

Obstetrical Emergencies

What follows is a discussion of problems relating to pregnancy in the order during the pregnancy when they may be encountered. This may help you determine the cause of the particular problem depending on how far along the woman is in her pregnancy.

Miscarriage

Miscarriage, or *spontaneous abortion*, is a very common occurrence during the first few weeks of a pregnancy. There may be none of the usual symptoms of early pregnancy. Many of these women do not even know that they are pregnant. In these instances the woman may have a slightly delayed, heavy period.

A miscarriage is a natural process that can usually take place without medical intervention even if the pregnancy is more advanced, although a physician may be able to shorten the process and reduce the amount of discomfort involved. The woman may begin to have midline menstrual-like cramps that occur in a regular pattern. These labor pains will increase in frequency and severity, and vaginal bleeding will begin. The bleeding will increase and the contractions intensify until, after one or two hours of hard cramps and heavier-than-menstrual bleeding, the woman will pass fetal tissue and the "hamburger-like" placenta. Prior to passing the placenta she may pass some smooth, dark colored, liver-like blood clots. Within minutes after passing the placenta, the cramping will diminish markedly and the bleeding will decrease to a very light flow.

Some women may have the placenta fail to pass within a reasonable length of time, and the blood loss may become excessive. In these cases, definitive medical intervention may be necessary to terminate the process and prevent further blood loss. Much of the blood lost during a miscarriage will be new blood that was made by the mother during the first few weeks of the pregnancy. If the woman's uterus can be made to contract forcefully, the miscarriage process may be accelerated. This is commonly done with a medication by her physician when the miscarriage process has begun. It is possible to accomplish the same effect in the wilderness by simulating breastfeeding. Having the woman lightly stroke her nipples for a minute out of every three or four minutes will cause her pituitary gland to release the hormone pitocin, which will augment her contractions, shorten the miscarriage process, and diminish the amount of blood lost during the process. She can stop the stimulation about thirty minutes after the tissue passes. The woman's uterus will be back to normal within two weeks following the miscarriage, and she could re-attempt pregnancy after her next normal menstrual period. This will usually occur about six weeks after the miscarriage.

Ectopic Pregnancy

While a miscarriage is a natural event that is usually a safe, uncomplicated process, an ectopic pregnancy is another matter. When the developing embryo implants in the fallopian tube rather than into the uterine cavity wall, it will begin invading into the wall of the tube, and the blood vessels in the tube will enlarge dramatically. (An ectopic pregnancy can occur in other pelvic sites, but the fallopian site is the most common.) Shortly after she first notices some of the symptoms of early pregnancy, as soon as a couple of weeks, the

woman may notice some mild cramping and vaginal bleeding. The pain will usually be on one side or the other, but it may be midline. The pain and bleeding will increase as the placenta continues to eat its way into the fallopian tube. Eventually it will destroy the enlarged tubal vessels, and the woman will begin to hemorrhage into her abdominal cavity. Emergency surgery will be required to stop the bleeding and repair the damage. An ectopic pregnancy is obviously not a problem that can be dealt with in a wilderness situation. The real problem is determining whether a pregnant woman's cramps and bleeding are due to an impending miscarriage or an ectopic pregnancy. Therefore, in order to be safe, a woman with symptoms of early pregnancy, and with vaginal bleeding, should be considered as having an ectopic pregnancy. She should be evacuated as soon as possible.

Placenta Previa

Bleeding during the last three months of pregnancy may signal a potentially serious problem with the placenta. If the placenta should implant right over the cervix then it may separate off the uterus when the cervix starts to thin and dilate prior to labor. This condition is known as *placenta previa*, and it is potentially fatal unless an emergency Cesarean Section is performed promptly. Bleeding from a placenta previa is usually painless, and may be profuse. A bleeding placenta previa is one of the causes of the rare "audible hemorrhage," bleeding so rapid that it can be heard, e.g., like a running faucet. Again, not a problem easily dealt with in the

wilderness. Fortunately, nowadays most women have an ultrasound scan early in their pregnancy, and know if they have a placenta previa before they make their wilderness plans. These women will be advised to minimize their activities during the last two months of their pregnancy, and will have a Cesarean Section delivery as soon as their baby's lungs are mature. If they start to bleed heavily they will have to have an emergency C-Section.

Placental Abruption

Another problem that may be signaled by bleeding during the last few months of pregnancy is a separation of the placenta off the uterine wall, known as a *placental abruption*. The separation may be partial or complete, the latter variety being catastrophic for the developing infant and potentially lethal for the mother. Partial abruptions may only result in a small amount of blood loss, or it may cause massive hemorrhage if it extends to involve more of the implantation site. Placental abruptions are more common when the woman has high blood pressure complicating her pregnancy, may be caused by trauma, and also may be caused by cocaine use during pregnancy. When the placenta separates from the uterus it will cause uterine irritability with contractions that increase in frequency and intensity. Within a fairly short time the uterus may contract continuously, called *tetanic contraction*, and cause constant, severe pain. If the placental implantation site is high in the uterus, or if the blood ruptures through the membranes into the amniotic sack, there may be no visible bleeding.

Note: Women suspected of either having a placenta previa or a placental abruption must be quickly transported to medical care, preferably where a surgical team and operating room are standing by. Transport should be as rapid and as smooth as possible. Any bumping or jostling may aggravate the bleeding.

Premature Labor

Since most pregnant women usually do not plan wilderness trips during the latter weeks of their pregnancy, there is a good chance that, if you are asked to assist with a delivery in a remote area, the woman will be in premature labor. When a woman goes into labor more than three weeks early (37 weeks or less into the pregnancy), the labor is con-

sidered to be premature. If the delivered infant weighs less than five pounds, then the infant is considered to be premature. Most of the causes of premature labor remain unknown. Most women just go into labor early, for no obvious reason. Premature rupture of the membranes, cervical and uterine infections, incomplete prenatal care, and trauma to the uterus are several of the known, but less common, causes of premature labor.

Premature labor, in itself, causes no problems for the woman. The infant, however, is at risk of several problems by being born early. First, and most significantly, the baby's lungs may not be mature and he or she may have varying degrees of respiratory distress depending on the degree of lung immaturity. The infant may also have diffi-

culty maintaining its temperature and meeting its requirements for food and water due to its immature organ systems. Premature infants are somewhat more fragile than their term pregnancy counterparts, and do not have their reserves of lung function and fat. In addition, the markedly premature infant, one born more than two months early, may not tolerate the stress of labor, suffering some degree of damage that would not have occurred to a term baby.

Except for paying particular attention to maintaining the premature infant's temperature, the method of delivery is the same as for the delivery of a term infant, and will be covered in the next section. The other complications of prematurity usually do not develop for several hours to days after birth.

Normal Childbirth

Any woman who suspects that she is going into labor should be encouraged to leave the wilderness and reach a hospital as soon as possible, where her condition can be evaluated and her delivery conducted in as safe an environment as possible. Although most deliveries occur without incident, a delivery away from facilities where the capability for an emergency Cesarean Section delivery, intravenous blood and fluid administration, and the administration of oxygen and medications to the mother and/or child unnecessarily jeopardizes the health and possible survival of either or both the mother and child.

Assessment: Pregnant Patient

How do you decide that a mother cannot possibly reach medical attention in time for her labor and delivery? You must estimate how long it will take to get her to a hospital or birthing center by whatever means available, versus how long you have before she delivers. Here are a few tips to estimate the time that might be available:
1. The more prior deliveries she has had, the quicker the labor will be. First pregnancies usually—but not always—have at least four to six hours of hard labor while the labor from a fifth and subsequent pregnancy may last only an hour. Women who have had short labors tend to

have shorter subsequent labors. Ask how long her last labor was and subtract an hour.
2. The smaller the infant, the quicker the labor will be. A premature labor that starts six weeks early may be several hours quicker than a labor at term for the same pregnancy.
3. Ask her if she had a "gush" of clear fluid and has been leaking fluid since. If her membranes have ruptured, her labor will be about 25 percent faster than if her membranes were intact.
4. A woman who is having regular contractions every two to three minutes, lasting 45 seconds or more, and has to stop walking during her contractions, will likely have her baby within an hour or two.

5. If she has the urge to push with the contractions, then you had better wash your hands.

Three Stages of Labor

Labor is divided into three stages. During the first stage, which lasts eight to twelve hours for the first pregnancy, and progressively less in subsequent ones, the cervix gradually *effaces* (thins) and dilates with each contraction of the uterus to allow the infant's head to pass through. The second stage, which takes from thirty minutes to two hours, commences as the woman starts to forcefully push the baby down the birth canal. It starts with the complete dilation of the cervix, and ends with the delivery of the baby. The third stage, which usually lasts five to ten minutes, involves the delivery of the placenta.

Delivery of the Baby

When you have decided that it will be impossible to reach a hospital, then your focus should switch from transporting the mother to preparing for the delivery. The best position for a mother in labor is lying on her side, and the left side is preferable. This takes the weight of the uterus, which will weigh ten to twelve pounds with the baby, placenta, and fluid, off the mother's vena cava, the large vein in the abdomen that is bringing blood back to her heart. Compression of the vena cava acts like a loose tourniquet around the middle of the mother's body. Blood continues to flow through her aorta to her legs and uterus, but it cannot return to her heart to complete the circuit. This blood that is "trapped" in the lower half of her body will cause a progressive decrease in her cardiac output, falling blood pressure, and decreased blood flow to the placenta, the lifeline for the fetus. Many women who lie on their backs during the last months of pregnancy will feel light-headed for this reason. Turning the mother on her side quickly solves the problem. The lateral recumbent position (side position) can also be used during delivery, and is a preferred position when the mother is lying on a flat surface, as opposed to a birthing bed or delivery table with her bottom at the foot of the bed. When the baby is delivered there will be space between its head and the "bed" which will keep his or her face out of the normal fluids that accumulate there during a delivery.

When planning on where you are going to deliver this baby you should consider several things. If possible, the mother should be elevated off of the ground to make your task of attending the delivery easier. A cot, bed, picnic table, or even a pile of brush covered with a tarp will serve to raise her body a little. If the weather is cold or raining, it would be best if you could fashion some sort of shelter for the delivery. Have her remove her undergarments and place some clean clothing beneath her buttocks to soak up the amniotic fluid and blood that will be passed during her labor and delivery. You will be placing the newborn baby on her bare chest and upper abdomen following the delivery so she should be wearing loose clothes on her upper body, and no brassiere. If possible, heat some clean water and wash your hands and the mother's hands and her perineal area (vagina and rectal area) with soap and water. Now, cover her lower body with sufficient insulation to keep her warm during the rest of her labor. If she prefers to walk about during labor that is fine, but have her lie down when she starts to feel the urge to push during her contractions. The delivery is near.

When she has the urge to push, you should begin inspecting her perineum to watch for the top of the baby's head to appear. If you gently stretch the opening of her vagina, between contractions, when the top of the baby's head becomes visible, you can reduce the amount of tearing that will occur with the delivery somewhat. Insert a couple of fingers along side the baby's head and gently run your fingers around the baby's head, stretching her tissues away from the head. The baby's head will descend a little with each contraction until, finally, the top of its head, down to its ears, is visible outside the mother's vagina. From this point on, due to the fact that the rest of the baby's head will be tapering down to its neck and getting smaller, it will be easier to expel.

At this point the mother will have a tremendous urge to push the baby out as rapidly as possible. Here your assistance can prevent damage to the baby. If the baby's head is allowed to "pop" out rapidly, the sudden change in pressure may cause the rupture of some small blood vessels in the baby's brain. You can prevent this by simply placing the palm of your hand on the top of the baby's head and *gently* slow the delivery of the head. Tell the mother to stop pushing, and you may have to be quite loud and forceful to overcome her tremendous urge to do so, and then have her bear down gently to complete the delivery of the head. Allow the head to come out at the same speed that it had been descending up to that point: *Slowly.*

The baby's head will usually come out face down, or more rarely, face up. Have the mother stop pushing so that you can clean some of the amniotic fluid and mucous from the baby's mouth. If the baby's face is down, gently rotate the head either direction until the head is facing sideways. It will rotate one direction quite easily as its shoulders align with the birth canal. When it is facing to the side, gently wipe the mucous and fluid from the baby's nose and mouth. Now ask the mother to push with the next contraction, and gently press down on the upper side of the baby's head and neck so that the frontmost shoulder of the baby passes beneath the front of the mother's pelvic bone. As the shoulder and chest start to come out, gently lift the baby's head and allow the rear shoulder to be delivered. Have the mother continue to bear down gently—the largest part is now out and you do not want her to force the baby out so rapidly that you cannot hang on to it—and finish the delivery. If the mother looks down between her legs, and watches the baby's body being delivered, she can control her pushing so that the delivery is slow and smooth.

As the body comes out, be planning how you are going to hold on to the slippery little body that has begun to squirm around. You want to wind up holding the baby with its head below the rest of its body so that the amniotic fluid within its airway will drain out its nose and mouth during the first few breaths. The easiest way to do this is to place your index finger and thumb around the baby's neck, with the rest of your hand supporting the baby's head, and then let the baby's body rest up your arm. This will leave your other hand free. Support the baby with its body inclined towards its head, and rotate the head towards the side so that secretions can run out its nose and mouth. Now have the mother lift up her shirt or jacket and place the baby against the skin of her chest and upper abdomen, keeping the baby warm and keeping baby's head lower than the rest of its body.

Wipe the baby's skin dry with the softest, cleanest clothing you have, paying particular attention to getting his or her hair and scalp dry. This drying process will not only serve to prevent critical heat loss, but also will stimulate the infant sufficiently to ensure that it is breathing adequately. You should be vigorous in the drying process, especially if the baby seems sleepy, limp, or is not breathing and crying loudly. Rubbing the baby's back is a particularly safe and effective way of stimulating it to breathe. As you finish the drying, you should feel the umbilical cord between your fingers and check the baby's pulse, which will be very easy to feel through the two umbilical arteries in the cord. It should be about 140 beats per minute, roughly twice as fast as yours would be if you were not just delivering a baby.

If the baby's pulse is less than 100, and it is still limp and not breathing vigorously, you should perform mouth-to-nose-and-mouth ventilation until the baby responds (SEE CHAPTER 4: AIRWAY AND BREATHING). Do this about 60 times per minute, or once each second, until the baby's pulse has increased to over 100, it has begun to breathe, and it begins to flex and squirm about. As the baby's brain begins to receive an adequate amount of oxygen it will start to wake up and fuss. The fussing and crying will serve to continue to provide adequate oxygen, which causes further awakening and the cycle continues upward.

Carefully tie the umbilical cord with a couple of pieces of wide string, e.g., clean shoelaces, several inches from the baby, and about one inch apart. Now cut the cord between the strings. Check for and immediately stop any bleeding that may occur from the umbilical cord. Baby has little blood to lose. If you are not the father then it might be nice to let dad cut the cord. It's quite a thrill to perform the ceremony of setting your son or daughter loose in the world.

Delivery of the Placenta

Several minutes (it may seem like hours though) will have passed by now, and the placenta should be separating off from the wall of the uterus. This is usually heralded by a gush of blood. Applying a little gentle traction on the umbilical cord will cause the placenta to be delivered. Again, do this slowly so that all of the placenta comes out, and so that the membranes do not tear off, leaving some inside to cause complications later. Grasp the delivering placenta and twist it continuously as it comes out. This will cause the membranes, which are trailing behind the placenta, to form a stronger rope-like strand as they are delivered and prevent them from tearing.

As soon as the placenta is delivered you should begin massaging the mother's uterus to make it contract. The blood vessels in the uterus that supply the site where the placenta was imbedded will bleed profusely until the uterus contracts. They run through the various layers of the uterine muscle, and when the uterus contracts they are pinched off. The bleeding will go from a heavy stream to just a trickle when the uterus contracts. Place the flat of your hand on the mother's lower abdomen, just above her pubic hair, and massage the uterus firmly—hard enough so that it is uncomfortable for mom. The uterus should contract down to the size of a small grapefruit, and the bleeding will slow to a minimal flow. Continue massaging the uterus for ten minutes or so, and then repeat the process anytime the mother starts bleeding heavily again. Another method that may be used in addition to uterine massage is to have the baby begin nursing at the mother's breast. The act of nursing causes the release of pitocin from the mother's pituitary gland. This hormone is necessary for the milk letdown reflex, but also causes uterine contractions. Newborns do not need any liquids at all for 24 hours, but they may try and nurse for the first hour or so after birth. The nursing also helps start the maternal-child bonding process that is so important for both the mother and child.

Care of Mother and Child

If the mother and child are doing well, your wilderness living situation is comfortable and warm, and you have sufficient food and supplies, then you should defer trying to travel any long distances for a couple of days so that the mother can have some time to recover from the delivery. She should nurse the baby every three hours, drink lots of liquids, and enjoy some well-deserved rest. If the above conditions are not met then you should probably attempt to transport the mother and child to a more tolerable environment several hours after her delivery. The infant will stay warm if she carries him/her against her breasts with some covering clothes for insulation.

Complications Of Delivery

Umbilical Cord Around Neck

If you see the umbilical cord wrapped around the baby's neck, gently attempt to slip the cord over the head. Usually the cord will be loose enough to slip over easily. If the cord is wrapped too tightly to move, it must be tied off securely, with two pieces of string a couple of inches apart, and cut between the ties. Delivery from that point should not be delayed.

Prolapsed Cord

When the umbilical cord slips down into the vagina before the baby, a complication called a *prolapsed cord* may occur. Once this happens, the descending baby may compress the cord against the bones of the woman's pelvis, cutting off all or part of the baby's blood supply.

If you can see the cord presenting before the baby, elevate the mother's hips, or place her in a knee-to-chest position, and attempt to lift the presenting part of the baby off the baby's life-sustaining cord. Instruct the mother to stop pushing. Usually rapid transportation to a facility capable of performing a Cesarean Section is all that saves mother and child.

If transport is delayed, attempts should be made to reduce the prolapsed cord. Use the techniques described above to relieve compression of the cord. Then attempt to push the cord above the presenting part of the baby. Keep cord manipulation to a minimum. Deliver the baby as rapidly as possible, and be prepared to resuscitate the newborn.

Breech Presentation

Should you encounter a *breech presentation*, where the baby's feet or buttocks are coming out first, you should initiate transport to a hospital as rapidly as possible. If transport is delayed, do not do anything until the mother has pushed the baby out beyond the point where the baby's belly button and umbilical cord are showing. At that point you should grasp the baby by the hips and pull gently until its armpit is visible. Put your finger in the vagina, behind the baby's back, and try to pull the baby's arm forward and down in front of its chest. Then rotate the baby one half turn and repeat the process for the other arm. If you cannot get the arms to come out, then rotate the baby until it is face-down and back-up. Put your index finger in the mother's vagina beneath the baby's head and place the tip of your finger in the baby's mouth. Have another person, or the mother, push down firmly on her lower abdomen while she bears down, and while

you lift upwards on the baby's body and pull down (outwards) with your finger in the baby's mouth. The idea is to "rock" the baby's head out of the vagina and keep the baby's neck flexed, with its chin on its chest. It is very important that the baby be delivered within a couple of minutes of when its belly button is visible. From this point on the baby will no longer be receiving any blood or oxygen from the mother since the umbilical cord will be pinched off. If you have difficulty delivering the head, which is the largest part and is coming last, then you will have to

push harder from above and pull harder from below. Just remember to keep the baby's neck flexed, using your finger in the baby's mouth to keep the chin down.

Note: It is beyond the scope of this chapter to describe all of the complicated positions the baby can assume during childbirth, and it would be extremely difficult to remember the ways of managing these abnormal fetal presentations. Fortunately, more than 98 percent of babies are born head first.

Evacuation Guidelines

It is recommended to evacuate for a check-up any woman assessed as possibly being pregnant if the woman did not know she was pregnant prior to the wilderness trip. All pregnant women should be evacuated if an assessment reveals the possibility of complications with the pregnancy. Should a baby be delivered in the wilderness, mom and child should be evacuated, speed being not especially relevant if both patients are doing well.

Richard Sugden, MD, contributed his expertise to this chapter.

Chapter 34:   *Psychological And Behavioral Emergencies*

You should be able to:

1. *Describe the difference between crisis stress and critical incident stress, and describe the management of each.*

2. *Define the basic psychological impairments including depression, mania, grief, anxiety, suicidal behavior, and assaultive behavior, and describe the management of each.*

Introduction

If it were a perfect world, every wilderness experience would proceed happily and without conflict. Indeed, many an account of expeditions paints a rosy picture of lifelong friendships forged on the way to a mountain top. It's inevitable, however, that stress in the wild outdoors will sometimes produce behavior which is less than impeccable. It's reasonable to call these types of situations psychological and/or behavioral emergencies, emergencies in which normal interpersonal interaction is negatively interrupted.

This chapter addresses psychological and behavioral emer-gencies from three points of view:

1. *The Responses of Healthy People to a Crisis:* Everyone in a group may experience certain reactions to a crisis, to unusual stress, which are perfectly normal responses to abnormal events, such as serious injury to a member of the group. A WFR should be able to recognize and deal with these responses.

2. *The Responses of Healthy People to a Critical Incident*: Everyone in a group may react in certain ways to a critical incident, an overwhelmingly stressful event, such as multiple and/or especially gruesome deaths. A

WFR should be able to recognize the need for critical incident stress management.

2. *Basic Psychological Impairment*: Less likely to occur in the wilderness, mental disorders, difficult to assess even by trained mental health workers, are especially difficult to assess by the average WFR. One important principle to remember is that behavioral changes are sometimes due to physical disease, and a WFR should be able to recognize at least the possibility of needing to evacuate the patient for professional help.

Normal Responses To Crisis

A *crisis* is an unstable period when people have to respond and adapt to unusual and possibly critical changes in the state of affairs. The changes could be as mild as running out of food, or as serious as a party member with a broken leg. People generally

have strong emotions and high expectations when their worlds are altered by unexpected events. Plans are disrupted, sometimes enough to seriously or permanently alter the expedition. An activity previously designed as enjoyable is transformed to one

requiring hard work to resolve. People are likely to harbor some intense, and often negative, feelings about this because many people do not know how to behave when faced with a crisis. They may have preconceived notions of what to do, but sometimes these are based on the unreality of television and cinema, not on good judgment and common sense.

People are initially affected, sometimes drastically, by the impact of adrenaline as it engages the "fight or flight" response to anything they perceive as a threat. They may get very excited, angry, even explosive, all solely due to this powerful hormone. The initial effects usually fade within a few minutes as the group adjusts to the idea that an emergency has occurred. Levels of adrenaline, however, may remain high enough after the initial surge to sustain everyone for quite some time, but eventually individual coping mechanisms will engage.

Wilderness leaders need to appreciate that there are varying normal responses to a crisis. Until there is time to regroup, behaviors may seem unusual when, in truth, they should be expected. Some behaviors which may emerge in the face of a crisis include:

1. *Regression*. Many grown people revert to an earlier stage of development. The theory is that, since their parents used to care for them as children, someone else may care for them now if they behave in a childlike manner. In particular, tantrums used to be very effective. Tantrum-like or very dependent behavior is not unusual.

2. *Depression*. Closing into one's inner world is another common tactic. This is where some people find the sources of strength to cope with an emergency. This is characterized as a shut-down effect: Fetal positioning, slumped shoulders, down-cast eyes, arms crossed over the chest, and unwillingness or difficulty in communicating.

3. *Aggression*. Some people lash out, physically or emotionally, at threats, including the vague threat of an emergency. High adrenaline levels may intensify the response, and so may the feelings of frustration, anger, and fear that commonly surround unexpected circumstances. This response is characterized by explosive body language, including swinging fists and jumping up and down.

What one should do about the various behaviors that surface during a crisis depends somewhat on the individual circumstances. As a general rule, open communication, acknowledgment of the emotional impact of the event, and a healthy dose of patience and tolerance will go far during resolution of the situation. Some basic procedures to consider in crisis management might include the following:

1. *Engage the patient in a calm, rational discussion.* You can start the patient down the trail that leads through the crisis.

2. *Identify the specific concerns* about which the patient is stressed. You both need to be talking about the same problems.

3. *Provide realistic and optimistic feedback.* You can help the patient return to objective thinking.

4. *Involve the patient in solving the problem.* You can help the patient and/or the patient can help you choose and implement a plan of action.

Note: Someone who completely loses control and becomes hysterical needs time to settle down in order to become an asset to the situation. Breaking through to someone who has lost control can be a challenge. Try *repetitive persistence*, a technique developed for telephone interrogation by emergency services dispatchers. Remain calm, but firm. Choose a positive statement which includes the person's name, such as "Syd, we can help once you calm down." (An example of a negative statement would be "Syd, we can't help unless you settle down.") Persistently repeat the statement with the *same* words in the *same* tone of voice. The irresistible force (you) will eventually overwhelm the immovable object (the hysterical person).

Surprisingly few repetitions are usually needed to pierce the haze of hysteria, as long as the tone of voice remains calm. Letting frustration or other emotions creep into the tone of voice, or changing the message, can ruin the entire effort. Over time, the overwhelming responses that generated the hysteria may occasionally re-surface. This is normal. Without being judgmental or impatient, regain control through repetitive persistence.

A crisis may bring out a humorous side (sometimes appropriately, sometimes not) among the group. When you wish to release the intensity surrounding a situation of crisis, *appropriate* laughter is one of the best methods.

It should also be noted that many people cope just fine with emergency situations and unexpected circumstances. They are a source of strength and an example of model behavior for the others.

Critical Incident Stress

There is an expectation that a trip into the wilderness—even just for the weekend—entails certain risks that one cannot find in daily life. A good trip entails a lot of physical effort and team work. People expect to be able to cope with the usual demands of the wilderness, and, thus, they develop unusual coping mechanisms. Sometimes, however, for some or all of the people on the trip, events surpass standard coping mechanisms. Then a wilderness-style critical incident has occurred.

A *critical incident* is almost any incident in which the circumstances are so unusual or the sights and sounds so distressing as to produce a high level of immediate or delayed emotional reaction that surpasses a person's normal coping mechanisms. Critical incidents are events which cause predictable signs and symptoms of exceptional stress in *normal* people who are having *normal* reactions to something *abnormal* that happened to them. A critical incident from a wilderness perspective may be caused by such events as the sudden death or serious injury of a member of the group, a multiple death accident, or any event involving a prolonged expenditure of physical and emotional energy.

People respond to critical incidents differently. Sometimes the stress is too much right away, and signs and symptoms appear while the event is still happening. This is *acute stress*, and this member of the group is rendered non-functional by the situation, and needs care. In more cases,

signs and symptoms of stress come later, once the pressing needs of the situation have been addressed. This is *delayed stress*. A third sort of stress, common to us all, is *cumulative stress*. In the context of the wilderness, cumulative stress might arise if multiple, serial disasters strike the same wilderness party.

The course of symptom development when a person is going from the normal stresses of day-to-day living into distress (where life becomes uncomfortable) is like a downward spiral. People are not hit with the entire continuum of signs and symptoms at once. However, after a critical incident, a person may be affected by a large number of signs and symptoms within a short time frame, usually 24 to 48 hours.

The degree of impairment an event causes an individual depends on several factors. Each person has life-lessons that can help, or sometimes hinder, the ability to cope. Factors affecting the degree of impact an event has on the individual include:

1. *Age*. People who are older tend to have had more life-lessons to develop good coping mechanisms.

2. *Degree of education.*

3. *Duration of the event*, as well as its suddenness and degree of intensity.

4. *Resources available for help*. These may be internal (a personal belief system) or external (a trained, local critical incident stress debriefing team).

5. *Level of loss*. One death may be easier than several, although the nature of a relationship (marriage partners or siblings, for example) would impact this factor.

Signs and symptoms of stress manifest in three ways: physical, emotional, and cognitive. Stress manifests differently from one person to the next. Signs and symptoms which occur in one person may not occur in another, who has responses of his or her own.

Signs and Symptoms of Critical Incident Stress

When an experience is an unusually powerful emotional event, there may be a series of reactions. These are both common and normal. Signs and symptoms of critical incident stress include:

Physical: Enduring fatigue, sleep dysfunction (either needing too much or insomnia), change of appetite (eating too much or too little), gastrointestinal upset, headache, backache, chills, nausea, muscular twitches or tremors, shock-like symptoms (especially in acute stress), hyper-activity or its opposite, under-activity.

Emotional: Anger, irritability, fear, grief, anxiety, guilt, depression, feeling overwhelmed, identification with the patient(s) in a rescue, emotional numbness, feelings of helplessness or hopelessness.

Cognitive: Memory loss, especially anomia (the inability to remember names); inability to attach importance to things other than the incident; concentration problems; loss of attention span; difficulties with calculations, decision-making, and problem-solving; flashbacks; nightmares (especially recurrent ones); amnesia for the event; violent fantasies; confusing the importance of trivial and major tasks.

Critical Incident Stress Management

The sooner the event is defused or debriefed, the faster the reactions will ease or disappear. Denial prolongs the pain, and can keep the event freshly in mind far longer than necessary. Once a situation has been identified as a critical incident, there are several options for managing the group's response. During a critical incident, watch for acute stress symptoms. Someone allowed to continue functioning when suffering acute stress can cause additional, if inadvertent, rescue burdens to arise.

Soon after the event, within a few hours, a *defusing* is likely to help the group. Everyone is brought together and the event is discussed informally. This is *not* a critique of how the event was handled. A defusing is a time for examining how people are responding to the situation emotionally, physically, and cognitively. It is an acknowledgment that something unusual happened, and that unusual responses may be occurring because of it. Defusing these intense reactions allows healing to begin.

As a WFR, you may be called upon to manage a defusing. It is generally best to form the group into a circle with no one hanging back "in the shadows." Establish guidelines for the defusing. Encourage everyone to speak, but do not allow anyone to cast blame or dwell on things he or she thinks were done wrong. Let no one interrupt while another is speaking. Ask each person to relate 1) his or her role during the incident, 2) how he or she felt and now feels, and 3) what he or she thought and now thinks.

A formal critical incident stress *debriefing* requires the assistance of a trained group. Many Critical Incident Stress Management (CISM) or Critical Incident Stress Debriefing (CISD) teams exist. You may wish to check for local availability even before leaving the trailhead.

A formal debriefing is conducted by a group composed of both peer counselors (in this case, the ideal would be wilderness-oriented peers) and mental health workers who have been specially trained in CISM. Only those who were involved are invited. The process usually takes two to four hours.

The relief of a properly-debriefed group is palpable. The ability for an untrained, or well-intentioned but naive, group to cause permanent damage to participants is also very real. Call in only an established, trained CISD group.

Basic Psychological Impairment

There is a wide range of potential for psychological impairment stemming from various causes. Although not common to wilderness expeditions, psychiatric (or behavioral disturbances of various sorts) may be encountered. This may be especially true for groups which use the wilderness as an experiential education forum for students with health or social challenges, including alcoholics, status offenders, and others.

It is important to recognize that apparent psychological emergencies may be due to organic causes, which means the root of behaviors that seem bizarre or deranged is not psychological at all, but physical. Medical conditions, such as meningitis or encephalitis, can cause significant behavioral changes, sometimes in the course of just a few days. Hypoxia, hypoglycemia, hyperglycemia, and hypothermia can all cause an alteration in a person's behavior. Trauma, e.g., a subdural hematoma, can do likewise. Substance abuse may be the culprit.

Deciding whether someone in the wilderness has a psychiatric illness is not the domain of untrained people, regardless of how well-intentioned. The goal in the field is to protect the patient, and those around him or her, from potentially dangerous behavior while access to proper help is arranged. In particular, dangerous behavior may occur as a result of depression, mania, grief, extreme anxiety or panic, suicidal feelings, and loss of control for some reason that leads to assaultive or menacing behavior.

Depression

Everyone gets the "blues" now and then. This is normal. Clinical depression is different because it is enduring. Depression is known as an "affective disorder." This means it is outwardly manifested by mood, feelings, or tone, in this case characterized by lowered or diminished actions and feelings. Two criteria are needed for identification of clinical depression: 1) A mood characterized by feeling blue, irritable, hopeless, depressed, or sad, and 2) at least four of the following symptoms present almost continuously *for at least two weeks*:

A. Sleep disturbance (too much or too little)

B. Eating disorder with significant weight loss or gain

C. Psychomotor agitation or retardation

D. Loss of interest or pleasure in usual activities

E. Fatigue and loss of energy

F. Feelings of worthlessness and guilt

G. Difficulty concentrating or paying attention

H. Preoccupying thoughts of death or suicidal feelings

Unless someone heads out on a shorter wilderness trip already feeling depressed, it would require a lengthy trip to encounter clinical depression in the backcountry. If it does present, however, it is easy to see that depression can have serious impact on the group's safety and enjoyment of the expedition. Furthermore, there is little room for preoccupation and difficulty concentrating, or for fatigue and poor self-care, in terms of getting adequate rest and nutrition. Since there are as many as 74 medical conditions that can present with a depressed mood, it remains essential to seek proper diagnosis of clinical depression when the signs and symptoms of it appear.

Note: People with a known history of depression may already have medication that masks its signs and symptoms. Although it can take up to three weeks for the effects of the medication to start, they allow a person to function in a relatively normal way.

Mania

Mania is a mood disorder characterized by excessive elation, agitation, accelerated speaking, and hyperactivity. Ideas may flood out so fast that none seems connected with the next, a phenomenon known as a "flight of ideas." Mania can be dangerous if the hyperactivity, which is hard to control, occurs in dangerous locations, such as precipitous terrain and whitewater.

Sometimes mania and depression combine in a cyclical pattern known as "bipolar disease." This patient experiences extreme and uncontrollable mood swings from the depressed end of the spectrum to the manic. This people can be difficult to be around, generating frustration and anger within the group, especially if the nature of the disease is not understood.

Grief

Grief is the emotional response to loss. Even something as simple as permanently losing one's favorite pocket knife in the grass can generate a small degree of grief. Sorrow and regret are sharp and painful. There may be times on a wilderness trip that unusual behavior, e.g., crying easily, unexplained sadness, arises in a person who is in mourning. Identifying the cause of the behavior might be a relief for everyone concerned.

If news must be given to the group that someone has just died, be prepared for any behavior. Some people lash out, others draw within, just as in any other personal crisis. The group leader must assess the group and decide the best means for breaking the news. There may be times to tell everyone together, and times to not. Use the words "dead" and "died" so there is no chance of misinterpretation.

The first response to news of a death is a "grief spike," a totally consuming period of time, usually five to 15 minutes, in which the world shrinks down to that single acute pain. Give the news, but do not expect anyone to hear anything else until after the grief spike passes. Expect both anger and guilt feelings to be prominent, depending on the circumstances surrounding the death. Grief dissipates over time through a course of mourning, which for major losses normally takes about one year.

Anxiety and Panic

Acute anxiety or panic attacks can be very disruptive, especially if they occur with poor timing, such as above tree line with an electrical storm fast approaching. These are characterized by a discrete but unpredictable onset of symptoms, often without warning or an apparent precipitant. Physical symptoms include rapid heartbeat or palpitations, light-headedness, sweating and shaking, and sometimes fainting. There are feelings of terror or apprehension, and fear of dying, losing control, or "going crazy."

If someone with the above symptoms has good contact with reality, the cause is likely to be a panic disorder—if not, there may be an affective disorder or organic cause. Other conditions associated with anxiety or panic include phobias, hyperventilation syndrome, and generalized anxiety disorder (characterized by persistent anxiety of at least a month-long duration).

Field care begins with close, careful assessment of the person's behavior, and identifying the apparent cause. Many people who have not had a panic attack believe they are dying of a heart attack. Anything that can help the person regain a sense of control will help. Because anxiety can be infectious, watch the rest of the group, and communicate in a supportive, calm fashion with everyone. If calm, patient support does not work after awhile, it may be necessary to be firmer and set limits, especially where the safety of the group is at stake.

Suicidal Behavior

Suicide was recently the ninth overall cause of death in the United States. About two-thirds of suicidal gestures or attempts are made by females, although males are successful twice as often, since they tend to use more definitive means. e.g., gunshots and hangings. Teen males are a high risk population, as are men over 45 and women over 55. It is believed that many single-person "accidents"—on the highways, but also in the wilderness—are actually suicide. Anyone who speaks of suicide or makes suicidal gestures should be taken seriously. It may or may not happen, but the group which ignores the suggestion may be unpleasantly surprised. Suicidal behavior, by the way, is *not* inherited.

It may seem difficult to broach the subject with someone who is causing concern, but if suicidal thoughts are suspected, inquire directly. There are numerous myths about suicidal behavior. One myth is that talking with someone about suicide will drive them to do it. After developing good trust and rapport, ask, "Are you thinking of suicide?" If the answer is "Yes," ask what method he or she is thinking about. The more concrete the plans, the more likely suicide is to happen. If a person who was previously seriously considering suicide seems suddenly much better emotionally and behaviorally, the "miraculous" recovery may instead mean a decision has been made to go through with it. The patient may feel the conflict has been taken out of the situation. Be careful.

A helpful approach is to let the patient talk, and avoid judgmental or opinionated replies. "Oh, you don't want to do that!" is not what a suicidal person needs to hear. Instead, try to generate questions that elicit more than single-word answers, such as "Can you explain what makes you interested in suicide?" In general, treat the person normally. Expect the person to continue doing a fair share of the group's tasks. But watch him or her carefully.

Assaultive Behavior

For many reasons, people sometimes become menacing or assaultive. In a time of crisis, people typically rely on old behavioral patterns for survival. Those who become aggressive may act on those feelings and become physically dangerous to others on the expedition. Sometimes a period of venting is helpful if the nature of the outburst is not threatening to the others. Wilderness life can be stressful, people live in close quarters, and eruptions of intense emotions are not unusual.

Resolving such a situation requires good rapport and tact. The goal is to calm the individual, not to trigger worse behavior. In some cases, it may be best not to intervene until later. At other times, someone who is out of control may need physical restraint. Evidence of homicidal intentions, for example, should be treated seriously and immediately. When enough people are available, use all the resources available, and coordinate the effort through good communication. One person per extremity is best; hold the elbows and knees, not the feet and hands. Let restraint accomplish its intended purposes without seeming punitive or brutal.

Evacuation Guidelines

Wilderness care of psychiatric and behavioral emergencies relies on good judgment and common sense among the group in deciding which states need professional help—and thus evacuation—and which can be tolerated until the trip is scheduled to end. These emergencies demand open, honest communication among group members.

Kate Dernocoeur, EMT-P, contributed her expertise to this chapter.

You should be able to:

1. *Describe the need for and write a pre-trip plan.*

2. *Describe the factors affecting the organization of a simple wilderness evacuation.*

3. *Prepare a written evacuation plan and medical report that could be sent out to request a wilderness evacuation.*

Introduction

Emergency and long term care of the patient is only one of the responsibilities of the Wilderness First Responder. Leadership of the evacuation—from shelter construction, communication, and group organization to planning and patient transportation—may also demand attention.

Wilderness evacuations are mental as well as physical challenges. Outdoor leader and educator Paul Petzoldt gave wise advice for any emergency: Step aside for a moment and review the situation. He was well aware of the crucial role that planning plays in wilderness emergency

procedures, and the dangers of haste. Consider: Forgotten maps have caused rescue teams to become lost. Misinformation has sent rescue teams hiking through the night for a patient with minor injuries. Verbal messages have been distorted from passing through several people or by misstatements by exhausted messengers. Errors in organization and technique may multiply over time, compounding the difficulty of the situation. The rescue team bivouacking without sufficient clothing, shelter, or a stove may themselves need rescue. The poorly constructed litter that falls

apart a mile down the trail slows and stresses both the group and the patient. A misdiagnosed medical problem can initiate an unnecessary wilderness rescue. Rescuers have been injured, and some have died, responding to non-emergencies.

Wilderness evacuations, involving rescuers in strenuous and potentially dangerous activities, need support via planning, organization, and leadership. This chapter presents a plan for organizing the management of a simple wilderness emergency, and discusses some of the options the leader should consider.

Pre-trip Plans

A pre-trip plan is the foundation of an effective wilderness evacuation. An organized expedition or rescue group should have a written pre-trip plan. In an ideal wilderness world, even a short personal trip with a few friends has a written pre-trip plan. This document should be adaptable to a wide variety of contingencies including a lost person, an ambulatory patient, and a non-ambulatory patient. It should cover situations requiring

a technical rescue. It should be frequently reviewed and updated.

As your pre-trip plan is written, consider possible scenarios and draft guidelines for their management. Investigate your options for response to a medical emergency on your expedition, or in your rescue area. Research and catalogue resources and evacuation options. Contact local rescue groups, and check out their capabilities. Know if helicopters, technical rescue teams,

and paramedical support is available. Know when self-rescue is an option, and when outside help must be utilized. Know who is responsible for rescue in your wilderness area. On a personal level, prepare for an emergency by always carrying water, shelter, map, compass, matches, spare clothing, extra food, and a first aid kit—as well as humility and competence.

```
┌─────────────────────────────────────────────────────────────┐
│                    Pre-Trip Plans:                          │
│  1.  Guidelines for how you will respond to emergency and non-│
│      emergency situations.                                   │
│  2.  Lost person and technical rescue protocols.            │
│  3.  Special instructions for serious injury, illness, or a fatality. │
│  4.  Resource lists—rescue services, etc.—with names, addresses, │
│      and telephone numbers.                                 │
│  5.  Maps with roadheads and location of nearest phones marked. │
└─────────────────────────────────────────────────────────────┘
```

Evacuation Organization

After immediate medical and safety needs have been addressed, many things begin happening simultaneously. Evacuations always have more tasks than people, and every task is important. Someone needs to assume leadership and delegate responsibilities, and it is recommended that the leader refrain from becoming involved in the details of emergency care. He or she needs to maintain a higher stance, a broader perspective. Your priorities are the safety of the rescuers, the care of the patient, and the organization of the rescue. Although they are discussed here separately and as a sequence, these tasks typically happen at the same time.

Safety

Review scene safety. This is as important as the initial scene survey. Look around, identify environmental hazards, and take steps to manage them. Inclement weather may make on-the-spot shelter a priority. Rockfall or avalanche danger may dictate an immediate move to a safer location. You may need to caution overzealous rescuers in steep terrain or on a slippery riverbank to be careful. Take care of immedi-

ate scene stabilization needs: Someone delegated to manage the patient/s. Someone to write the SOAP note. Someone to gather equipment. Stop and make eye contact with everyone: Slow down, be thoughtful, be careful.

Evacuation Organization

Develop a plan for the evacuation, and delegate the tasks necessary to accomplish the plan. These often include: Briefing the group, selecting and briefing a messenger team who will go for help, writing an evacuation plan, building a fire, finding and organizing a campsite, feeding the group, preparing the evacuee's pack, building a litter, scouting a route, breaking trail through snow, finding and marking a landing site for a helicopter, or packing soft snow for a landing pad. To make the best plan you will need an inventory of all available resources. Gather and inventory all your equipment: Maps, first aid kits, food, water, stoves, shelters, technical outdoor gear.

When planning the evacuation consider: The severity (urgency) of the medical problem, the distance to the roadhead, the terrain difficulty, the strength and stam-

ina of the group, the weather, communication, and rescue possibilities (SEE CHAPTER 36: WILDERNESS TRANSPORTATION OF THE SICK OR INJURED).

Severity of Medical Problem

It is fundamental to determine the severity of the medical situation. How soon does the patient need to be in the hospital? Minor medical problems may be well-handled by a group walking out or carrying out a patient. Life- or limb-threatening problems may require utilizing helicopters, fixed-wing aircraft, radios, and other means of outside support.

Distance to the Roadhead

Consider how far it is to the roadhead, and to the nearest telephone. Do not underestimate the time it will take to travel the distance, initiate your evacuation plan, and have help return. Messengers in good physical shape on a good trail can hike approximately three miles an hour. Paddlers must negotiate rapids and portages. Rescuers burdened with litters and medical gear hike slowly. Darkness, deep snow, boulders, weather, river crossings, and other technical obstacles must be factored into the time estimate. Speed on litter carriers is often less than one-half mile an hour.

Terrain Difficulty

Think about the terrain difficulty. The time of day when you reach the rough country can be as important as its difficulty. Crossing rough or technically demanding terrain is best when you are fresh, rather than later in the trek when you're exhausted.

Strength, Stamina of Group

Consider the group's physical strength and stamina, and their technical abilities and experience. They must be strong enough for the hard physical work, and skilled and experienced enough to be safe when crossing rivers, glaciers, scree, boulders, or other technically demanding terrain.

Weather

Consider the weather. Will you be able to deal with deteriorating weather? Will it slow, stop, or alter your time table or your chosen evacuation method or route?

Communication

In many cases radio or telephone communication is not available and/or not reliable from remote areas. Messages must be delivered on foot. If there is no chance to talk to a rescue group, the written message must be accurate, concise, and complete.

Determine if messengers should be sent. Designate the leader and a large enough messenger group to be safe and effective. Four is typically considered an appropriate number for safety and traveling efficiency, but four messengers is often not practical.

When deciding on the composition of the messenger group consider: Physical stamina, first aid skills, night travel and navigation skills, foul weather experience, and any experience in the technical terrain that may be encountered.

The messenger group should carry written instructions including copies of the evacuation plan (SEE BELOW) and the SOAP note. They should be prepared for extenuating circumstances with food, clothing, sleeping bags or bivouac gear, and maps marked with the accident site, the desti-

nation roadhead, and the intended line of travel.

Written Reports

Written reports should include both a SOAP note (SEE CHAPTER 3: PATIENT ASSESSMENT), detailing the patient's condition, and the evacuation plan, detailing considerations for getting the patient out.

Evacuation plan should include:

- Type of evacuation, e.g., walking, helicopter, litter
- Marked maps showing:
- Location of accident
- Present location of group and patient
- Anticipated route out of mountains
- Roadhead destination
- Any special requests, e.g., doctor, litter, helicopter
- Plans for messenger group returning to expedition
- Plans for the group remaining in the field
- Always have an alternate plan included in your report. This allows any rescue party to anticipate and support your actions if the initial plans go awry.

Tod Schimelpfenig, WEMT-I, contributed his expertise to this chapter.

Chapter 36: *Wilderness Transportation*
Of The Sick Or Injured

You should be able to:

1. *Describe the possibilities for transporting sick or injured patients from the wilderness including walk-outs, carries, horse transports, and vehicle transports.*

2. *Demonstrate the improvisation of various means of transporting sick or injured patients from the wilderness including improvised one-rescuer carries, two-rescuer carries, and litters.*

Introduction

On the streets, patients are rushed in a speedy vehicle to a hospital where expert medical advice and care are immediately available. In the wilderness, transporting a sick or injured patient requires time to plan, organize, and prepare. Everyone benefits, especially the patient, when as much as possible of the preparation has been done pre-trip (SEE CHAPTER 35: EMERGENCY PROCEDURES FOR OUTDOOR GROUPS).

Once the critical decision to evacuate a patient has been made, the next decision may be just as important: How? In general, the choices are 1) do it yourself, 2) go for help, or 3) a combination of one and two when you have a larger group that can begin an evacuation while sending out messengers who request additional person-power to meet the evacuation enroute.

Wilderness Transportation Possibilities

Walk-out/ski-out

The ambulatory patient is the easiest evacuation. Patients with upper extremity injuries or stable athletic injuries to the knee or ankle can often carry their own weight. The best person to make the decision is often the patient who knows how he or she feels compared to how he or she used to feel. The patient knows best how usable an injury is. Improvised crutches and canes can be of assistance. The patient's gear may need to be distributed to other members of the group.

An optimum group size for a walking patient is at least four including the patient. If the patient becomes unable to continue walking, one person can remain with the patient while the others press on to the roadhead.

One-rescuer Carries

For disabling yet still relatively minor injuries, such as sprained ankles or knees, or a fractured but stable lower leg, the group may evacuate the patient by sharing not only the weight of the patient's gear but also the weight of the patient. The simplest techniques involve one rescuer carrying one patient, and require nothing more than physical strength and, perhaps, a few materials.

Patients can be moved short distances with the age-old piggy-back method. Carrier and carried soon tire, and longer distances will ask for a better system of holding the patient in place than strength of arm and back.

Backpack Carry: Internal frame packs, the kind with a sleeping bag compartment in the bottom, can be slipped on the patient like a pair of crude shorts allowing the patient to be "worn" out of the wilderness in relative "comfort." If the pack must be cut to fit, discussion over whose pack to use may last a long time.

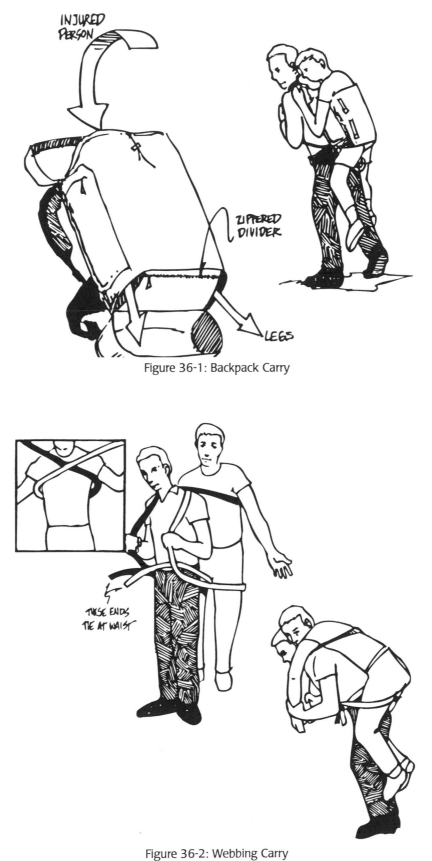

INJURED PERSON

ZIPPERED DIVIDER

LEGS

Figure 36-1: Backpack Carry

THESE ENDS TIE AT WAIST

Figure 36-2: Webbing Carry

Webbing Carry: With 15 to 20 feet of nylon webbing, a carrying system can be improvised. The center of the length of webbing should be placed at the center of the patient's back, brought under his or her arms, and crossed over the chest. The webbing then passes over the rescuer's shoulders, and back around the rescuer and between the patient's legs. When brought around the patient's legs and tied in front of the rescuer, a seat is formed. When slack develops, in the system, the webbing can be untied, the patient hitched up, and the webbing tied again. Pressure points in the system, such as the armpits of the patient, the shoulders of the rescuer, and the legs of the patient, should be padded to increase the distance the system can be utilized before both participants collapse in pain.

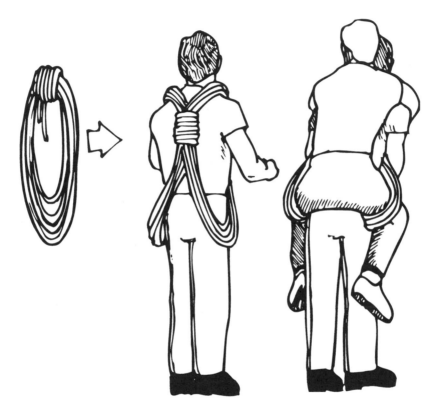

Figure 36-3: Split coil carry

Split-Coil Carry: If a climbing rope is available, it can be tied in a mountaineer's coil and split into two approximately equal halves connected at the knot of the coil. When laid on the ground, a split-coil looks something like a ropey butterfly. The rescuer sticks one arm through each of the "wings" of the butterfly, wearing the coil like a rucksack. The patient legs go through the lower part of each "wing," allowing the patient to be carried like an awkward backpack. Once again, padding at the pressure points adds comfort to the system.

Two-rescuer Carries

When the strength of two people is required to move a heavier patient, the weight can be distributed evenly by the rescuers standing on both sides of the patient. Each rescuer reaches for the other rescuer's hand under the patient's arms and behind the back. With the other hand, each rescuer reaches under the patient's knees. Using their legs and not their backs, the rescuers stand with the patient seated in a temporary chair.

If one rescuer is obviously stronger than the other, the weight of the patient can be distributed unevenly by having one rescuer stand at the patient's head and the other rescuer at the patient's feet. The first rescuer reaches beneath the patient's arms, and the second beneath the patient's knees. Although useful for short distances, this position is not especially comfortable for the patient over long distances.

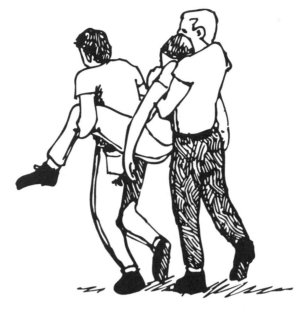

Figure 36-4: Two-rescuer carry

Two-Rescuer Pole Carry: Easier on both rescuers and patient is the two-rescuer pole carry (or ice axe carry). If two rescuers are wearing backpacks, a pole or long ice axe can be shoved into the strap system or tied to the bottom of each pack. When the pole is well padded, the patient can sit with relative comfort with his or her arms over the shoulders of the rescuers. The rescuers can carry in relative comfort, but this system is awkward when the carriers are of significantly different height.

Note: None of these carrying techniques demanding only one or two rescuers are recommended for seriously injured patients, and neither do they represent all the possible ways for one or two rescuers to move a patient. You are limited only by your imagination and the needs of patient and rescuers.

Litters

Patients unable to walk are often best treated by camping and attending to their needs while a team goes for help, even though the patients may be seriously ill or injured, e.g., myocardial infarction, injuries to the spine, multiple fractures that are difficult to stabilize, any condition that is exacerbated by movement. These patients will be endangered by moving them without adequate means.

The most important situation in which to consider moving someone immediately, even when the only mode of transportation falls short of ideal, involves a patient whose condition is steadily deteriorating, e.g., increasing difficulty breathing, persistent acute abdominal pain, heat stroke, unconsciousness for an unknown reason.

You may also choose to move any patient under less than ideal conditions when the method for transporting the patient promises to do no further harm.

Litter evacuations are slow, safe, and effective. Litters may be commercially made, or improvised in the field (SEE BELOW). In any case, the litter must be well constructed, the patient must be packaged appropriately, and the carry must be well organized and properly managed.

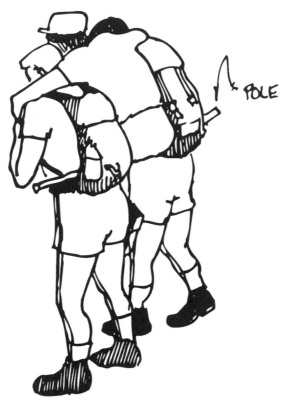

Figure 36-5: Two Rescuer pole carry

Commercial Litters

Several manufacturers offer litters made from metals, plastics, fiberglass, or combinations. They are all the same general shape. Many of them can be attached to large wheels and pushed like a cart, or converted into sleds and pulled over snow, or attached to a rope system and lifted by a helicopter or hauled up/lowered down a vertical slope. Commercial litters are much easier to handle and carry than improvised litters, and they eliminate the risk of the litter falling apart during patient transport. In other words, they offer a huge advantage over any litter you can make in the wilderness: They provide better patient care.

Pole Litter

As old as injuries, a pole litter, made from materials provided by the wilderness, probably represents the first litter ever improvised. It starts with two poles longer than the patient, and preferably of dry dead wood. Green wood flexes, making the carry difficult for litter bearers and miserable for the patient who bounces up and down with each flex. Shorter pieces of wood are lashed parallel to the longer poles until a "bed" is created. Materials for lashing include vines, grasses, rope, cord, string, boot laces, or anything else long and flexible enough. For patient comfort, the "bed" needs lots of padding.

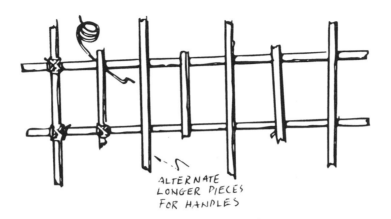

Figure 36-6: Pole Litter

Blanket Litters/Tarp Litter

With the advent of weaving, large pieces of cloth became available to improvise litters. Blankets seldom appear in wilderness areas these days, but tarps and tent flys do. A simple wrap around two long poles creates a workable litter when the patient's weight binds the tarps to the poles by way of friction. Cross braces lashed to the ends of the poles add stability and ease to carrying.

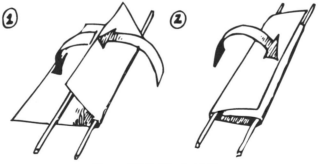

Figure 36-7: Blanket Litter

Rope-and-Pole Litter

Something like a hammock can be woven between two poles if you have enough rope on hand. Start by laying two long poles on the ground about shoulder width apart. Cross braces are needed at each end to give the litter stability. The cross braces can be sticks, ice axes, tent poles, or anything else available. With one end of the rope, lash one end of one cross brace into place. Wrap the rope around and around one pole, pulling the loop formed by each wrap out to an imaginary center line between the two poles. Finish one side by tying one end of the second cross brace into place. You can cut the rope and lash the second cross brace into place, or continue with the rope whole. As you work your way down and around the second pole, run the rope through the loops you've already made on the first pole. Tie off the second end of the first cross brace. The number of loops is completely relative to the length of your rope, but the more loops, the more solid the patient's "bed." Take all the slack out of the system. Pad the "bed" well.

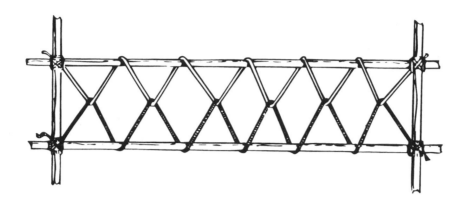

Figure 36-8: Pole and Rope Litter

Rope Litter

When poles aren't available, say above treeline, but a rope is, a non-rigid litter can be woven using only the rope. There are numerous ways to weave a rope into a litter, but they all have two things in common: They are the least easy to carry, and the most uncomfortable for the patient to ride in.

One method of constructing a rope litter requires a length of rope of approximately 150 feet (50 m). Find the center of the rope, and stack the two halves 10 or 12 feet apart. From the center, make 14 to 18 bends in the rope, seven to nine of them on either side of the center point. The bends should be about as wide as the patient. If you have a full length sleeping pad, lay it on the ground first, beneath the bends, to serve as a guide for the size of the litter. Bring the rope down past each bend tying a clove hitch in the rope at end bend and pulling the loop of the bend through the clove hitch until all the bends have a loop through a clove hitch. Weave the remainder of both ends of the rope around the litter and through the loops that extend through the clove hitches. Tighten the hitches, and tie off the ends of the rope. Pad the "bed" of the litter.

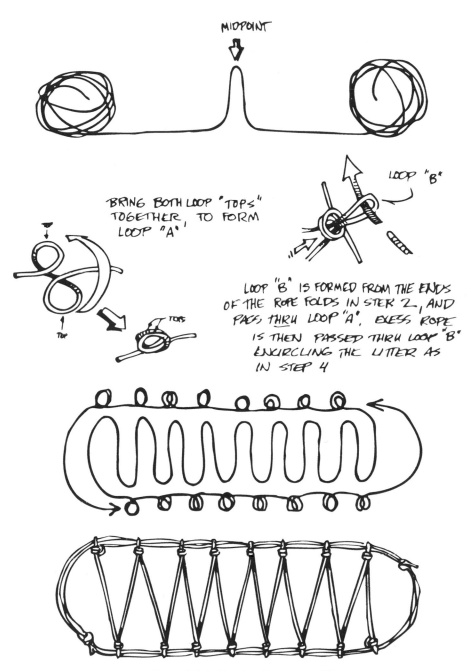

MIDPOINT

BRING BOTH LOOP "TOPS" TOGETHER, TO FORM LOOP "A"

LOOP "B"

TOPS

TOP

LOOP "B" IS FORMED FROM THE ENDS OF THE ROPE FOLDS IN STEP 2, AND PACS THRU LOOP "A". EXESS ROPE IS THEN PASSED THRU LOOP "B" ENCIRCLING THE LITTER AS IN STEP 4

Figure 36-9: Constructing a rope litter

Pack Litter

With three or four external frame packs, you can improvise a fairly substantial litter. Since the frames are molded to fit the shape of the wearer's back, they should be placed together in a way that best matches the shape of the person who will be carried. Take time to ensure the lashings are secure. Duct tape works well for lashing pack frames. Once again, adequate padding is required to create patient comfort.

Internal frame packs can be strapped to two long poles to form a litter, often by using the abundance of straps attached to the packs themselves. In an extreme situation, you can slit holes in the bottoms of the packs, slipping them over the poles and adding cross braces at the ends of the poles for stability.

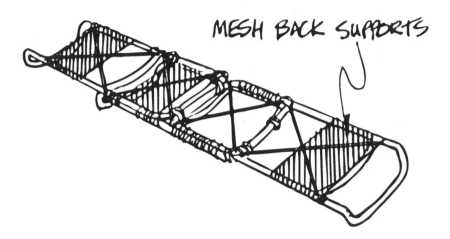

MESH BACK SUPPORTS

Figure 36-10: Pack litter

Litter Packaging

Riding in a litter is at best an uncomfortable experience for the patient. All the attention you can pay to the details of packaging a patient for a carry is time well spent.

If you have a sheet of plastic, a tarp, or tent fly, place it spread out in the litter first. It can be rolled up against the side of the patient, providing extra padding, and it can be quickly rolled out and wrapped around the patient in case of rain, wind, and/or cold. In most situations, you will package a patient on his or her back because 1) it is easier, in general, to provide care, and 2) it is easier to fit the patient in the litter. Pad-

ding in the "bed" of the litter is essential. Soft pads behind the knees and the small of the back help ease discomfort. Create a pillow when a neck injury is not suspected, and place a slim pad beneath the head when a neck injury is suspected.

Sometimes a patient will require packaging on his or her side. This patient is usually unconscious, and you are concerned about maintaining an adequate airway, something a stable side position offers.

All patients need to be secured in a litter, and that means straps. Straps should be placed on the bony structures of the patient: lower leg, upper leg,

pelvis, chest. Do not place straps across the abdomen or neck. Straps across the chest must not impede breathing. The arms should be left free if the patient is conscious. Freeing the arms increases the patient's feeling of security while decreasing the claustrophobia inherent inside a litter. The tightness of the straps will depend partially on patient comfort and partially on the ruggedness of the terrain to be crossed. Straps can be loosened or tightened as the evacuation proceeds, depending on need. Pad well beneath the straps where they press on the patient.

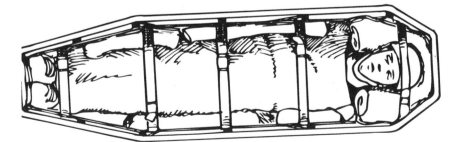

Figure 36-11: A patient packaged in litter

Litter Carrying

The carry of a litter provides an excellent opportunity to create a second patient. When it's time to move the loaded litter, remind the bearers to lift with their legs, not their backs. Space the bearers out evenly, preferably three to a side. The National Association for Search and Rescue (NASAR) recommends at least three teams of six to eight people for litter carries. Experience suggests that a group of at least 10 to 12 is necessary for litter carries of more than a few miles. Ease of carrying can be increased if eight to 10 feet of rope or webbing is attached to the litter for each bearer. This strap is thrown over the shoulder and across the back of the bearer, and held in the hand away from the litter. Use of the carrying strap allows each bearer to shift the weight of the litter to a shoulder, easing the stress on the hand holding the litter. The carrying strap also allows bearers of different heights to adjust the attitude of the litter.

One or two people walking in front of the litter can route find and clear obstacles for the litter party. People following behind the litter can carry the food, fuel, shelter, and clothing of the litter bearers.

In awkward situations such as carrying in boulders or deadfall, or across streams, stop the carry and move the free members of the party to the front of the litter. The litter can then be passed hand to hand over obstacles. In caves and other tight passages, the litter can be slid on the ground (pulled by a line attached to one end) or passed caterpillar style over rescuers lying in the passageway. In technical terrain, litters are lowered, belayed, and slung across ravines and rivers in with rope systems.

Care of the Littered Patient

It is very lonely inside a litter. There is pain and discomfort, and sometimes darkness, and the inability to move around to find just the right spot. The muffled sounds that come from the people carrying you are often unintelligible. You feel terrible to cause this much trouble, but there's nothing you can do about it.

As a litter bearer assume the responsibility for the mental as well as the physical comfort of your patient. Talk to the patient, especially when the litter is not being carried. Lean down near the patient's face, and speak quietly and confidently. If someone else is talking to the patient don't butt in. It's difficult to carry on two conversations under normal circumstances, impossible for an injured person. Ask about the injury: What can be done to make it more comfortable? Is it better, worse, the same? Ask about the amount of warmth inside the litter: Too little? Too much? Answer the patient's questions honestly and to the best of your ability.

If the patient is unconscious talk to them anyway. Reach inside the covering of the litter to check for warmth. Listen to the breathing and check the quality of the pulse gently at the carotid artery in the neck. Unless it is blistering cold, you may choose to periodically uncover an unconscious patient to make sure any splints you've put on are not cutting off circulation.

In terms of bodily needs, the basic rule of the rescue is: If you gotta, they gotta. When you drink, offer the patient a drink, if the injury or illness allows. When you eat, try to get the patient to eat, again if the injury or illness allows. If you feel a chill coming on, even more so the possibility that the patient is cold. If you are too hot, check the patient's comfort. If you need sunglasses, or sunscreen, or a toothbrushing, consider the needs of the patient, too.

When nature calls you to the bushes for a break, it's time to check in on your patient's need to urinate. He or she is often too embarrassed or too unwilling to cause a commotion to ask. You might have to unwrap your neat litter package to accommodate the patient, but that's part of the game. The job can usually be accomplished for a man by turning the litter on its side if the day is warm and he isn't too deep in coverings. He may be able to stay on his back and use a water bottle as a urinal. The problem is less easily solved for a woman, but she can sometimes catch most of her urine in a wide-mouth water bottle. If something absorbent is placed between her legs first, any spill can immediately be caught. In the least easily managed scenario, you have to take your patient out of the litter for urination or defecation, and repack him or her when the job is done.

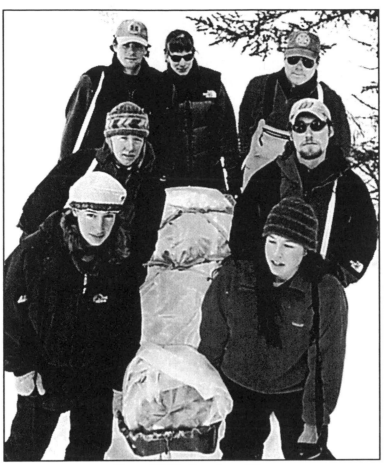

Figure 36-12: Carrying a litter

Horse Transports

Evacuation by horse is an option in some areas. The patient must be conscious and able to sit on the horse without falling off. This method is injury dependent. Lower leg, foot, and upper extremity injuries can be transported this way, while pelvic, hip, thigh, or back injuries are less likely to. The patient with a splinted leg may be unable to avoid striking the limb against trees, rocks, and other obstructions, and have difficulty controlling the horse. The chance of the patient falling off the horse must be considered. Horses have limits in steep and rocky terrain.

Vehicle Transports

You may be able to utilize a four wheel drive vehicle, snowmachine, fixed wing airplane, boat, helicopter, or other vehicle to transport a patient if there is a suitable loading/landing site nearby, or if the patient can be moved by person-power before transferring into a vehicle.

Snowmachines

In some winter situations, a large snowmachine with an enclosed cabin may be able to access and transport a patient. Even though limited by unpacked snow and steep terrain, it is far more common to find a snowmobile used for patient transport.

For the patient unable to sit behind the driver of a snowmobile, there are sleds designed specifically to be pulled by the machine in order to haul cargo and people. The patient has to be well protected from wind and cold, and the ride is not especially smooth.

The Wilderness First Responder

Boats and Airplanes

Boat evacuations can range from paddling a sick person in a double kayak to flagging down a larger vessel. Airplanes are options in many areas. The patient must first be moved, of course, to an adequate airstrip.

Helicopters

Nothing has done more to change the face of wilderness rescue than helicopters. They land in remote areas on spots on the earth inaccessible to aircraft only a few years ago. If the spot isn't flat enough, they've been known to land on one skid while a patient is quickly loaded. When there is no spot to land, they have hovered with a rescuer hanging from a rope or cable, a rescuer equipped to attach the patient to the hauling system for evacuation.

Helicopters go where the pilot wants because of the rapid spinning of two sets of blades. The large overhead blades create lift by forcing air down. The pilot can vary the angle at which the blades attack the air and the speed at which they rotate in order to vary the amount of lift. The entire rotor can be tilted forward, backward, or sideways to determine the direction of travel. Without a second set of blades spinning in an opposite direction the helicopter would turn circles helplessly in the air. Some large helicopters have two large sets of blades spinning in opposite directions, one fore and one aft, but most of the helicopters used in the wilderness maintain stability with a small tail rotor.

When they are close to the ground the spinning blades build a cushion of air that helps support the helicopter. This cushion of air varies in its ability to work depending on its density. Rising air temperatures and increasing altitude reduce air density. So trying to land on a mountain top on a hot day is dangerous for a helicopter, and the weight of one person may eliminate lift-off.

Air density is also altered by the nearness of a mountainside. The downward shove of air by the blades can recirculate off the mountainside and reduce lift.

One of the greatest fears of mountain flying is a sudden downdraft of air that can slam a helicopter toward the ground. Downdrafts are not only dangerous but also unpredictable.

Add to air density and downdrafts the possibility of darkness and fog and wind, and you will understand that even if a helicopter is available it may not be able to come to your rescue.

When you're in need of a rescue the approaching thump-thump-thump of rapidly rotating blades is a joyous sound. To give the helicopter rescue the greatest chance of success, a suitable landing zone (LZ) will have to be found. The ideal LZ should not require a completely vertical landing or take off, both of which reduce the pilot's control. The ground should slope away on all sides allowing the helicopter to immediately drop into forward flight when it's time to take off. Landings and take offs work best when the aircraft is pointed into the wind which gives the machine the greatest lift. The area should be as large as possible, at least 60 feet across for most small rescue helicopters, and as clear as possible of obstructions such as trees and boulders. Clear away debris (pine needles, dust, leaves) which can be blown up by the wash of air with the possibility of producing mechanical failure. Light snow can be especially dangerous if it fluffs up dramatically to blind the pilot. Wet snow sticks to the ground but also sticks to the runner of the helicopter and adds dangerous weight. If you have the opportunity, pack snow flat well before the helicopter arrives—the night before would be ideal—in order to harden the surface of the LZ. Tall grass can be a hazard in an LZ since it disturbs the helicopter's cushion of supporting air and hides obstacles such as rocks and tree stumps.

To prepare an LZ clear out as much of the debris as possible including your equipment and all the people except the one who is going to be signaling the pilot.

Mark the landing zone with weighted bright clothing or gear during the day or with bright lights at night. In case of a night rescue, turn off the bright lights before the helicopter starts to land. They can blind the pilot. Use instead a low-intensity light to mark the perimeter of the LZ, such as chemical light sticks, or at least turn the light away from the helicopter's direction. Indicate the wind's direction by building a very small smoky fire, hanging brightly colored streamers, throwing up handfuls of light debris, or signaling with your arms pointed in the direction of the wind.

The greatest danger to you occurs while you're moving toward or away from the helicopter on the ground. *Never approach from the rear and never walk around the rear of a helicopter.* The pilot can't see you, and the rapidly spinning tail rotor is virtually invisible and soundless. In a sudden shift of the aircraft, you can be sliced messily to death. Don't approach by walking downhill toward the helicopter where the large overhead blade is closest to the ground.

It is safest to come toward the helicopter from directly in front where the pilot has a clear field of view, and only after the pilot or another of the aircraft's personnel has signaled you to approach. Remove your hat or anything that can be sucked up into the rotors. Stay low since some helicopter's blades sink closer to the ground as their speed diminishes. Make sure nothing is sticking up above your pack such as an ice axe or ski pole. In most cases someone from the helicopter will come out to you to remind of the important safety measures.

One-skid landings or hovering while a rescue is attempted are solely at the discretion of the pilot. They are a high risk at best, and finding a landing zone and preparing it should always be given priority. The factors may simply add up to the impossibility of air rescue and alternatives need to be considered in all cases.

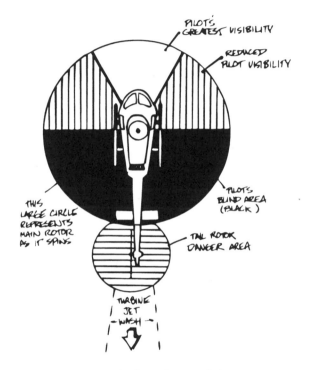

Figure 36-13: Helicopter Safety

Conclusion

Wilderness transportation of the sick or injured is at best a risky business for everyone involved. Litter bearers may stumble and end up a patient. Improvised carrying systems can fall apart, causing injury to bearers and/or further injury to the patient. Helicopters may crash. When an evacuation is necessary, choose a method that provides the least possibility of harm to all participants.

Chapter 37: *Wilderness Medical Kits*

You should be able to:

1. *Describe the general guidelines for packing a wilderness medical kit.*

2. *List the possible contents of a general wilderness medical kit.*

Introduction

The choice of contents for a wilderness medical kit can vary from the minimalist kit—a roll of duct tape and a roll of sterile gauze—to the maximalist kit that could alone burden the back of a strong porter. Every kit carried by a Wilderness First Responder should at least be the result of much forethought.

General Guidelines

1. Accept the fact that there is no such thing as the perfect wilderness medical kit. Many factors will determine your choices of specific contents, and, eventually, no matter how much you plan and prepare, some day you'll want something that isn't there and/or discover you've carried an item for years and never used it. When considering the contents of a kit, take into account: a) The environmental extremes you will face, e.g., altitude, cold, heat, endemic diseases; b) The number of people that may require care; c) The number of days the kit will be in use; d) The distance from definitive medical care; e) The availability of rescue, e.g., helicopter; f) Your medical exper-tise and/or the expertise of other group members; and g) Pre-existing problems of group members, e.g., diabetes.

2. Choose specific items for the wilderness medical kit, whenever possible, that are versatile rather than particular. For example, a wide variety of sizes and shapes of Band-Aids® is nice, but wound coverings can be improvised from pads of gauze and strips of tape. Triangular bandages are useful, but safety pins and T-shirts can be used to improvise slings. Medical adhesive tape has limited usefulness compared to duct tape.

3. Be familiar with the proper uses of all the items in the wilder-ness medical kit *before* you need to use them.

4. Evaluate and repack the wilderness medical kit before every trip. Renew medications that have reached expiration dates. Replace items that have been damaged by heat, cold, or moisture. Remove items that are unnecessary for the proposed trip, e.g., insect repellent on win-ter trips, and add items that may be useful on the upcoming adventure.

5. Encourage each group member to pack and carry a per-sonal first aid kit in order to reduce the size and weight of the general wilderness medical kit.

Specific Considerations

Specific considerations for a wilderness medical kit can be divided into four categories: trauma care supplies, tools, miscellaneous supplies, and medications. Keep in mind that these are suggestions and not requirements.

Trauma Care Supplies

1. Adhesive strips, e.g., Band-Aids®.
2. Sterile gauze pads and/or sterile gauze rolls.
3. Athletic tape, one inch by ten yards, and/or duct tape.
4. Tincture of benzoin compound.
5. Wound closure strips.
6. Microthin film dressings, e.g., Tegaderm®, Opsite®.
7. Large trauma dressings and/or an individually wrapped sanitary napkins.
8. Moleskin and/or molefoam.
9. Gel wound coverings, e.g., 2nd Skin®.
10. Soap-impregnated cleaning sponges, e.g., Green Soap Sponges®.
11. Antimicrobial towelettes and/or alcohol wipes.
12. Lightweight splint, e.g., SAM Splint®.
13. Elastic wraps and/or Coban®.
14. Rubber gloves.

(SEE CHAPTER 12: FRACTURES, CHAPTER 14: ATHLETIC INJURIES, CHAPTER 15: SOFT TISSUE INJURIES, AND CHAPTER 31: COMMON SIMPLE WILDERNESS MEDICAL PROBLEMS).

Tools

1. Trauma shears.
2. Forceps (tweezers).
3. Irrigation syringe.
4. Disposable scalpels.
5. Safety pins.

Miscellaneous Supplies

1. Pad and pencil.
2. Sawyer Extractor® (SEE CHAPTER 21: NORTH AMERICAN BITES AND STINGS).
3. Stethoscope.
4. Blood pressure cuff.
5. Pocket rescue mask.
6. Thermometer.
7. Sunscreen and lip protection.
8. Insect repellent.
9. Insect bite treatment, e.g., StingEze®.
10. Water disinfection system (SEE CHAPTER 30: COMMUNICABLE DISEASES).
11. Small flashlight.

Medications

1. Analgesic, e.g., aspirin, acetaminophen, ibuprofen—available over-the-counter for mild to moderate pain, and Percocet®, Vicodin®—narcotics available by prescription only for moderate to severe pain.
2. Anti-inflammatory, e.g., aspirin, ibuprofen, ketoprofen, naproxen—available over-the-counter (see Chapter 14: Athletic Injuries).
3. Antipyretic, e.g., aspirin, acetaminophen, ibuprofen.
4. Antihistamine, e.g., Benadryl®—available over-the-counter (see Chapter 28: Allergic Reactions and Anaphylaxis and Chapter 31: Common Simple Wilderness Medical Problems).
5. Antibiotic, e.g., cephalexin (e.g., Keflex®), erythromycin, ciprofloxacin (Cipro®)—all available by prescription only.

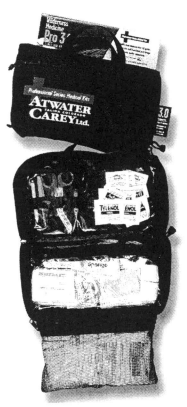

Figure 37-1:
Commercial first aid kit.

6. Anti-diarrheal, e.g., Imodium®—available over-the-counter (SEE CHAPTER 31: COMMON SIMPLE WILDERNESS MEDICAL PROBLEMS).
7. Anti-emetic, e.g., prochlorperazine (Compazine®)—available by prescription only.

8. Antifungal, e.g., Tinactin®, Monistat®—available over-the-counter (SEE CHAPTER 31: COMMON SIMPLE WILDERNESS MEDICAL PROBLEMS AND CHAPTER 32: GENDER-SPECIFIC EMERGENCIES).

10. Anti-vertigo, e.g., meclizine (e.g., Antivert®)—available over-the-counter (SEE CHAPTER 31: COMMON SIMPLE WILDERNESS MEDICAL PROBLEMS).

11. Decongestant, e.g., Afrin®, Sudafed®—available over-the-counter (SEE CHAPTER 22: DIVING EMERGENCIES AND CHAPTER 31: COMMON SIMPLE WILDERNESS MEDICAL PROBLEMS).

12. Antacid, e.g., Mylanta®—available over-the-counter.

13. Disinfectant solution, e.g., povidone-iodine—available over-the-counter.

14. Throat lozenges and/or hard candy.

15. Anti-altitude medications, e.g., acetazolamide (e.g., Diamox®), dexamethasone (e.g., Decadron®), nifedipine (e.g., Procardia®)—available by prescription only (SEE CHAPTER 18: ALTITUDE ILLNESSES).

16. Anti-anaphylaxis medication, e.g., injectable epinephrine (e.g., Ana-Kit®)—available by prescription only (SEE CHAPTER 28: ALLERGIC REACTIONS AND ANAPHYLAXIS).

17. Antibiotic ointment—available over-the-counter (SEE CHAPTER 15: SOFT TISSUE INJURIES).

Note: Use of all over-the-counter medications should follow directions on the label and/or directions from a physician. Use of all prescription medications should follow the directions of a physician.

Conclusion

Unless you are able to acquire medical supplies in bulk and/or free of charge, most Wilderness First Responders will save time and money by purchasing one of many excellent, commercially prepared wilderness medical kits. In addition, well-made kits offer durability, organization of supplies, easy access to supplies, and space to add on and take away from the included supplies.

Remember that the wilderness medical kit that saves lives rarely comes from a bag but, instead, from a brain packed with medical expertise. Aside from a few emergencies, e.g., anaphylaxis (SEE CHAPTER 28), your use of a medical kit is primarily to ease pain, speed healing, and prevent further injury, but it is knowledge and the ability to use that knowledge that makes the difference between life and death in a critical situation. Learn what you can do for the seriously hurt or sick person, and carry that information with you all times.

Appendix A: Leave No Trace

You should be able to:

1. *Explain the importance of leaving no trace in the wilderness.*

2. *Describe the six general principles of the Leave No Trace program.*

Introduction

Leave No Trace (LNT) is a national educational program that promotes and inspires responsible outdoor recreation through education, research, and partnership. LNT unites the U. S. Forest Service, National Park Service, Bureau of Land Management, U. S. Fish and Wildlife Service, educational programs, and the outdoor industry in teaching the public to enjoy the outdoors without harming it. "Leave no trace" is also an attitude, a philosophy that says you can move and live, even rescue patients from the wilderness, without leaving evidence of your activities. Without a predominance of a "leave no trace" approach to wilderness use, the foreseeable future may bring an end to a need for Wilderness First Responders because there may no longer be wilderness in which to respond.

Leave No Trace Principles

Plan Ahead and Prepare

Know the regulations, inherent risks, and special concerns for the area in which you'll be active. Travel the area in small groups. Avoid popular areas, whenever possible, during times of high use. Choose equipment and clothing in subdued colors. Repackage food and medical gear, whenever possible, into reusable containers.

Camp, Travel on Durable Surfaces

On the trail stay on designated trails. Walk in single file in the middle of the path. Do not shortcut switchbacks. When traveling cross-country, choose the most durable surfaces available: rock, gravel, dry grasses, or snow. Use a map and compass to eliminate the need for rock cairns, tree scars, and ribbons. Step to the downhill side of the trail and talk softly when encountering pack stock.

At camp choose an established, legal site that will not be damaged by your stay. Restrict activities to the area where vegetation is compacted or absent. Keep pollutants out of water sources by camping at least 200 feet (70 adult steps) from lakes and streams.

Pact It In, Pack It Out

Pack everything that you bring into wild country back out with you. Protect wildlife and your food by storing rations securely. Pick up all spilled foods.

Properly Dispose What You Can't Pack Out

Deposit human wastes in catholes dug six to eight inches deep at least 200 feet from water, camp, or trails. Cover and disguise the cathole when finished. Use toilet paper or wipes sparingly, and pack them out. To wash yourself or your dishes, carry water at least 200 feet away from streams or lakes, and use small amounts of biodegradable soap. Scatter strained dish water. Inspect your campsite before you leave, and pack out all trash—yours and others.

Leave What You Find

Treat our natural heritage with respect. Leave plants, rocks, and historical artifacts as you find them. Good campsites are found, not made. Altering a site should not be necessary. Let nature's sound prevail. Keep loud voices and noises to a minimum. Control pets at all times. Remove dog feces. Do not build structures or furniture or dig trenches.

Minimize Use, Impacts of Fire

Campfires can cause lasting impacts on the wilderness. Always carry a lightweight stove for heating water and/or cooking. Enjoy a candle lantern instead of a fire. Where fires are permitted, use established fire rings, fire pans, or mound fires. Don't scar large rocks and overhangs. Gather sticks no larger than an adult's wrist. Do not snap branches off live, dead, or downed trees. Put out campfires completely. Remove all unburned trash from fires and scatter the cool ashes over a large area well away from camp.

For information and materials on Leave No Trace call: 1-800-332-4100.

Appendix B: *Oxygen and Mechanical Aids To Breathing*

You should be able to:

1. *Describe how to safely use supplemental oxygen.*
2. *Demonstrate the correct use of oropharyngeal and nasopharyngeal airways.*
3. *Demonstrate how to set up oxygen delivery equipment and correctly deliver supplemental oxygen using a nasal cannula, simple mask, mask and reservoir, pocket mask, bag-valve-mask, and demand valve.*
4. *Demonstrate the use of suction equipment.*

Introduction

There are times when the patient treated by the Wilderness First Responder will benefit greatly from the administration of supplemental oxygen. An understanding of oxygen and its associated delivery equipment is fundamental, therefore, to providing optimum care to many patients.

Oxygen And Respiration

Oxygen is an odorless, colorless gas which makes up approximately 21 percent of the atmosphere. You inhale this atmosphere, use approximately five percent of the oxygen, and exhale about 16 percent of the oxygen.

At rest, most adults have a total inspired volume of about 500 ml/breath. This amount is referred to as "tidal volume." The respiratory system can use about 350 ml of this at the alveolar level, where gas exchange takes place. The remaining 150 ml is contained within the bronchi and bronchioles, an area known as "dead air space" since none of the air is used for gas exchange. One person may take great gasps of air much larger than 500 ml and another may take very shallow breaths of 200 ml. In either case the "dead air space" remains approximately 150 ml.

Safety

Since oxygen promotes combustion, it should never be used near an open flame, and petroleum products should not be used with oxygen equipment. Petroleum products include any sort of tape with petroleum-based adhesives in them, greases, or oils.

The rapid escape of oxygen from a tank, combined with the petroleum products, could create friction heat and start a dangerous fire.

Oxygen cylinders are potentially dangerous since the oxygen is stored in them under great pressure. They should always be kept laying flat, both when in use and in storage. If the neck should be accidentally cracked and the pressure rapidly escape, the tank could become a deadly missile.

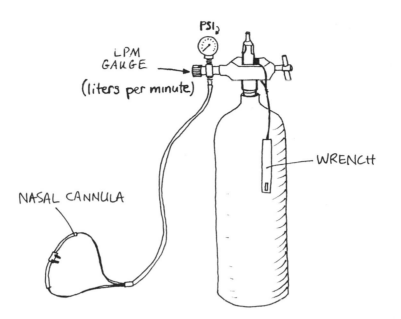

Appendix B-1: Oxygen Delivery System

The Tank

Oxygen is stored for use in special tanks (cylinders), and under a pressure, when the tank is full, of 2,000 psi (pounds per square inch). These cylinders are normally green, or shiny aluminum with a green label, for ease of identification. Portable tanks are available for use in the field and are conveniently sized to fit in backpack-like carrying cases. These are known as either C, D, or E tanks, depending on size. Even larger tanks are found on board ambulances and aeromedical units.

Oxygen cylinders must be inspected every five years for the presence of corrosion or damage that might affect safe delivery of oxygen to patients. In order to prevent corrosion resulting from moisture in atmospheric air, oxygen cylinders need to be maintained with a small amount of pressure within them at all times. This amount is referred to as "safe residual" and is usually 200 psi. Oxygen is very drying, and a small amount left in the tank will prevent atmospheric air from entering the tank, thus preventing moisture from corroding the interior of the tank.

The Regulator

Oxygen tanks are fitted with special regulators that reduce the pressure of the gas as it leaves the cylinder, normally to between 40 and 75 psi. An important safety feature of these regulators is a system of pin fittings. All cylinders used for gases have specific pin settings, and regulators for one gas cannot be attached to a tank used for another gas. When fitting a regulator onto an oxygen tank, it is important to check for the correct pin setting. Another feature of regulators is the plastic gasket, or washer, that is used to provide a seal onto the tank. It is important to check that the washer is present and in good condition before fitting the regulator onto the tank.

Before securing a regulator onto a tank, open the tank slightly to allow for a small amount of oxygen to escape. This will blow any dust or particulate matter away from the pin sites, keeping the regulator clear of obstructions. The regulator is then secured in place—finger tight only—and the tank can be opened one full turn to allow for oxygen delivery. All regulators have a gauge which tells the current pressure within the tank. When opening the regulator, the pressure gauge should be facing away from the WFR and/or patients. This prevents any danger should the gauge come apart due to the sudden change in internal pressure.

In addition to a pressure gauge, regulators will have a flow meter that allows the WFR to dial in the amount of oxygen to be delivered to the patient. This flow meter measures the amount of delivered oxygen in liters per minute (lpm). Regulators will deliver up to 15, sometimes 25, liters per minute.

Once you have finished using a tank and regulator, the tank should be shut off and any remaining pressure bled from the regulator and lines. This is done by either pressing the button on the demand valve or opening the liter flow gauge. Once the needle on the pressure gauge returns to zero, liter flow is shut off and the tank is secured.

Oxygen Therapy

Assessment of the patient will determine the type of oxygen therapy that is needed in each situation. During the initial survey, the WFR discovers if the patient has a *patent* (open) airway, and if measures are needed to maintain the airway in an open position. Further assessment will determine the patient's level of consciousness, the best indicator of oxygen perfusion to the brain. In addition to level of consciousness, a knowledge of the mechanism of injury will aid you in determining the most appropriate method of oxygen therapy. For example, a rock climber who has fallen and broken a rib may need only a low level of supplemental oxygen. A caver trapped with little or no ability to move her or his chest may need a much greater level of oxygen in order to maintain adequate oxygen perfusion to the brain.

Frequent checks on the patient's respiratory rate, tidal volume, and respiratory effort are also important. Can the patient, for instance, speak in full sentences or only in short phrases? An ongoing assessment of the patient is necessary in order to insure optimum oxygen therapy.

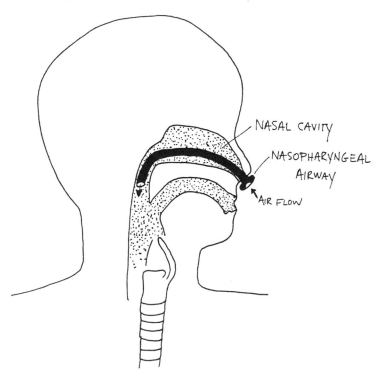

NASAL CAVITY

NASOPHARYNGEAL AIRWAY

AIR FLOW

Appendix B-2: Nasopharyngeal Airway

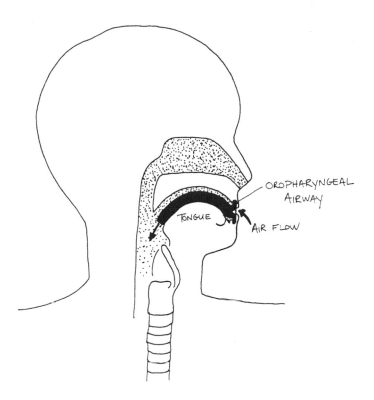

Appendix B-3: Oropharyngeal Airway

Airway Maintenance

The Oropharyngeal Airway

A short, curved oropharyngeal airway (OPA), also known as an oral airway, is used to keep the tongue away from the back of the throat, and thus keep the airway patent. They come in sizes from infant to large adult. The oropharyngeal airway is constructed so that it is possible to suction either through or alongside the OPA (SEE BELOW). Correct sizing is measured either from the center of the mouth to the angle of the jaw, or from the corner of the mouth to the earlobe. Either way is acceptable.

Oral airways should be used only with patients who are unconscious and have no gag reflex. When used with patients who have a gag reflex, there is danger of vomiting and aspiration, and of vocal cord spasm.

Insertion of the airway is performed first by opening the mouth with a jaw thrust or the *cross-finger technique* (placing your thumb and index finger between the patient's front teeth and pushing in opposite directions to open the mouth). The airway is inserted initially with the curved tip facing the roof of the patient's mouth. Once it is halfway in, the airway is rotated 180 degrees and placed so that the flange rests on the patient's lips. Should the patient have dentures, they may be left in place. Dentures provide for better maintenance of a patent airway since the OPA will stay in place easier.

The Nasopharyngeal Airway

Soft and flexible, nasopharyngeal airways are for use with conscious patients and those who may be unresponsive but have an intact gag reflex. They are of value where the patency of an airway is threatened or compromised. They will not, however, insure that the tongue will stay out of the back of the throat. Correct sizing is measured from the tip of the nose to the earlobe.

The airway should be lubricated with a sterile, water-based material, preferably containing a topical anesthetic. Do not use petroleum-based lubricants which may damage nasopharyngeal mucosa. Check to see if one nostril is noticeably larger, and utilize the larger one. If both nostrils appear the same size, it doesn't matter which one you use. The airway is inserted curved side down, gently pushing along the normal curvature of the nose. If resistance is met, do not force the airway further. Try the other nostril. The airway is inserted until the flange is flush with the outside of the nostril. It is normal for a small amount of bleeding to occur during insertion of the airway. If cerebrospinal fluid is leaking from the nose, or other signs of skull fracture are present (SEE CHAPTER 9: HEAD INJURIES), it is considered unsafe to insert a nasal airway since it may introduce infection into the brain cavity.

Passive Delivery

Passive delivery describes the process in which oxygen is brought to a patient who must be breathing adequately for the gas to be of benefit.

Nasal Cannula

The nasal cannula is soft tubing with two prongs which curve into the patient's nostrils. It is fastened around the ears and cinched up under the chin in a fashion similar to a bolo tie. It is used at a flow rate of between two and six lpm, and can deliver up to 40 percent oxygen at six lpm. A patient is free to talk while using a cannula, and it is relatively comfortable. The oxygen can be drying to nasal mucosa which may cause some itching. The cannula is used most often with patients in mild to moderate respiratory distress. It is especially useful with a patient who may vomit since it doesn't block the patient's mouth.

Simple Mask

The simple mask is made of plastic; comes in adult, child, and infant sizes; and is seldom seen these days on rescue scenes. An adult size can always be adapted to a smaller person. When properly fitted, the mask is snugged down over the bridge of the nose by pinching a small metal piece into place, and the strap is placed around the back of the head, above the ears. It is used at a liter flow rate of between six and 12 lpm, and can deliver up to 60 percent oxygen at 12 liters per minute. A disadvantage of the mask is that it can be claustrophobic to some patients. It may also be difficult to understand a patient who speaks inside the mask. There is also a danger of aspiration of vomitus which may be trapped in the mask.

Mask and Reservoir

A mask with a reservoir uses the simple mask with an oxygen reservoir bag attached. There may be thin rubber gaskets at the exhalation ports to prevent intake of any "room" air. The reservoir is filled with 100 percent oxygen through the liter flow connection at the tank. These may be Partial- or Non-Rebreather Masks, depending on the presence of outside gaskets. With a good seal, the Non-Rebreather (NRB) will deliver about 95 percent oxygen. The liter flow setting must be high enough to insure that the reservoir bag does not fully deflate when the patient inhales. A setting between 10 and 12 lpm is usually sufficient for this. This mask is excellent for patients with lowered tidal volume or decreased respiratory effort.

Positive Pressure Delivery

Pocket Mask

There are several types of lightweight barriers available to the Wilderness First Responder for use in ventilating patients who are not breathing on his or her own. The principle behind these devices is that the rescuer is protected from contact with the patient's exhaled breath and/or secretions or blood. These devices fit directly over the patient's mouth and nose. Oropharyngeal or nasopharyngeal airways are appropriate in many cases where a pocket mask will be used. Good head position of the patient, one that keeps the airway open, must be maintained by the rescuer while using the mask. Pocket masks are available with oxygen inlet ports that allow for delivery of up to 50 percent oxygen to the patient at a liter flow rate of 10 lpm. One advantage of a pocket mask is that the rescuer is able to tell when the patient's lungs are fully inflated by the back pressure felt with mouth-to-mask ventilation. Pocket masks come in adult sizes but can be used with children or infants.

Bag-Valve-Mask

The bag-valve-mask (BVM) device uses a semi-rigid bag, filled with either ambient air or supplemental oxygen, and a transparent mask that fits tightly onto the patient's face. These devices come in adult, child, and infant sizes. There are reservoir tubes or bags that fit onto most BVMs which increase the potential for delivery of up to almost 100 percent oxygen to the patient. They may be used on patients who need respiratory assistance or on non-breathing patients.

When used as a respiratory assist device, the WFR synchronizes squeezing the bag with the beginning of the patient's inspirations. The use of a BVM allows you to feel lung resistance as the lungs reach full, preventing overflow of air into the stomach.

Proper technique of the BVM allows the WFR to maintain an open airway on the patient and ventilate adequately at the same time. While holding the transparent mask in the fleshy area between the thumb and forefinger, a good mask seal can be maintained by pressure onto the patient's face. At the same time, the other fingers of the hand can hold along the patient's jaw line, maintaining good head position. This technique is called the "anesthesiologist grip." With the bag firmly attached to the mask, you can ventilate the patient with the other hand by squeezing the bag. If your hands are small, the bag can be swiveled so that it is near the forearm, and pressed against the body to fully deflate the bag for each desired ventilation.

Demand Valve

The demand valve is a fitting that attaches to the oxygen tank via a length of sturdy tubing. It has within it a special valve which will allow oxygen to be released with a slight amount of

negative pressure. Therefore, a patient can self-administer oxygen simply by inhaling through the mask, the oxygen being delivered on "demand." Oxygen can also be delivered via a demand valve by depressing a button on the device. Thus it is frequently used with non-breathing patients, as in CPR. An OPA is inserted in order to maintain a patent airway, and the patient is ventilated as is appropriate to the situation.

Since the demand valve works directly off pressure through the regulator (between 40 and 75 psi, remember, depending on the regulator), there is danger of too great a pressure entering the patient's respiratory system. For this reason a demand valve is never used with patients under 12 years of age. There is less ability to feel when the lungs are fully inflated with a demand valve, therefore more danger of overflow into the stomach. This overflow promotes vomiting, a dangerous situation with an unconscious patient.

Suction

The Wilderness First Responder knows that airway patency is of paramount importance in patient care. Whether it be bleeding, vomiting, broken teeth, food particles, or buildup of saliva, potential problems exist in maintaining the patient's airway. At times a patient can be positioned so that potential complicating fluids can flow out, i.e., on his or her side. When this is not possible, as with suspected spinal injuries, you must carefully protect the patient's airway. A knowl-

edge of suction devices and technique can be lifesaving for the patient.

There are numerous portable suction devices available for use in wilderness rescue. Some are battery powered, some work from the oxygen in a portable tank, others are hand-operated. As with anything taken into the wilderness, weight and durability must be taken into account when choosing equipment. You may even choose a simple turkey baster for use as a suction device.

Suction devices use either a rigid or soft *catheter* (a tube inserted into the body) in order to collect materials threatening the airway. The rigid, or tonsil tip, catheter attaches onto suction tubing. The soft catheter is sometimes part of suction tubing or may need to be attached onto the tubing. In either case, the catheter is inserted only to the back of the throat. Once the catheter has been inserted through the mouth and to the back of the throat, suction is then initiated. You must not suction a patient for more than 15 seconds, unless greater time is needed, in order to clear an airway for ventilation. If possible, pre-oxygenate the patient before suctioning by assisting ventilations or providing supplemental oxygen. Suction devices have their limits, and large particulate matter or thick secretions require rolling a patient and/or the use of finger sweeps in order to clear the airway. A conscious patient who must remain supine may even help to suction themselves.

Dan De Kay, RN, WEMT, contributed his expertise to this chapter.

Appendix C: Automated External Defibrillation

You should be able to:

1. *Describe the advantages of automated external defibrillation.*

2. *Describe the use of an automated external defibrillator.*

Introduction

Ventricular fibrillation (v-fib) is rapid, quivering, incomplete contractions of the muscle fibers of the ventricles of the heart. V-fib often results from blockage in coronary blood vessels, but it may also be the result of other causes such as a substantial electric shock or certain drugs. A patient in v-fib is in cardiac arrest: pulseless and breathless. V-fib typically converts to *asystole* (the absence of all heart activity) within a few minutes. Asystole cannot be converted back to a normal rhythm with a defibrillator, but v-fib can be converted back to a normal rhythm. Electrical *defibrillation* stops fibrillation by stopping the heart via a shock through electrodes placed on the chest wall. If the shock is applied in time, the heart will sometimes start again under its own electrical impulse and in a normal rhythm. V-fib is the most common rhythm encountered by bystanders initiating CPR, and electrical defibrillation gives a patient in ventricular fibrillation the single most important chance of survival.

Although wilderness medicine situations today seldom offer patients in cardiac arrest an opportunity to be defibrillated, that fact is changing. Shipboard clinics, rural clinics, aeromedical units, even some remote camps are acquiring a defibrillating device and the skills to defibrillate. It is recommended that the Wilderness First Responder carry at least a basic understanding of the easiest form of defibrillation, the automated external defibrillator.

Survival Rates for Patients with a Witnessed Cardiac Arrest

Care	Survival Rate
No CPR, delayed defibrillation	0-2 percent
Early CPR, delayed defibrillation	2-8 percent
Early CPR, early defibrillation	20 percent
Early CPR, very early defibrillation	30 percent

The Device

Conventional defibrillators require a relatively high degree of skill in heart rhythm recognition and device operation. An automated external defibrillator (AED) only requires the operator to recognize cardiac arrest in the patient, properly attach the device to the patient, and memorize a short treatment sequence. An AED interprets the cardiac rhythm for the rescuer, recommending a shock when appropriate. Learning to use an AED is much easier than learning CPR, but CPR skills remain critical. Patients in cardiac arrest for up to ten minutes have been resuscitated via electrical defibrillation when CPR was performed in the interim. It seems that CPR extends v-fib.

Although something of a generic term, all "automated external defibrillators" utilize a cardiac rhythm analysis system. All AEDs attach to the patient with cables connected to two adhesive pads which are stuck to the patient's chest. When the device is turned on, the patient's cardiac rhythm is analyzed. If the device reads ventricular fibrillation—or ventricular tachycardia above a certain rate—it will charge its capacitors and deliver, or recommend the rescuer deliver, an electric shock.

Operational Procedures

Four simple steps are followed in using all AEDS: 1) turn the device on, 2) attach the device to the patient, 3) initiate the analysis of the patient's heart rhythm, and 4) deliver the shock if a shock is indicated.

Since CPR seems to extend v-fib, CPR should be initiated immediately on pulseless, breathless patients. If possible, it is recommended that CPR be performed from the patient's right side while one rescuer sets up the AED on the patient's left side. The left side gives the AED operator better access to the patient. When the device is in place beside the patient's head, the AED operator activates the device. The cables are attached to the device and to the adhesive pads. The two pads are stuck to the patient, one on the chest wall beneath the right shoulder (the upper right sternal border), the other on the chest wall beneath the left nipple (the lower left ribs over the apex of the heart). When the pads are attached, CPR is halted, and the analysis control button is pressed. All rescuers must avoid contact with the patient during the five to 15 seconds it takes the machine to do the analysis. If a shock is indicated, the device will so indicate in one of several ways including a written message or a synthesized voice command, depending on the model of AED.

If the device indicates a shock, the AED operator must loudly remind everyone to remain clear of contact with the patient, usually by saying "Clear" or something similar, before pressing the shock delivery button or before the device automatically delivers the shock. After the first shock, rescuers do *not* resume CPR. The analysis control button should be pressed a second time for an immediate check on the patient's heart rhythm. If the patient remains in v-fib, the device will recharge and indicate a second shock. The same sequence may be repeated, and a third shock delivered if necessary. The sequence of three shocks takes about 90 seconds. Most AEDs will deliver the first two shocks at 200 joules, and the third at 360 joules. Some devices require the operator to increase the joules manually.

If the third shock does not resuscitate the patient, CPR should be resumed for 60 seconds before the AED is activated for a second round of analyses and shocks. The three shock sequences should be repeated until the machine gives a "no shock recommended" message. Local protocols, however, may require immediate transport of the patient, if available, after the first round of shocks. In most cases, CPR should be continued during transport, but use of the AED during transportation is not acceptable since movement interferes with heart rhythm analysis.

If the rescuer is alone, CPR should be performed for one minute first. After a minute of CPR, assistance should be summoned, e.g., dial 911, if help is available. Then the AED should be utilized.

Glossary

abandonment: leaving a patient in need of medical care after initiating care.

ABCDE: airway, breathing, circulation, disability, environment.

abduction: movement away from the midline of the body.

abrasion: wound in which one or more layers of skin are scraped away.

acclimatization: process of physiologically adjusting to a new environment, e.g., altitude.

acetabulum: hip socket.

Achilles tendon: tendon connecting the heel bone to the muscles of the lower leg.

acidosis: condition produced by the accumulation of acid or the reduction of base in the body.

ACL: anterior cruciate ligament.

acute mountain sickness: a range of physiological problems caused by a failure to acclimatize to higher altitudes.

acute: an immediate problem with a short duration, not chronic.

adduction: movement toward the midline of the body

AED: automatic external defibrillator.

AEIOUTIPS: common causes of an altered level of consciousness: alcohol, epilepsy, infection, overdose, underdose, trauma, insulin, psychosis, stroke.

afterdrop: continued lowering of core temperature after a patient has been removed from a cold environment.

AGE: arterial gas embolism.

alkalosis: condition produced by the accumulation of base or the reduction of acid in the body.

allergen: allergy causing substance.

ALS: advanced life support.

alveoli: sacs of the lungs where gas exchange takes place.

ambulatory: able to walk.

ambulatory: walking.

amenorrhea: absence of a menstrual cycle.

AMI: acute myocardial infarction; heart attack.

amnesia: loss of memory.

amniotic sack: thin membrane covering the fetus and placenta and containing amniotic fluid.

amputation: separation of a body part from the body.

AMS: acute mountain sickness.

analgesic: pain reliever.

anaphylaxis: severe allergic reaction to a foreign protein characterized by bronchoconstriction and vasodilation.

anesthetic: agent that produces a partial or complete loss of sensation.

aneurysm: abnormal widening of a blood vessel, usually an artery.

angina pectoris: pain in the chest.

angioedema: swelling of the mucous membranes of the lips, mouth or other part of the respiratory system.

ankle hitch: an anchor at the sole of the foot from which traction can be pulled for a traction splint.

anomia: inability to remember names.

anorexia: loss of appetite.

anovulatory cycle: no ovulation.

anterior: front.

anti-diarrheal: substance used to prevent or treat diarrhea.

anti-emetic: substance used to prevent or treat vomiting.

anti-inflammatory: substance used to counteract inflammation.

antibiotic: substance that inhibits growth of or destroys microorganisms.

anticholinergic: agent that blocks parasympathetic nerve impulses.

antihistamine: drug that counteracts the effects of histamines.

antipyretic: agent that reduces or relieves fever.

antivenin: serum containing antitoxin for animal or insect venom.

aorta: main artery that leaves the heart and travels to the body.

aortic valve: valve between the left ventricle and the aorta.

apnea: absence of breathing.

appendicitis: inflammation of the appendix.

aqueous humor: salty fluid that fills the cornea.

arachnoid: web like membrane surrounding the brain and spinal cord, the middle of the three meningeal layers.

arterial gas embolism: air bubble in the arterial blood stream.

arteriole: small artery.

arteriosclerosis: thickening, hardening and loss of elasticity of the arteries.

artery: vessel carrying blood from the heart.

asphyxia: condition of insufficient intake of oxygen.

aspirate: to draw in or out by suction.

asthma: condition resulting in shortness of breath and wheezing due to swelling of bronchi and swelling of their mucous membranes.

asystole: absence of all activity in the heart.

ataxia: loss of muscle coordination leading to difficulty in maintaining balance.

atherosclerosis: clogging of the arteries from fatty deposits and other debris.

atrium: upper chamber of each half of the heart.

auscultate: listen.

AVPU: alert, verbal, pain, unresponsive; scale for determining level of consciousness.

avulsion: forcible tearing away of a part or structure.

axial: along the side of the body.

bacteria: single cell microorganisms.

baroreceptors: nerve endings sensitive to changes in pressure.

barosinusitis: pain or inflammation of nasal sinuses due to pressure changes; sinus squeeze.

barotitus media: inflammation of the middle ear due to changes in pressure; middle ear squeeze.

barotitus: inflammation of the ear due to changes in pressure.

barotrauma: injury caused by a change in pressure, as in SCUBA diving.

basal cell carcinoma: skin cancer affecting the basal cells of the epidermis.

basal metabolic rate: the constant rate at which a human body consumes energy to drive chemical reactions and produce heat to maintain an adequate core temperature.

Battle's sign: bruising behind the ears indicating a fracture to the base of the skull.

BEAM: body elevation and movement; technique for lifting spinally injured patients.

biliary duct: duct carrying bile to the small intestine.

bipolar disease: cyclical pattern of depression and mania.

bleb: a fluid filled blister.

BLS: basic life support.

BMR: Basal metabolic rate.

BP: blood pressure.

brachial: arm from the shoulder to the elbow.

bradycardia: slow heart rate, typically less than 60 beats per minute.

brain stem: part of the brain connecting the cerebral hemispheres to the spinal cord.

breech presentation: baby presents feet or buttocks first during birth.

bronchiole: small bronchus; small airway of the lung.

bronchitis: inflammation of the mucous membranes of the bronchi.

bronchospasm: spasms in the muscles of the bronchi.

bronchus: one of the two large airways branching off from the trachea.

BSI: body substance isolation; universal precautions against communicable disease.

buboe: inflamed, enlarged lymph node.

bursae: fluid filled sac or cavity commonly found in joints that reduces friction.

BVM: bag valve mask.

calcaneo-fibular ligament: ligament connecting the heel and the fibula.

calcaneous: heel bone.

capillary: minute blood vessel where gas exchange occurs between the bloodstream and the tissues.

cardiac arrest: the cessation of heart muscle activity.

cardiogenic: originating in the heart.

cardiovascular system: relating to the heart, the blood vessels and the blood.

carotid artery: primary blood vessel supplying the head and neck.

carpopedal spasms: muscular spasms in the hands and feet.

cartilage: tough elastic tissue forming protective pads where bone meets bone.

catheter: tube inserted into the body for the addition or removal of fluids.

CC: chief complaint.

Centruroides: particularly potent species of scorpion found in the SW US.

cerebellum: part of the brain that helps control movement.

cerebral: relating to the cerebellum.

cerebrovascular accident: interruption of normal blood flow to a part of the brain.

cerebrum: largest part of the brain consisting of two hemispheres.

cervical vertebrae: first seven bones of the spinal column.

cervix: lower narrow end of the uterus.

CHF: congestive heart failure.

chondromalacia: disintegration of cartilage under the kneecap.

chronic obstructive pulmonary disease: a collection of diseases sharing the common symptoms of airway obstruction in the small to medium airways, excessive secretions, and/or constriction of the bronchial tubes.

chronic: slow progression or of long duration, not acute.

cilia: hairlike processes.

CISD: critical incident stress debriefing.

CISM: critical incident stress management.

clavicle: collar bone.

closed pneumothorax: tear in the lining of the lung resulting in air accumulating the pleural space with no open wounds.

cnidoblast: capsule containing the stinging nematocyst of Coelenterates.

cnidocil: trigger on a cnidoblast.

CNS: central nervous system; brain and spinal cord.

CO: carbon monoxide.

coccyx: last bone of the spinal column consisting of 4 fused vertebra; tail bone.

cochlea: cone shaped tube in the inner ear that aids in hearing.

Coelenterates: phylum of sea creatures including jellyfish, fire coral, stinging medusa, Portuguese man-of-war, sea wasp, hairy stinger, stinging anemone.

collateral ligament: ligament on the inside of the knee (medial collateral ligament) or on the outside of the knee (lateral collateral ligament).

comminuted fracture: fracture in which the bone is splintered or crushed.

commission: an act.

conduction: heat lost from a warmer object when it comes in contact with a colder object.

congestive heart **failure:** process in which blood and tissue fluids congest due to the heart's inadequacy.

conjunctiva: membrane lining the eyes.

constipation: infrequent or difficult bowel movements.

contusion: ruise. convection: heat lost directly into the air.

COPD: chronic obstructive pulmonary disease.

coronary artery: vessel that supplies the heart muscle with blood.

CPR: cardiopulmonary resuscitation.

crackle: abnormal breath sound heard by listening to the chest, produced by air passing through small airways filled with secretions.

cranium: skull.

crepitus: sound or feel of broken bone ends grating against each other.

critical incident: incident so distressing it surpasses an individual's normal coping mechanisms.

crown: area of a tooth above the gum.

CRT: capillary refill time.

cruciate ligaments: cross shaped ligaments that hold the knee joint together. Anterior cruciate ligament attaches to the rear of the femur and the front of the tibia, posterior cruciate ligament attaches to the front of the femur and the rear of the tibia.

Cryptosporidium: protozoa found in surface waters.

CSF: cerebrospinal fluid; fluid cushioning the brain and spinal cord.

CSM: circulation, sensation and motion.

cuboid: one of the instep of the foot.

cuniforms: small bones of the foot.

CVA: cerebrovascular accident; stroke.

cyanosis: blue hue to the skin indicating a lack of oxygen in the blood.

DAN: Divers Alert Network.

DCS: decompression sickness.

decompression sickness: accumulation of nitrogen bubbles in the tissue after breathing compressed air and ascending too quickly.

DEET: N,N-diethyl-meta-toluamide; insect repellent.

defibrillation: stopping fibrillation of the heart using electricity or drugs.

defusing: informal discussion of a critical incident, not a critique.

deltoid ligament: ligament attaching the tibia to bones on the inside of the ankle.

dentin: calcified area surrounding the pulp of a tooth.

dependent lividity: discoloration of the skin, as from a bruise, where non-circulating blood has settled via gravity

depression: altered mood characterized by lack of interest in pleasurable things.

dermatitis: inflammation of the skin.

dermatophytes: fungi that grow on skin.

dermis: skin.

diabetes mellitus: disease in which the pancreas secretes an insufficient amount of insulin.

diabetic ketoacidosis: production of ketones during hyperglycemic complication of diabetes.

diaphoresis: profuse sweating .

diaphragm: large muscle separating the abdominal and thoracic cavities, used in breathing.

diarrhea: frequent passage of unformed watery bowel movements.

diastolic pressure/diastole: pressure measured during the relaxation phase of the heart between contractions.

DICC: disoriented, irritable, combative, comatose.

dislocation: the complete or partial disruption of the normal relationship of a joint.

distal: away from the center.

diuretic: drug that causes increased urination.

DKA: diabetic ketoacidosis.

DNR: Do Not Resuscitate

dorsalis pedis pulse: pulse located on the top of the foot.

ductus deferens: excretory duct of the testicle.

dura mater: outer membrane of the meninges covering the brain and spinal cord.

dysentery: bacterially caused diarrhea that may produce blood and mucus in the stool.

dysmenorrhea: pain associated with menstruation.

dyspnea: difficulty breathing.

ecchymosis: bruising.

ectopic pregnancy: pregnancy that implants outside of the uterus, commonly in the fallopian tube.

edema: swelling.

efface: thin, as in the cervix during labor.

electrolytes: solution containing acids, bases and salts that conducts an electrical current.

embolism: obstruction of a blood vessel by a clot of blood or other foreign substance.

emetics: vomit inducers.

emphysema: chronic pulmonary disease characterized by destruction of the alveoli.

enamel: hard covering of the crown of a tooth.

endometrium: lining of the uterus.

envenomation: introduction of poison into the body by a bite or sting.

epidermis: outer layer of the skin.

epididymis: organ lying behind the testicle that stores sperm.

epididymitis: inflammation of the epididymis.

epidural: above the dura mater.

epigastric: upper abdomen.

epiglottis: structure overlying the larynx that prevents food or liquid from entering the airway.

epistaxis: nosebleed.

eschar: scab.

esophagus: tube carrying food and liquid from the mouth to the stomach.

ETOH: alcohol.

eugenol: oil of cloves.

eustachian tube: tube extending from the middle ear to the back of the throat.

evaporation: the process of changing liquid into vapor.

eversion: turning outward.

evisceration: abdominal contents exposed and protruding from an open wound.

expiration: exhaling.

fallopian tube: tube extending from the ovary to the uterus.

fascia: membrane which covers muscle.

febrile: feverish.

fecal impaction: hardened feces forming a blockage in the descending colon preventing passage of fecal material.

femoral: relating to the femur.

femur: thigh bone.

fibrin: protein that helps clotting and scabbing occur.

fibula: small lower leg bone.

fimbria: finger-like structures at the end of the fallopian tube.

flail chest: two or more ribs fractured in two or more places creating a floating section of rib.

FOAM: free of any movement.

foramen magnum: large opening at the base of the skull through which the spinal cord passes.

Fowlers position: semi-reclined position used to transport patients.

fracture: a break in the normal continuity of a bone.

frostbite: localized tissue damage caused by freezing.

frostnip: superficial frostbite.

fungus: primitive life-form that feeds on living plants, decaying organic matter and animal tissue.

Fx: fracture.

gallstone: concretion formed in the gall bladder or bile duct.

gastric distention: air overinflating the stomach.

gastritis: inflammation of the stomach.

gastrocnemius: calf muscle.

gastrocolic: relating to the stomach and colon.

gastroenteritis: inflammation of the gastrointestinal tract.

germ: microscopic organism that might infect a human and cause disease.

Giardia: protozoa with flagella found in surface water.

gingiva: gum.

glottis: the vocal cords and space between them.

glucagon: hormone that increases the concentration of glucose in the blood.

gluteals: muscles of the buttocks.

greenstick fracture: fracture that does not extend all the way through the bone.

grief: emotional response to loss.

gross negligence: extreme deviation from the accepted standard of care.

guarding: protecting an area of injury through muscle tension or physical positioning.

HACE: high altitude cerebral edema.

hamstrings: muscles in the back of the leg.

hantavirus: virus transmitted by inhaling aerosolized microscopic particles of dried rodent saliva, urine or feces causing severe respiratory distress.

HAPE: high altitude pulmonary edema.

heat cramps: painful spasm of major muscles being exercised; caused by dehydration and electrolyte depletion.

heat exhaustion: weakness produced by fluid loss from excessive sweating.

heat stroke: life threatening condition produced by exposure to hot environments or excessive heat production characterized by an elevated core temperature.

hematemesis: blood in the vomit.

hematoma: pooling of blood.

hematuria: blood in the urine.

hemiparesis: weakness affecting one side of the body.

hemiplegia: paralysis affecting one side of the body.

hemoptysis: coughing up blood.

hemorrhage: bleeding.

hemostasis: control of bleeding.

hemothorax: blood in the pleural space.

high altitude cerebral edema: fluid collecting around the patient's brain.

high altitude pulmonary edema: fluid shifting from the pulmonary capillaries and filling the alveolar spaces.

histamine: natural substance in the body released from the immune system in response to an injury or foreign protein.

HR: heart rate.

humerus: upper arm bone.

Hx: history.

hydrophobia: fear of water.

Hymenoptera: bees, hornets, wasps, yellow jackets and fire ants.

hyperbaric: high pressure.

hyperglycemia: high blood sugar.

hypertension: high blood pressure.

hyperventilation syndrome: breathing fast without another cause.

hyperventilation: breathing unusually fast and/or deep.

hypoglycemia: low blood sugar.

hypostome: feeding apparatus of a tick.

hypothalamus: portion of the brain responsible for controlling certain metabolic activities, including temperature regulation.

hypothermia: lowered core temperature.

hypovolemic: low blood volume.

hypoxia: low oxygen level.

ICP: intracranial pressure.

ICS: incident command system.

ilio-tibial band: long tendon from the buttock, down the thigh, across the knee and attaching to the outside of the tibia.

IM: intramuscular.

immersion foot: a non-freezing cold injury from prolonged contact with cold and moisture that causes inadequate circulation and tissue damage.

immersion syndrome: sudden death following immersion in cold water.

impacted fracture: fracture in which bone ends are wedged together.

impingement: inflammation and pain in a tendon.

implied consent: legal assumption that an unconscious or unreliable patient would desire treatment if they were conscious or reliable enough to make a decision. Also applies to minors when a parent or guardian is unavailable to offer consent.

incision: smooth laceration often made by a knife.

incontinence: loss of bowel and/or bladder control.

inferior: below.

inferior vena cava: large vein carrying blood to the heart from the pelvis, abdomen and lower limbs.

inflammation: protective tissue response to injury.

informed consent: consent to treat obtained after a patient has been informed of the risks and benefits of a proposed treatment.

inguinal hernia: piece of intestine protruding into the groin or scrotum.

insomnia: inability to sleep.

inspiration: inhaling.

insulin shock: a diabetic condition resulting from excessive insulin or inadequate blood sugar.

insulin: hormone required to move sugar out of the bloodstream and through cell walls.

integumentary system: skin.

intercostal muscles: muscles between the ribs

interstitial space: space between cells.

inversion: turning inward.

ischemia: lack of blood supply.

IV: intravenous.

JVD: jugular vein distention.

keratin: hard protein in skin, nails and hair.

kidney stone: concretion formed in the kidney and excreted through the urinary tract.

laceration: a cut through the skin.

lacrimal: relating to tears.

LAF: look, ask, feel.

laryngospasm: a constriction of the muscles of the upper airway.

larynx: upper end of the trachea.

lassitude: psychological weariness.

lateral: side.

LCL: lateral collateral ligament.

ligament: connective tissue holding bone to bone.

LLQ: left lower quadrant of the abdomen.

LNT: leave no trace.

LOC: level of consciousness.

lumbar vertebrae: five bones of the spine found between the thoracic vertebrae and the sacrum.

LUQ: left upper quadrant of the abdomen.

lymphadentitis: inflammation of the lymph nodes.

lymphangitis: inflammation of the lymph channels or vessels.

LZ: landing zone.

malaise: general feeling of discomfort or indisposition.

malleolus: rounded distal end of the tibia or fibula.

mania: mood disorder characterized by excessive elation, agitation, accelerated speaking and hyperactivity.

MAST: medical anti-shock trousers.

MCL: medial collateral ligament.

medial: near the midline.

medical advisor: a licensed physician who advises an unlicensed medical practitioner.

medulla: lower portion of the brain stem.

melanocytes: cells of the skin that control pigmentation.

melanoma: form of skin cancer.

menarche: initial menstrual period.

meninges: three membranes surrounding the brain and spinal cord including the dura mater, the arachnoid and the pia mater.

meniscus: crescent shaped fibrocartilage in the knee joint.

metacarpophalangeal joint: where the finger or thumb joins the hand.

MI: myocardial infarction; heart attack.

miscarriage: spontaneous abortion.

mitochondria: intracellular "furnaces" where food is burned in the presence of oxygen to create energy.

mitral valve: valve between the left atrium and the left ventricle of the heart.

mittelschmerz: pain and bloody discharge associated with ovulation.

MOI: mechanism of injury.

mucous membranes: membrane that lines passages and cavities that air passes through.

mucus: fluid secretion that acts as a lubricant in the mucous membranes.

myocardial infarction: heart attack.

myocardium: heart muscle.

NASAR: National Association of Search and Rescue.

nasopharynx: part of the pharynx above the soft palate.

navicular: bones at the base of the wrist and ankle.

necrosis: tissue death.

negligence: the careless, unintentional act which harms another

person to whom you owe a duty of care.

nematocyst: stinging cell.

neurogenic: originating in the nervous tissue.

nitrogen narcosis: increased concentration of nitrogen gas in body tissues from SCUBA diving that produces a sensation of euphoria and impaired judgment.

NOLS: National Outdoor Leadership School.

NPA: nasopharyngeal airway.

NRB: non-rebreather oxygen mask.

NSAID: non-steroidal anti-inflammatory drug.

N/V/D: nausea/vomiting/diarrhea.

oblique fracture: diagonal break in a bone.

odontoid process: bony projection of the second cervical vertebra that the first cervical vertebra rotates upon.

olecranon: bony upper end of the ulna.

omission: failure to act.

OPA: oropharyngeal airway.

open pneumothorax: open wound causing a tear in the lining of the lung resulting in air accumulating the pleural space.

operculum: trap door on a cnidoblast.

OPQRST: onset, provokes, quality, radiation, severity, time.

ophthalmic: relating to the eye.

organelle: specialized structure within a cell that performs special functions for that cell.

oropharynx: part of the pharynx between the soft palate and the epiglottis.

orthopnea: difficulty breathing lying down.

orthostatic vitals: dizziness, change in heart rate, or change in blood pressure that result from sitting or standing up from a supine position.

otitis externa: inflammation of the outer ear, a.k.a., swimmer's ear.

otitis media: inflammation of the middle ear.

ovary: gland that produces eggs in the female reproductive system.

ovulation: release of an egg from an ovary.

ovum: egg.

P: pupils.

palliate: to reduce pain or make feel better.

palpate: to feel.

paradoxical respiration: asymmetrical chest wall movement associated with a flail chest.

paraparesis: partial paralysis of the lower portion of the body.

paraplegia: paralysis of the lower portion of the body.

parasite: organism that lives on or within another organism.

paresthesia: loss of or unusual sensations.

parietal pleura: membrane lining the thoracic cavity.

PASG: pneumatic anti-shock garment.

patella: kneecap.

patellar compression syndrome : created by too much pressure on the back of the kneecap by too much walking, especially downhill.

patent: clear and open, as in an airway.

pathogen: microorganism capable of producing disease.

PCL: posterior cruciate ligament.

PE: pulmonary embolism.

pedal: relating to the foot.

pelvic inflammatory disease: inflammation of the fallopian tubes, ovaries and/or uterus.

perfusion: fluid passing through an organ or tissue, typically well oxygenated blood.

pericardial sac: sac surrounding the heart.

pericardial tamponade: filling of the pericardial sac with fluid.

perineal: area between the vagina and anus.

periodontal abscess: area of infection and pus formation found on the gum.

peripheral: away from the center.

peritonitis: inflammation of the abdominal lining, the peritoneum.

permethrin: insect repellent spray applied to clothing; an insecticide.

PERRL: pupils equal round and reactive to light.

PFD: personal flotation device.

phalanges: bones of the fingers or toes.

pia mater: inner membrane of the meninges covering the brain and spinal cord.

PID: pelvic inflammatory disease.

placenta previa: placenta implants over the cervix.

placenta: organ that provides nourishment to the fetus.

placental abruption: separation of the placenta from the uterine wall.

plague: disease caused by the bacteria Yersinia pestis.

pleura: lining of the lungs.

pleural space: potential space between the parietal and visceral pleura.

PMS: premenstrual syndrome.

pneumonia: infection or inflammation in the lungs.

pneumonic: concerning the lungs.

pneumothorax: tear in the lining of the lung resulting in air accumulating the pleural space.

PNS: peripheral nervous system; nerves except the brain and spinal cord.

polyuria: increased volume of urine output.

POS: pulmonary overinflation syndrome.

posterior: back.

postictal: period of recovery following a seizure.

premenstrual syndrome: cluster of symptoms that occur prior to menstruation.

priapism: painful, constant, emotionally unprovoked erection of the penis due to damage to nerves that control the genitals.

prolapsed cord: cord presents before the baby in the vaginal canal during birth.

prone: face down.

prostatitis: inflammation of the prostate.

proximal: near the center.

psychogenic: originating in the mind.

pulmonary edema: fluid in the lung.

pulmonary embolism: clot in a pulmonary artery or arteriole.

pulmonary overinflation syndrome: rapid increase in pressure within the lung, caused by too rapid an ascent when SCUBA diving.

pulmonary valve: valve between the right ventricle and the pulmonary artery.

pulp: soft portion in the center of a tooth containing nerves and blood vessels.

pulpitis: inflammation of tooth pulp.

pulse pressure: difference between the systolic and diastolic pressures.

puncture: wound made by a sharp, pointed object.

Px: prevention.

quadriceps: thigh muscles.

quadriplegia: paralysis of all four extremities.

rabies: virus transmitted from the saliva of infected mammals that travels in the nervous system.

raccoon eyes: bruising around the eyes indicating a skull fracture.

radial: pertaining to the radius bone.

radiation: heat given off by a warm object as infrared energy.

radius: shorter lower arm bone.

reduction: a return to normal bone to bone relationship.

respiratory arrest: cessation of breathing.

rhinoviruses: group of viruses that cause the common cold.

RICE: rest, ice, compression, elevation; technique for limiting swelling.

rigor mortis: stiffness that occurs in a body after death.

RLQ: right lower quadrant of the abdomen.

root: area of a tooth below the gum.

rotator cuff muscles: supraspinatus, infraspinatus, subscapularis, teres minor; keep the head of the humerus in the shoulder socket.

RR: respiration rate.

RUQ: right upper quadrant of the abdomen.

sacrum: five fused bones of the vertebrae between the lumbar and the coccyx.

SAMPLE: symptoms, allergies, medications, past relevant history, last oral intake, events.

scapula: shoulder blade.

sclera: fibrous tissue covering the white of the eye.

scrotum: sac containing the testicles and the spermatic cord.

SCTM: skin color, temperature and moisture.

SCUBA: self contained underwater breathing apparatus.

seizure: a sudden electrical discharge in the brain.

separation: enlargement of the spaces between bones.

sepsis: condition resulting from a buildup of microorganisms or toxins in the blood.

septicemia: blood poisoning from buildup of bacteria or toxins in the blood.

serum: the watery portion of blood.

shin splints: persistent pain in the shin area.

shin: front of the lower leg.

sinusitis: infection of the sinuses.

SOAP: subjective, objective, assessment, plan.

SOB: short of breath.

sphygmomanometer: a blood pressure cuff.

spirochete: spiral-shaped bacterial microorganism.

spontaneous pneumothorax: tear in the lining of the lung resulting in air accumulating the pleural space that occurs spontaneously.

sprain: stretching or tearing of ligaments.

sputum: substance coughed up from the airway.

squamous cell carcinoma: skin cancer affecting the cells of the epidermis.

S/S: signs and symptoms.

status asthmaticus: a prolonged asthma attack unrelieved by conventional treatment.

status epilepticus: a persistent seizure or series of seizures with no time for adequate breathing.

sternum: breastbone.

stoma: artificial opening created in the trachea to assist breathing.

strain: stretching or tearing of muscle fibers or tendons.

stridor: high pitched sound created by constrictions in the airway.

sub-acute: somewhat acute.

subarachnoid: the space between the arachnoid and the pia mater.

subcutaneous emphysema: air bubbles underneath the skin.

subcutaneous: under the skin.

subdural: below the dura mater.

subungual: under a finger or toe nail.

sucking chest wound: open pneumothorax.

superior: above.

superior vena cava: large vein carrying blood to the heart from the head neck, upper limbs and thorax.

supine: face up.

syncope: fainting.

synovial fluid: clear lubricating fluid, as in a joint.

systolic pressure/systole: pressure measured during the contraction phase of the heart.

T: body core temperature.

tachycardia: increased heart rate, typically greater than 100 beats per minute.

talo-fibular ligament: ligaments connecting the talus to the fibula.

talus: ankle bone.

TBSA: total body surface area.

tendon: connective tissue holding muscle to bone

tendonitis: inflammation of a tendon, also spelled tendinitis.

tension pneumothorax: build up of air in the lung that eventually completely collapses the injured lung and begins to exert pressure on the uninjured lung and the heart.

testis: gland that produces sperm.

tetanic contraction: continuous uterine contraction.

thermoregulation: heat regulation.

thoracic vertebrae: 12 vertebra between the cervical vertebrae and the lumbar vertebrae, with ribs attached.

thorax: chest cavity.

TIA: transient ischemic attack; temporary stroke.

tibia: large lower leg bone.

tibio-fibular ligament: ligament holding the tibia and fibula together.

tidal volume: volume of air inhaled during normal inhalation.

TIL: traction in line.

tinnitus: ringing in the ear.

torsion of the testis: twisting of the testis within the scrotum.

ToSTOP: things that cause the brain to stop--changes in toxins, sugar, temperature, oxygen, pressure.

toxic shock syndrome: infection caused by the bacterium Staphylococcus aureus.

trachea: windpipe.

transient ischemic attack: temporary stroke with signs and symptoms lasting less than 24 hours.

transverse fracture: horizontal break in a bone.

traumatic asphyxia: compression of the chest from a crush injury.

Trendelenburg position: position in which the patient's head is low and the feet are elevated; typical position for the treatment of shock.

triage: sorting of patients to determine the order of treatment.

tricuspid valve: valve between the right atrium and the right ventricle of the heart.

TSS: toxic shock syndrome.

tularemia: illness caused by a tickborne bacteria.

Tx: treatment.

tympanic membrane: eardrum.

ulcer: open sore or lesion in the lining of the stomach or intestine.

ulna: longer lower arm bone.

umbilical cord: cord with two arteries and one vein connecting the fetus to the placenta.

ureter: tube connecting the kidney to the bladder.

urethra: tube from the bladder to the outside.

urethritis: inflammation of the urethra.

URI: upper respiratory infection.

urinary tract infection: infection of the urethra, bladder, ureters, and/or kidneys.

urticaria: hives.

urushiol: oil found in plants such as poison ivy, oak, and sumac that causes contact dermatitis.

uterus: organ of the female reproductive system that supports a fetus.

UTI: urinary tract infection.

UV: ultraviolet.

UVA: ultraviolet A.

UVB: ultraviolet B.

UVC: ultraviolet C.

UVR: ultraviolet radiation.

vagina: birth canal.

Valsalva maneuver: forced exhalation with a closed mouth, nose and glottis which causes the pulse to slow down.

vasoconstriction: a narrowing of the vessels.

vasodilation: a widening of the vessels.

vasogenic: originating in the vessels.

vein: vessel carrying blood from the tissues to the heart.

ventricle: lower chamber of each half of the heart.

ventricular fibrillation: rapid, uncoordinated, quivering of muscle fibers in the ventricles of the heart.

venule: small vein.

vertigo: dizziness caused by a disturbance in equilibrium.

vestibular system: middle part of the inner ear that helps determine balance.

VF: ventricular fibrillation.

virus: microorganism that depends on another organism for survival.

visceral pleura: membrane covering the lungs.

vitreous humor: clear fluid that fills the eye.

VT: ventricular tachycardia.

WFR: Wilderness First Responder.

xiphoid process: sword-shaped cartilaginous protuberance at the lower end of the sternum

Index